ATLAS OF STANDARD SURGICAL PROCEDURES

ATLAS OF STANDARD SURGICAL PROCEDURES

Atlas
of Standard Surgical
Procedures

William V. McDermott, Jr., M.D.

David W. and David Cheever Professor of Surgery
Harvard Medical School
Chairman, Department of Surgery
New England Deaconess Hospital, Boston, Massachusetts

ARTWORK BY

Pam Alexander and Kathryn Sisson

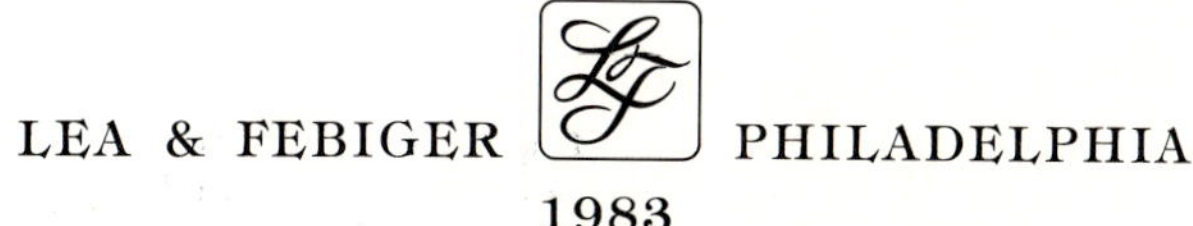

LEA & FEBIGER   PHILADELPHIA
1983

Lea & Febiger
600 South Washington Square
Philadelphia, Pa. 19106
U.S.A.

Library of Congress Cataloging in Publication Data
McDermott, William V., 1917-
    Atlas of standard surgical procedures.
    Bibliography: p.
    Includes index.
    1. Surgery, Operative—Atlases.   I. Title.
[DNLM: 1. Surgery, Operative—Atlases.   WO 517
M478a]
RD41.M38   1983   617'.91'028   82-12714
ISBN 0-8121-0842-6

Printed in the United States of America

Print Number: 2 1

To my wife, Mary, and to our children

PREFACE

The concept of this atlas evolved from many discussions concerning the rather complex residency training program in this department. Until 1973, the seat of the department had been at the Boston City Hospital and then, owing to a number of problems in that institution, it was moved to the New England Deaconess Hospital. The structure of the program involves other hospitals—the Faulkner, Mount Auburn, Cambridge, Manchester Veteran's Administration Medical Center, and the Lahey Clinic Medical Center—all of which were included for specific reasons, since no one institution alone provided the volume and diversity which we felt were required for the total education of a surgeon. The value of this type of consortium of hospitals was obvious as we reviewed the type and number of operative procedures performed by our residents during their training period, but their training also lacked the uniformity characteristic of a program in which the majority of a trainee's experience is derived from one institution and often heavily influenced by one individual. In this environment, the young surgeons work in several different institutions under the guidance of several excellent surgeons. They learn that there are different but equally effective methods of performing both the ordinary and the more complex surgical procedures. This variety contributed to the breadth of their education and, we felt, provided them with unusual opportunity for the development of versatility. On the other hand, this variety brought with it a certain degree of insecurity, particularly in the earlier stages of training. With this in mind, we frequently discussed the possibility of a simplified syllabus to which each of the residents could refer as he embarked on new procedures.

From this beginning and after an exploration of a possible need for a formalized atlas of the common surgical procedures carried out during residency training programs in general surgery, we finally decided to expand the syllabus into a more formalized atlas.

In the design of the atlas it has been obviously difficult to determine which procedures should be included or omitted, since the resident in a general surgical program is exposed to many specialty areas and to the subspecialties of general surgery which may become a part of his later surgical life. However, it would be impossible to extend the number of procedures into all the areas in which a general surgical resident might be involved; thus, certain limitations have been arbitrarily imposed. Another area that presents problems relates to the introduction of stapling techniques into the procedures of surgery. It was decided to omit specific details of any of these procedures relative to closures of anastomoses since they are so well described in the information that accompanies the instruments. Certainly, they have proved to be extremely useful, and each surgeon must arrive at his own decision as to how widely he will utilize the instrumentation and the technology in his own application to the various procedures described herein.

In this atlas, only one particular technique is shown for each procedure. No implication is intended that each technique described is the only approach to a given surgical problem. Rather, each is one that is acceptable to the authors and to the surgeons in the department who have been given the opportunity to review, criticize, and suggest alterations in the original standardized format.

The book is intended only as an atlas of technique and no more than occasional passing references have been made to surgical philosophy, indications, preoperative management, or postoperative care. It is hoped that this will prove useful to young surgeons in training and possibly to their preceptors. Obviously, every surgeon in the evolution of his career introduces frequent alterations and variations in every procedure with which he becomes increasingly involved. This is to be encouraged, and the presentation of techniques in this book is intended only as a foundation on which each young surgeon can continually build his own individual approach to his craft.

The author is grateful to the many surgeons in this department who have contributed to the text of this atlas and to the ultimate pictorial representations. Formal contributions have been recognized in specific chapters.

In addition, surgeons in other university departments have presented helpful criticisms, suggestions, and revisions. To Dr. Paul Nora and Dr. William P. Graham I wish to express my appreciation.

Ms. Barbara Kern, Ms. Marguerite Norton, and Ms. Ann Erickson have worked closely with the author on the review, editing, and construction of the text and deserve full recognition for their role in the completion of the book.

Finally, the collaborating artists, Mrs. Pam Alexander and Ms. Kathryn Sisson, are fully recognized on the title page, but sufficient emphasis cannot be placed on their innovative and imaginative contributions which went far beyond the ordinary role of medical artists.

Boston, Massachusetts WILLIAM V. McDERMOTT, JR.

CONTRIBUTORS

The following members of the faculty of the Harvard Medical School and the Department of Surgery at the New England Deaconess Hospital have been of great assistance to the author in reviewing, commenting, and criticizing the composition and contents of this atlas. In three instances, specific individuals are given reference in chapter headings because of the degree of responsibility assumed in the areas of renal transplantation and vascular surgery.

To all these contributors, the author is most grateful.

ALBERT BOTHE, JR., M.D., Assistant Professor of Surgery
F. HENRY ELLIS, JR., M.D., PH.D., Clinical Professor of Surgery
GARY W. GIBBONS, M.D., Assistant Clinical Professor of Surgery
CARL HOAR, M.D., Assistant Clinical Professor of Surgery
ANTHONY P. MONACO, M.D., Professor of Surgery
MELVIN P. OSBORNE, M.D., Clinical Professor of Surgery
JOHN V. PIKULA, M.D., Associate Professor of Surgery
CORNELIUS E. SEDGWICK, M.D., Clinical Professor of Surgery
MALCOLM C. VEIDENHEIMER, M.D., Lecturer on Surgery
FRANK C. WHEELOCK, JR., M.D., Associate Clinical Professor of Surgery.

CONTENTS

ATLAS OF STANDARD SURGICAL PROCEDURES

CHAPTER ONE

INCISIONS, CLOSURES, AND HERNIAS

Perhaps, surprisingly, this initial chapter has presented the most difficulty in deciding how much should be encompassed under the general procedure of initiating and concluding an operation.

In terms of an anatomic description of various incisions, it became obvious at the outset that few if any general principles could be included and that proliferations of drawings concerning the exposure of a wide variety of anatomic fields would be unrewarding.

Therefore, this general area will be covered by only a few broad statements. First, the incision should be tailored specifically to the proposed operation and designed to provide maximum exposure, which is the key to the swift and efficient completion of any operation. Second, some consideration should be given to the cosmetic results of the ensuing scar formation. The incision may be tailored toward following skin lines, creases, including previous operations, and other such features provided this does not interfere unduly with the initial and primary principle of exposure. Third, the size of the incision depends, as indicated initially, not only on the extent of the planned operative procedure, but also on the body build and relative obesity of the patient. A few generalizations may be made, but these clearly will not cover all the possible variations. In a patient who has an asthenic configuration and a lean body build, one usually finds a high costal arch; adequate exposure for biliary surgery is probably accomplished with a right paramedian incision. In a mesomorph, however, with a flat costal arch and a low xiphoid, a transverse incision accomplishes the principle of exposure more satisfactorily. As another generalization, surgical orthodoxy has long maintained that a transverse incision is stronger and less uncomfortable in the postoperative period than a midline, paramedian, or pararectus incision, though with the basic principles of closure to be described, this assumes less importance. In certain areas, such as the neck, the elevation of flaps for adequate exposure permits placement of the incision for the maximal cosmetic effect, whereas this same principle applied to hernias or lower abdominal operations might end with the accomplishment of little and the addition of probable complications.

Throughout the atlas, incisions are considered relative to the operations described rather than under any set of principles or guidelines.

The same approach is followed for the principles of drainage and surgical anastomoses. Overall, it has been thought best to cover these general areas under the more specific anatomic headings of individual procedures or groups of procedures rather than together.

One particular area—abdominal wound closure—has been thought worthy of a specific description both in text and drawings. This area relates particularly to closure of abdominal wounds since it is in this area that the surgeon is most likely to encounter wound dehiscence, one of the more distressing and probably totally avoidable complications of the postoperative course. The sequence concerned with disruption of abdominal wound prior to removal of the skin sutures is characterized by the rather sudden appearance of a diffuse discharge of thin serosanguineous liquid from the incision sometime after the first postoperative week. If the skin sutures are removed, then the more dramatic and serious complication of evisceration is added.

Standard treatment consists, of course, in the return of the patient to the operating room and a resuture of the disrupted wound using retention sutures through all layers. Providing one leaves the wound, now solidly closed with retention sutures, for at least three weeks, secondary dehiscence is almost unheard of.

Earlier techniques based on Halsted's principle of layer closure with interrupted silk sutures were accompanied by an unacceptably high incidence of wound dehiscence. Recognition of the solidity of closures based on the "all-layer" concept, initiated techniques of utilizing a buried layer of nonabsorbable material which incorporated both fascia and peritoneum, or heavy reinforcing removable sutures through all layers of the abdominal wall. Both techniques protected against disruption, but both carried inherent disadvantages. With the former, either an aseptic foreign body reaction or any type of wound infection led to a prolonged period of extrusion of suture material. With the latter, the heavy sutures, even with protecting "boots," tended to cut through skin if the nature of the problem required a prolonged period prior to removal, and resulted in an ugly and uncomfortable superficial wound.

The ultimate answer to wound closure came with the advent of polyglycolic acid suture material which provides the best of all solutions. An all-layer "buried" closure can be utilized with full confidence that the material will remain intact during the critical period of wound healing but will ultimately be resorbed so that extrusion, sinuses, and chronic annoying superficial infections will be avoided. I use this sequence almost entirely in closure of abdominal wounds. The same principles have been applied to closure of thoracic wounds.

Because of the importance of this closure, more specific details are provided. First, retention sutures of No. 1 polyglycolic acid material are placed through both fascial and peritoneal layers at intervals between 1.0 and 2.0 cm. Next a running suture of the same material is used to close the peritoneum. As this closure is being effected, the individual loops of the retention sutures are picked up in the running suture (Fig. 1-1) to prevent any abdominal viscera or contents from being incarcerated as these retention sutures are tied at a later point in closure. These various fascial layers (depending on the location and direction of the incision) are then closed with a running suture of the same size and material (Figs. 1-1, 1-2). When the final fascial suture has been positioned, the retention sutures are then tied snugly, designed to buttress the closure (Fig. 1-3).

Inguinal hernias may be either indirect, direct, or combined. *Inguinal Hernia*
The indirect hernia is the result of a congenital defect due to failure of closure of the processus vaginalis, an outpouching of peritoneum drawn down through the inguinal ring into the scrotum together with the descent of the testicle. Under normal circumstances this narrow sac becomes completely obliterated leaving the spermatic cord and its contents in the male, or the round ligament in the female, as the contents of the inguinal canal. If, however, there is failure of obliteration of the sac, the contents of the peritoneal cavity may enter the inguinal canal through the internal ring and descend as far as the peritoneal sac is patent; if there is complete failure of obliteration, the hernia may become scrotal by descending down to the testicle in the scrotum itself. If the peritoneal sac obliterates at the internal ring but the internal surfaces fail to adhere and fibrose at any point along the line of descent of the processus, an isolated cystic dilatation may occur resulting in a hydrocele of either the scrotum or the canal.

A direct inguinal hernia is referred to as an acquired rather than a congenital defect and tends to occur later in life, although it should be emphasized that the first appearance of peritoneal contents in a congenital sac may not occur until the middle or

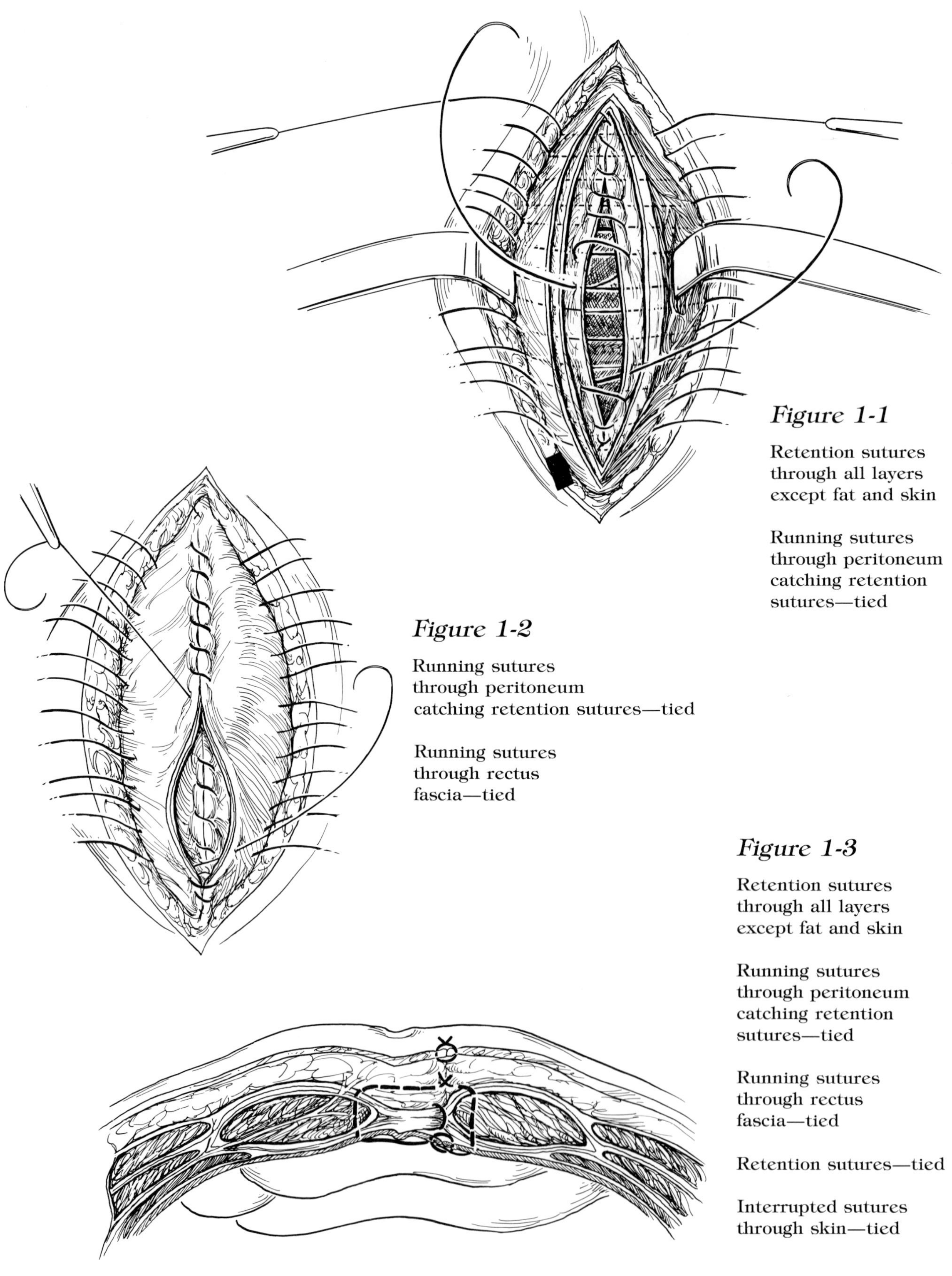

Figure 1-1

Retention sutures
through all layers
except fat and skin

Running sutures
through peritoneum
catching retention
sutures—tied

Figure 1-2

Running sutures
through peritoneum
catching retention sutures—tied

Running sutures
through rectus
fascia—tied

Figure 1-3

Retention sutures
through all layers
except fat and skin

Running sutures
through peritoneum
catching retention
sutures—tied

Running sutures
through rectus
fascia—tied

Retention sutures—tied

Interrupted sutures
through skin—tied

even the later decades. In the acquired defect, the floor of the canal consisting primarily of the transversalis muscle and fascia becomes weakened, and with continued strain a bulge of peritoneum protrudes into the floor of the canal stretching the transversalis fascia and muscle. As this becomes progressively larger with time, the transversalis fascia and muscle may be so attenuated as to be almost unrecognizable.

On physical examination alone it may be difficult to determine whether the obvious protrusion in the inguinal region is a direct or an indirect hernia, particularly in obese individuals. As a generalization, however, the appearance of the reducible bulge in the groin is indirect if it descends along the line of the canal and direct if it protrudes directly forward. Either hernia may descend into the scrotum, but a large scrotal hernia is more likely to be indirect in origin.

Both types of hernias may coexist and should be sought during the dissection.

In the ensuing descriptions of the technique for repair of inguinal hernias, the reader should recognize that innumerable techniques have been developed and described over several decades. Perhaps more important than the exact technique of repair is the recognition of the anatomy, and thus only the long-standardized Halsted or Bassini types of repair are described in this text. A recently popularized version of herniorrhaphy known as the Shouldice repair varies primarily in the utilization of polyglycolic acid suture material in continuous rows and emphasizes the careful dissection of the various muscular and fascial layers in the inguinal canal.

The incision for a repair of an inguinal hernia begins at the pubic tubercle on the appropriate side directed upward for 4.0 to 6.0 cm toward the anterior superior iliac spine and positioned 2.0 to 4.0 cm above the inguinal ligament. The incision is carried down through skin and subcutaneous fascia which exposes the thin layers referred to as the fascia of Scarpa and Camper. Further extension of the incision exposes the aponeurosis of the external oblique muscle that is a glistening white structure in the depths of the incision. This is incised for 1.0 to 2.0 cm in order to permit dissection beneath the aponeurosis and identification of the ileoinguinal nerve (Fig. 1-4). Once the nerve has been identified, the external oblique fascia is divided along the length of the incision. The nerve is dissected free and retracted over the lateral portion of the external oblique so that it is held out of the field by hemostats appropriately placed during the dissection of the hernia itself (Fig. 1-5). The contents of the inguinal canal come into view, and by dissecting laterally down on the undersurface of the external oblique to the shelving edge of Poupart's ligament, one exposes the floor of the inguinal canal. On the medial side, dissection, using the border of the internal oblique muscle and the conjoined tendon as an

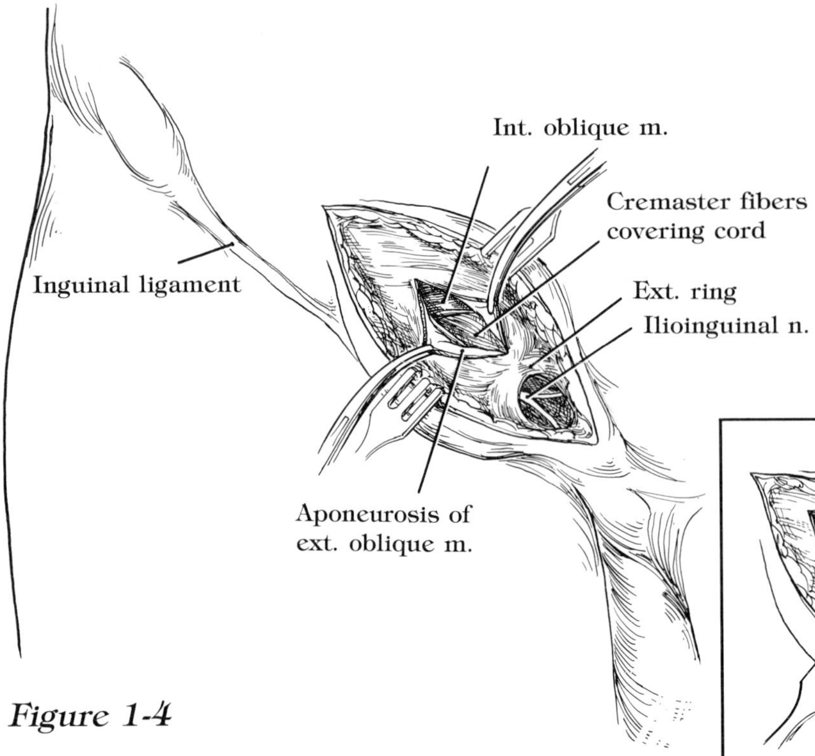

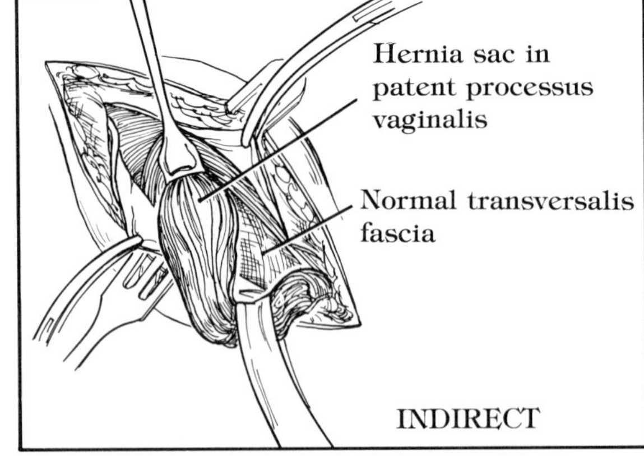

Figure 1-4

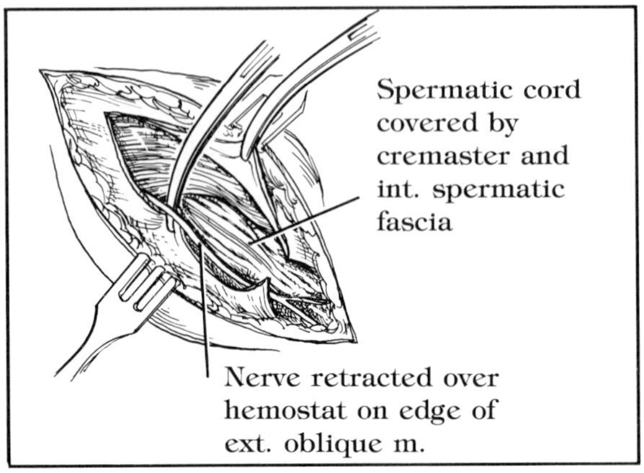

Figure 1-5

Figure 1-6

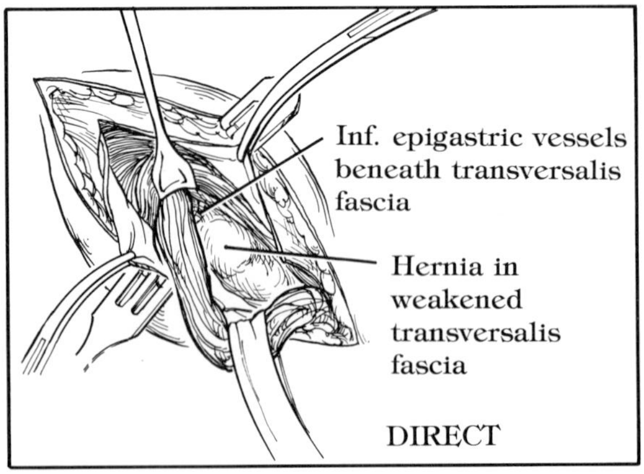

Figure 1-7

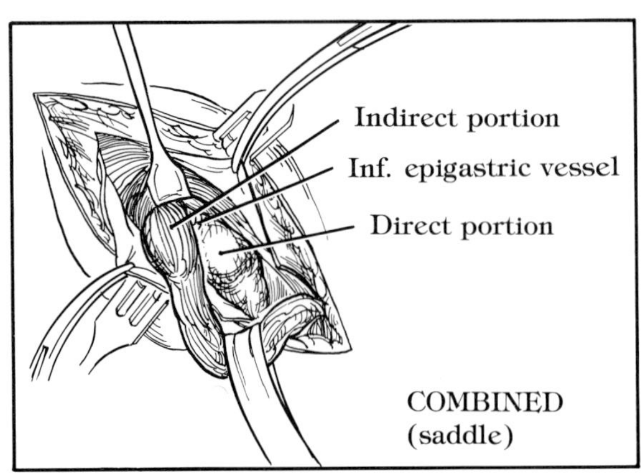

Figure 1-8

identifying point, also exposes the floor of the canal. These two dissections are then joined beneath the spermatic cord which is encircled with a holding tape or piece of rubber dam (Fig. 1-6). As the cord is dissected free through its entire length in the inguinal canal, the inferior epigastric vessels are identified at the lower border of the internal ring and the cord is freed inferiorly down to the pubic spine (Fig. 1-7). At this point, the floor of the canal is inspected to determine whether the transversalis fascia is intact or whether there is a bulging defect characteristic of a direct inguinal hernia. The cord itself is then thoroughly inspected by dividing the cremaster muscle along the length of the cord and dissecting through the structures in order to ascertain the presence or absence of the sac of an indirect inguinal hernia. In a significant number of cases one can identify both an indirect sac and a defect in the floor of the canal, thus forming a combined or "saddle" hernia (Fig. 1-8).

CAUTION

Although thorough inspection and dissection of the cord are important to avoid failure to recognize the presence of a sac, care should be taken to preserve the major vascular components of the sac such as the deferential artery to the testicle, the pampiniform plexus or veins, and direct venous return from the testicle in order to prevent infarction of or, at the least, painful ischemic swelling of the testicle in the postoperative period.

If a hernial sac is present, it should lie on the anterior surface of the cord beneath the cremaster muscle fibers, and can be separated and opened, permitting the insertion of a finger into the peritoneal pouch (Fig. 1-9). Using sharp and blunt dissection, one frees the sac from the cord up to the internal ring at which point the neck of the sac can be closed with a transfixing suture and the redundant portion cut free (Fig. 1-10). Prior to transfixion and division of the sac, a finger should be introduced into the peritoneal cavity to palpate the floor of the canal for identification of a direct hernial defect and also into the internal orifice of the femoral canal to determine the presence or absence of a femoral hernia (Figs. 1-11, 1-12).

In the young child, adolescent, or young adult with normal anatomy of the inguinal canal, little repair is needed following transfixion and excision of the congenital indirect inguinal sac. In older individuals and in particular those in whom a defect can be identified in the floor of the canal, one should begin the repair by reconstructing the transversalis fascia in the floor of the canal with interrupted or continuous nonabsorbable suture ma-

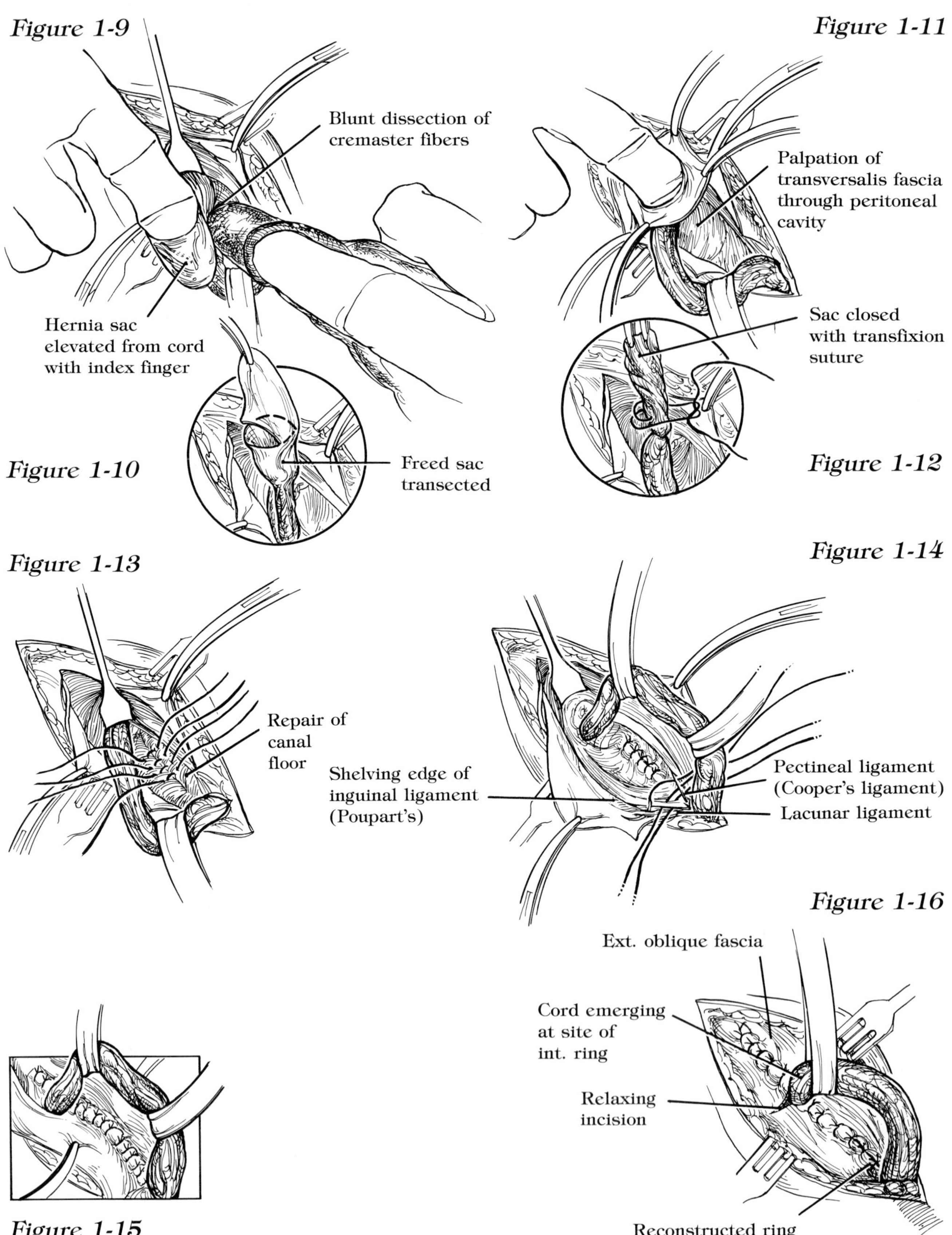

Figure 1-9
Blunt dissection of cremaster fibers
Hernia sac elevated from cord with index finger
Figure 1-10
Freed sac transected
Figure 1-11
Palpation of transversalis fascia through peritoneal cavity
Sac closed with transfixion suture
Figure 1-12
Figure 1-13
Repair of canal floor
Shelving edge of inguinal ligament (Poupart's)
Figure 1-14
Pectineal ligament (Cooper's ligament)
Lacunar ligament
Figure 1-16
Ext. oblique fascia
Cord emerging at site of int. ring
Relaxing incision
Reconstructed ring
Figure 1-15

terial (Fig. 1-13). The significant portion of the repair is then begun by placing a suture through the fascia overlying the pubic spine and then through the distal portion of the conjoined tendon near its attachment. This layer is continued with interrupted nonabsorbable sutures, bringing the conjoined tendon down to the lacunar (Gimbernat's) ligament, to Cooper's ligament up to the femoral vein, and then carrying the repair upward to Poupart's ligament. Reconstruction is completed by approximating the conjoined tendon and the internal oblique muscle to the shelving edge of Poupart's ligament up to the internal inguinal ring (Fig. 1-14).

CAUTION

Postoperative bleeding can be significant from damage to the external iliac vein, resulting in significant hematomas of the wound and even extensive retroperitoneal dissection. Arteriovenous fistulas and false aneurysms have been reported secondary to injury of the iliac artery.

The superior portion of the internal ring is closed above the entrance of the cord by bringing the muscular portion of the internal oblique to the shelving edge of Poupart's in such a fashion that the tip of the little finger can just be introduced into the newly reconstructed internal inguinal ring (Fig. 1-15). The remainder of the repair is generally considered relatively unimportant, depending on the surgeon. The so-called Halsted repair approximates the divided edges of the external oblique ligament beneath the cord whereas the Bassini repair places the cord beneath the reapproximated external oblique fascia (Fig. 1-16). The incision is then closed in layers for completion of the operation.

CAUTION

A significant proportion of recurrent hernias have been attributed to failure to provide a tight closure of the internal ring. There is probably an undue amount of apprehension about postoperative testicular swelling secondary to an overly tight closure since this complication is insignificant if mild and transient. When severe degrees do occur with infarction, it is more likely due to damage to the testicular artery and venous return in the core during dissection than to tight closure of the internal ring.

Sliding Hernia   The most important aspect of the management of the *sliding hernia* is the recognition of the nature of the defect. The abnormality occurs as either the sigmoid colon or the cecum begins to evert or "roll out" beneath the lateral reflection of the peritoneum and eventually protrudes through a defect in the internal ring in such a fashion that a portion of the wall of the sac is formed by the bowel itself. The major risk is that lack of recognition of the existence of the sliding hernia might lead the surgeon to open into the sac directly through the bowel wall. With recognition of the anatomic defect, however, the hernia can be easily repaired. Years ago, Roscoe Graham recommended a separate laparotomy incision with reduction of the everted sigmoid colon or cecum by traction and closure of the peritoneum up to the inguinal ring followed by ordinary hernia repair. In general, this is not considered necessary today and is perhaps an overcomplicated approach to the problem. The surgeon can open the sac after identifying the peritoneum, reperitonealize the everted bowel (Fig. 1-17), reduce the viscus, and then close the residual ring with a purse-string suture (Fig. 1-18). The inguinal canal is then reconstructed as indicated as in any direct inguinal herniorrhaphy.

Femoral Hernia   Several introductory generalizations can be made about *femoral hernias.* First, while they may occur in the male, the femoral hernia is by far the most common cause of a reducible bulge in the region of the inguinal canal and groin crease in the female. Secondly, an obscure and almost occult femoral hernia should always be suspected in the presence of acute small bowel obstruction because the deeper location of the defect and the tightness of the ring may make an incarcerated hernia more difficult to recognize on physical examination, particularly in obese patients. Certainly, as in the case of inguinal hernias, the recognition of the anatomic defect and the restoration of normal anatomy are more important than variance on the approach or the technique of repair. Thus, only the approach from above through the floor of the inguinal canal is described, although on occasion a small reducible defect may be easily corrected by a femoral approach from below the inguinal ligament. In addition, there are certainly times when a laparotomy may be the wisest approach, particularly in the presence of extensive and prolonged small bowel obstruction with a serious suspicion of infarction in an incarcerated femoral hernia.

Although there are surgical descriptions of repair of a femoral hernia by longitudinal incision in the upper thigh below the inguinal ligament, it is in general wiser to approach this defect from above the inguinal ligament and through the floor of the canal. This gives direct access to the neck of the hernia and control of the contents of the hernial sac in the event that it is necessary to inspect them and possibly resect any devitalized

Figure 1-17

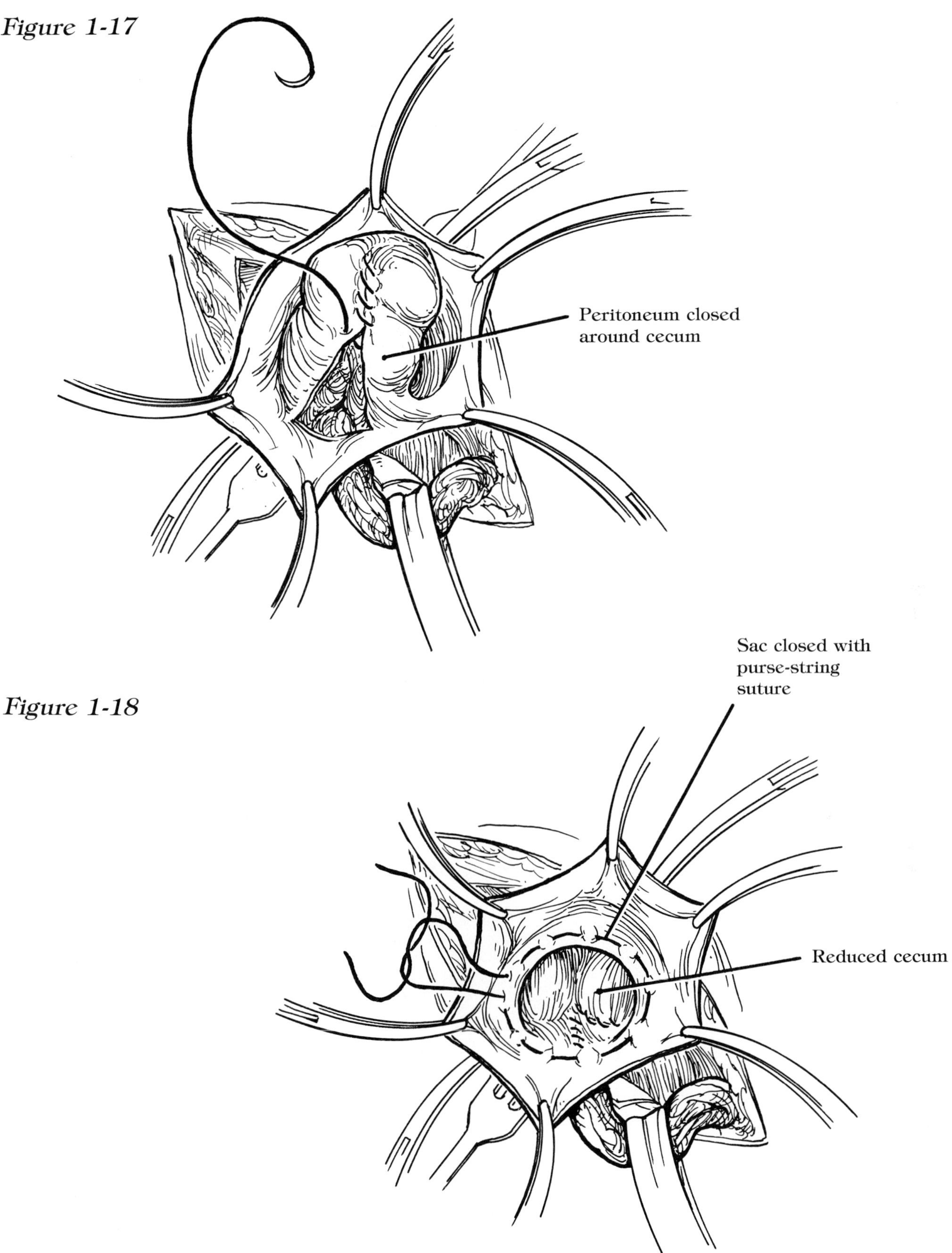
Peritoneum closed
around cecum

Sac closed with
purse-string
suture

Reduced cecum

Figure 1-18

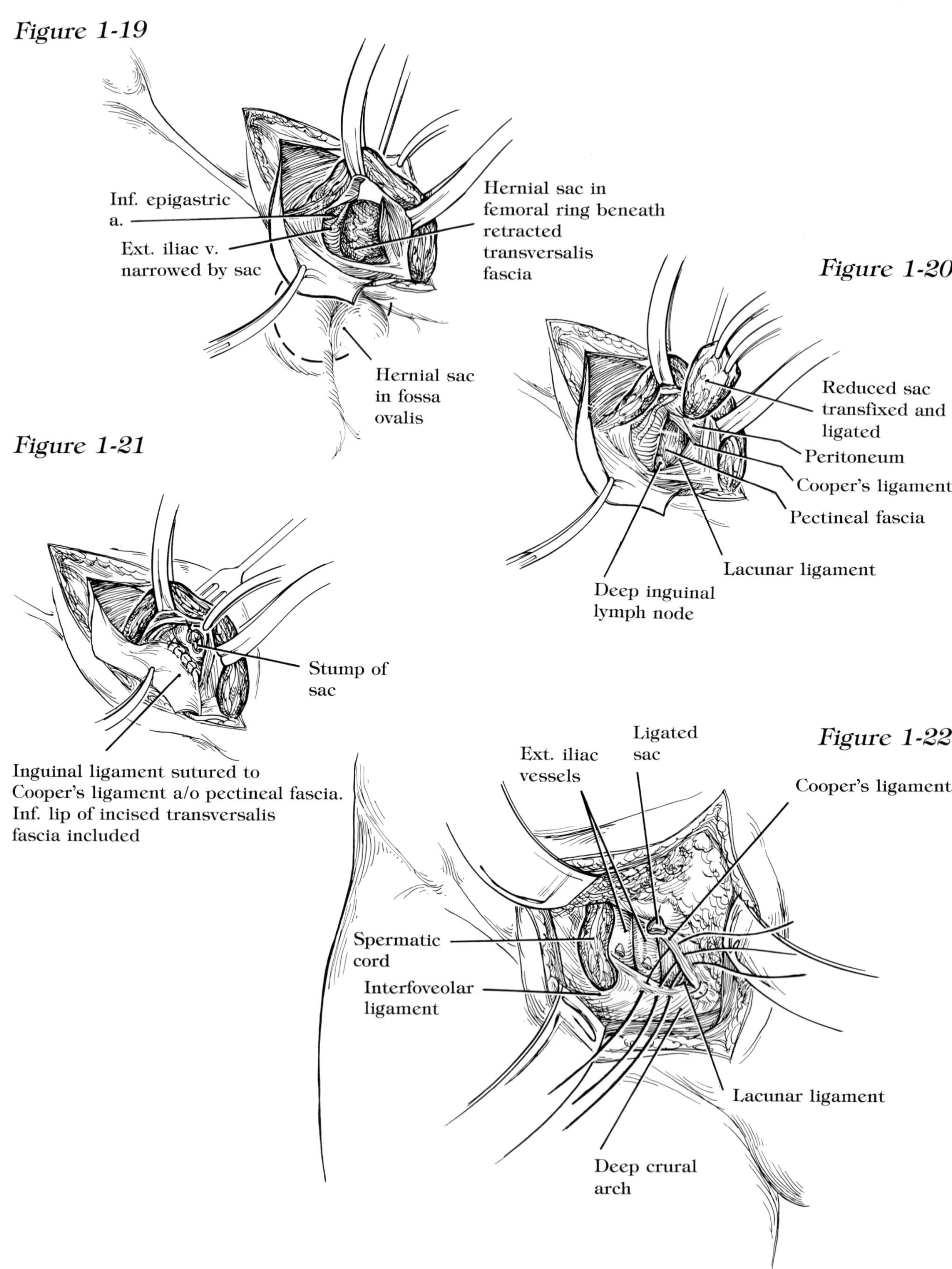

Figure 1-19
Inf. epigastric a.
Ext. iliac v. narrowed by sac
Hernial sac in femoral ring beneath retracted transversalis fascia
Hernial sac in fossa ovalis
Figure 1-20
Reduced sac transfixed and ligated
Peritoneum
Cooper's ligament
Pectineal fascia
Lacunar ligament
Deep inguinal lymph node
Figure 1-21
Stump of sac
Inguinal ligament sutured to Cooper's ligament a/o pectineal fascia. Inf. lip of incised transversalis fascia included
Figure 1-22
Ext. iliac vessels
Ligated sac
Cooper's ligament
Spermatic cord
Interfoveolar ligament
Lacunar ligament
Deep crural arch

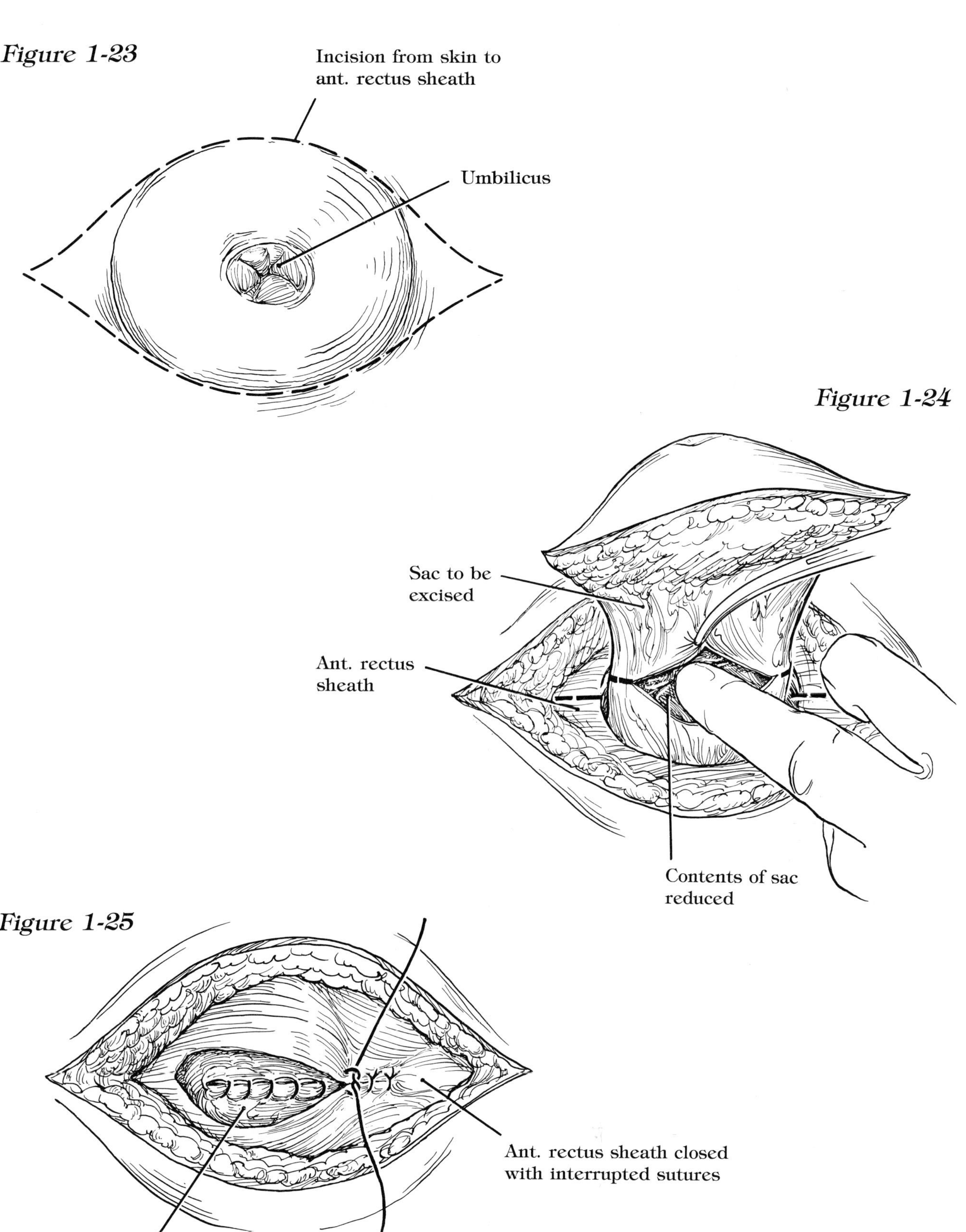

Figure 1-23
Incision from skin to
ant. rectus sheath
Umbilicus
Figure 1-24
Sac to be
excised
Ant. rectus
sheath
Contents of sac
reduced
Figure 1-25
Ant. rectus sheath closed
with interrupted sutures
Peritoneal sac closed
with continuous sutures

bowel (Fig. 1-19). The peritoneum can be opened and the contents of the sac reduced directly or, if there are no viscera contained within the sac, it can be dissected free, transfixed, and ligated (Fig. 1-20). The femoral canal is then obliterated by suturing the inguinal ligament to Cooper's ligament and to the pectineal fascia (Fig. 1-21). The inferior margin of the incised transversalis fascia may be included for added strength of the repair. The entire canal is then reconstructed as in a direct herniorrhaphy, but somewhat medial to the usual direct approach for an inguinal hernia (Fig. 1-22).

Umbilical Herniorrhaphy

An *umbilical hernia* is a common and often innocuous defect. Although it is not essential to remove the umbilicus in order to correct a defect in the fascia, it is in general wise and more satisfactory to approach repair in this way after apprising the patient of the necessity for this type of excision. With an elliptical transverse incision (Fig. 1-23), the umbilicus is dissected free including the hernial sac which can then be opened at the fascial level (Fig. 1-24) and trimmed in a circumferential manner so that the entire umbilicus and excess sac can be removed. When the sac is first opened, any incarcerated omentum or viscera contained therein can be reduced by splitting the sac longitudinally. The peritoneum is then closed and the fascial defect repaired with interrupted sutures (Fig. 1-25).

CHAPTER TWO

UPPER GASTROINTESTINAL SYSTEM

Despite the introduction of vagotomy procedures with or without associated drainage operation, distal, subtotal, or partial gastrectomy (to include the terms applied to indicate variations in the extent of the procedure) is still one of the standard operations of the general surgeon, applicable to the treatment of not only peptic ulcer disease but also other malignant or benign processes involving the stomach.

The incision is usually midline or left paramedian, carried from just above the umbilicus to the xiphoid in order to allow maximum exposure of the upper stomach in the event that favored radical resection is indicated. The procedure is begun by entering the lesser omental sac and starting the repetitive individual clamping, cutting, and ligating of the branches of the gastroepiploic system along the greater curvature of the stomach (Fig. 2-1). (In some instances, particularly when malignant disease of the stomach is known or suspected, it may be more appropriate to enter the lesser omental sac by separating the omentum from the transverse colon and mobilizing the greater curvature of the stomach in this fashion.) When dissection has been carried high on the greater curvature of the stomach to a point beyond the attachments of the vasa brevia (see Fig. 2-1), attention can then be directed distally along the greater curvature of the antrum and pylorus. The branches of the gastro-epiploic system are divided in this direction, eventually ligating the main vessels. The stomach can then be drawn anteriorly and

*Distal Partial
Gastrectomy*

upward. By division of an avascular attachment to the pancreas and retroperitoneal area, the celiac axis can be exposed and the major branches identified (Fig. 2-2). The left gastric artery may be clamped, cut, and ligated, or the partially mobilized stomach replaced and dissection begun in the area of the celiac axis by opening the lesser omentum along the lesser curvature. The right gastric vessels can be identified just beyond the pylorus and divided. Carrying the dissection up the lesser curvature allows one to identify and ligate the left gastric vessels (if they have not been divided posteriorly) (Fig. 2-3).

> CAUTION
>
> Whether the celiac axis is approached posteriorly with the stomach drawn upward or anteriorly by opening the lesser omentum along the lesser curvature, preservation of the hepatic artery is important. Although it has been recognized that ligation of the main hepatic artery may be surprisingly free from any evidence of hepatic ischemia or hepatocellular dysfunction, there are circumstances under which damage to or occlusion of this vessel could be disastrous.

The surgeon's choice at this point is whether the stomach should be transected first and the dissection carried distally into the paraduodenal area or whether the latter part of the dissection should be begun as an initial step in the removal of the stomach. In the second sequence, the dissection is carried beyond the pylorus along the duodenum using small straight hemostats and ligating the multiple small vessels encountered with fine silk. This maneuver is particularly difficult when there is a posterior penetrating ulcer. In this situation, the duodenum must be carefully mobilized around and beyond the ulcer crater to permit distal duodenal turn-in. An Allen-Kocher clamp is then placed across the duodenum just distal to the pylorus and an ordinary Kocher clamp on the gastric side of the pylorus for transection as shown in Figure 2-4. A number of methods have been described for turning in the duodenal stump, but one of the most satisfactory was one popularized by Dr. Arthur W. Allen. It consists of a continuous 3-0 chromic catgut stitch placed loosely around the clamp which is then removed as the suture is pulled down snugly over the duodenal mucosa (Fig. 2-5A). A second row is then placed, using the same stitch after turning in the end of the initial closure (Fig. 2-5B). The layer is completed by turning in the second end of the suture line in a similar fashion (Fig. 2-5C). An outer layer of interrupted silk sutures gives additional strength to the closure which is prone to disruption when ulcer

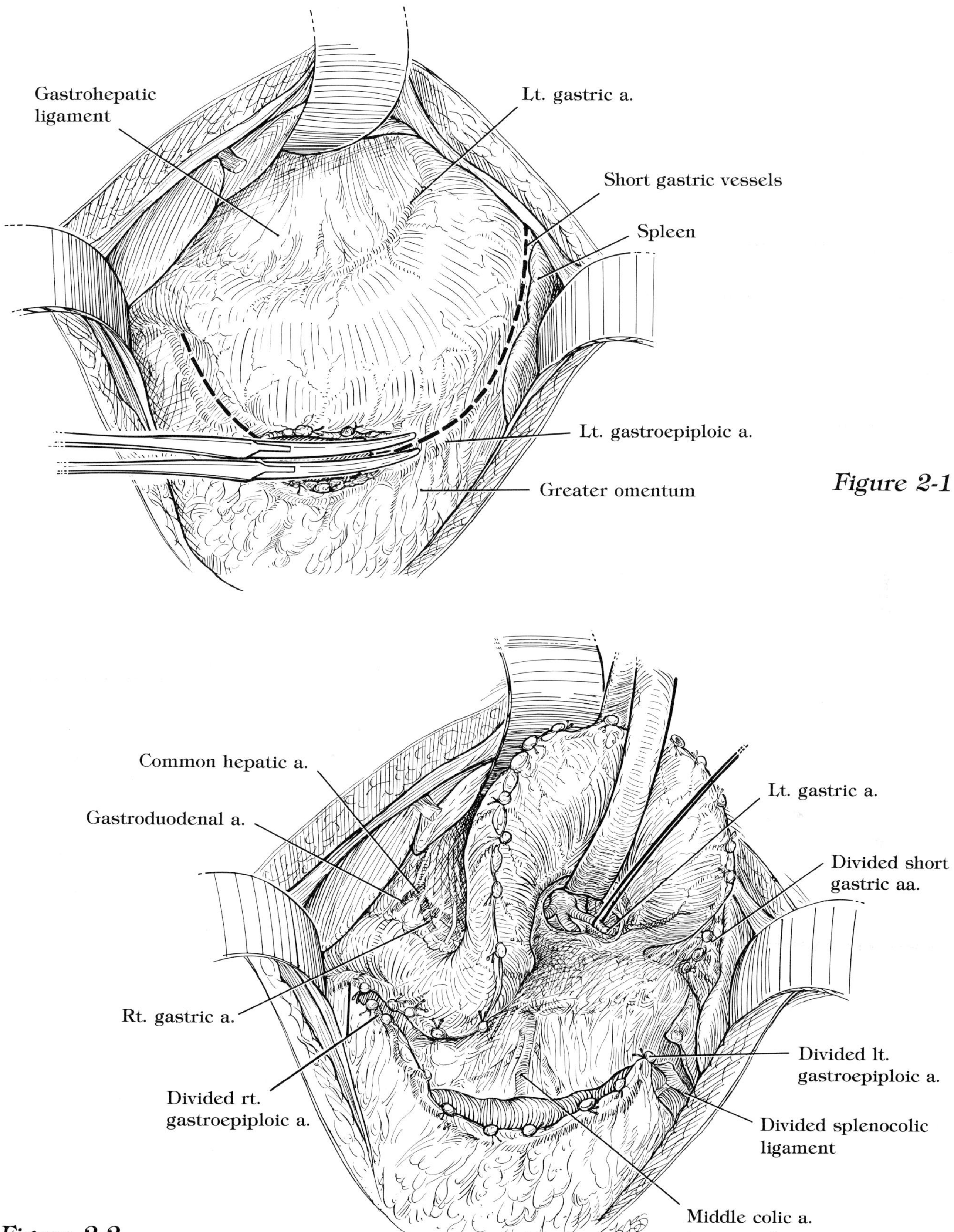

Gastrohepatic ligament
Lt. gastric a.
Short gastric vessels
Spleen
Lt. gastroepiploic a.
Greater omentum
Figure 2-1
Common hepatic a.
Gastroduodenal a.
Lt. gastric a.
Divided short gastric aa.
Rt. gastric a.
Divided rt. gastroepiploic a.
Divided lt. gastroepiploic a.
Divided splenocolic ligament
Middle colic a. in mesocolon
Figure 2-2

Figure 2-3
Rt. gastric a.
Divided lt. gastroepiploic a.
Rt.
gastroepiploic a.

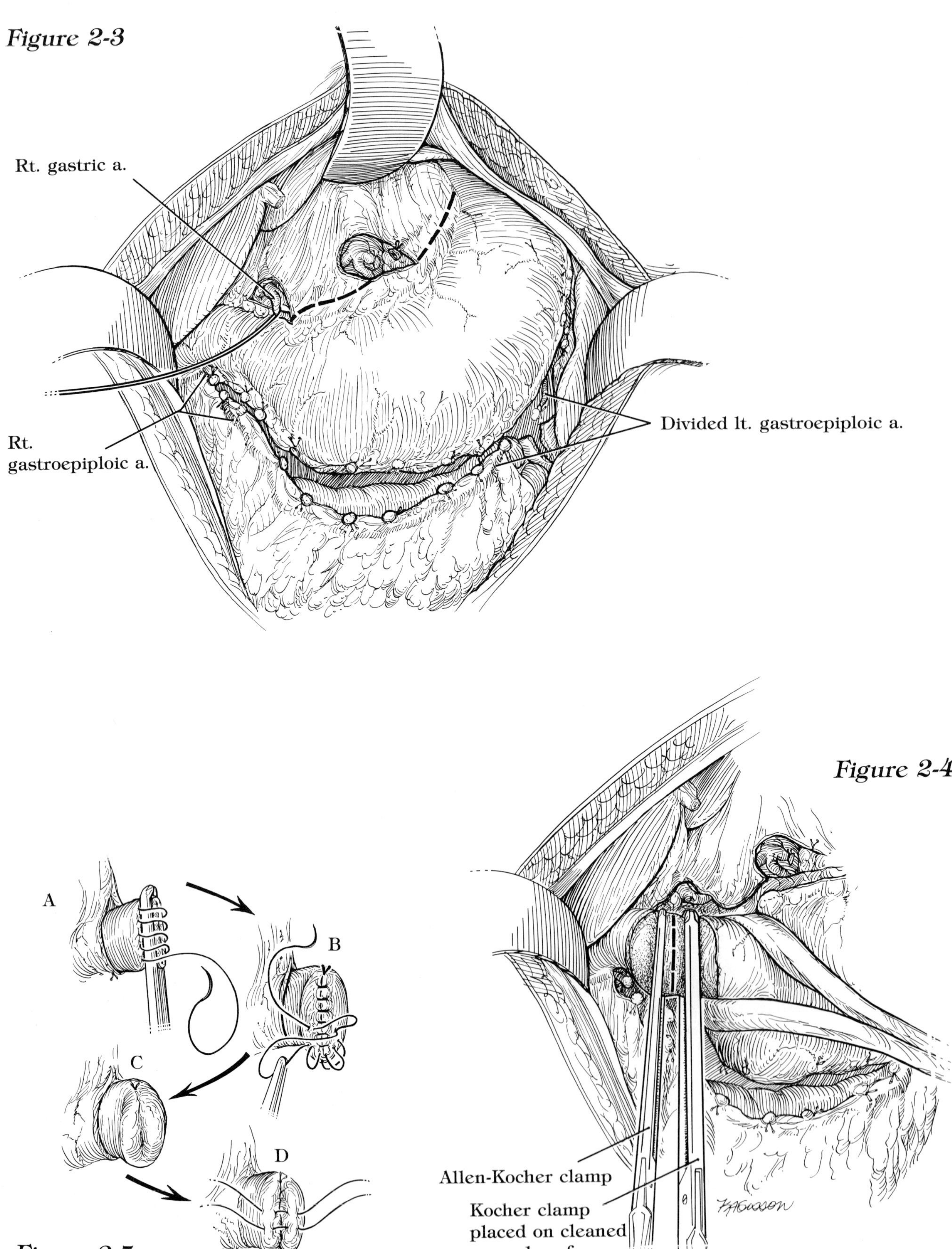

A
B
C
D
Figure 2-5
Figure 2-4
Allen-Kocher clamp
Kocher clamp
placed on cleaned
serosal surface

disease involves the duodenum with inflammation, edema, and fibrosis (Fig. 2-5*D*).

Gastric mobilization is then continued to a point high up on the lesser curvature above the level of the major arborization of the left gastric vessels. Depending on the surgeon's judgment as to the extent of the gastrectomy required, Payr or Allen-Kocher clamps are then placed across the stomach and the wall is divided (Fig. 2-6).

Gastroenterostomy is carried out as shown in Figure 2-7 in two continuous layers of 3-0 chromic catgut. The initial layer approximates the serosa of an antecolic loop of proximal jejunum to the posterior serosa of the stomach just beyond the point of transection. If a Hofmeister rather than a Polya type of closure is elected, a portion of the stomach is turned in with a previously placed double layer of chromic catgut. When the posterior continuous suture is placed, the ends are held with identifying clamps and an incision is made on the antemesenteric border of the jejunal loop of a size selected for the gastric stoma. The inner layer of the anastomosis is begun by approximating posterior mucosa and serosal layers of the stomach and jejunum with a continuous chromic catgut suture (Fig. 2-8) which is then continued around to make up the inner posterior and anterior layers of the anastomosis (Fig. 2-9). The gastroenterostomy is then completed with another anterior layer of chromic catgut sutures tied to the initially placed posterior layer which is identified by holding clamps (Fig. 2-10).

The anastomosis should then lie in such a way that the afferent limb to the lesser curvature is not so tense that it either obstructs or is obstructed by the transverse colon, and the efferent limb should not be kinked at the outer corner.

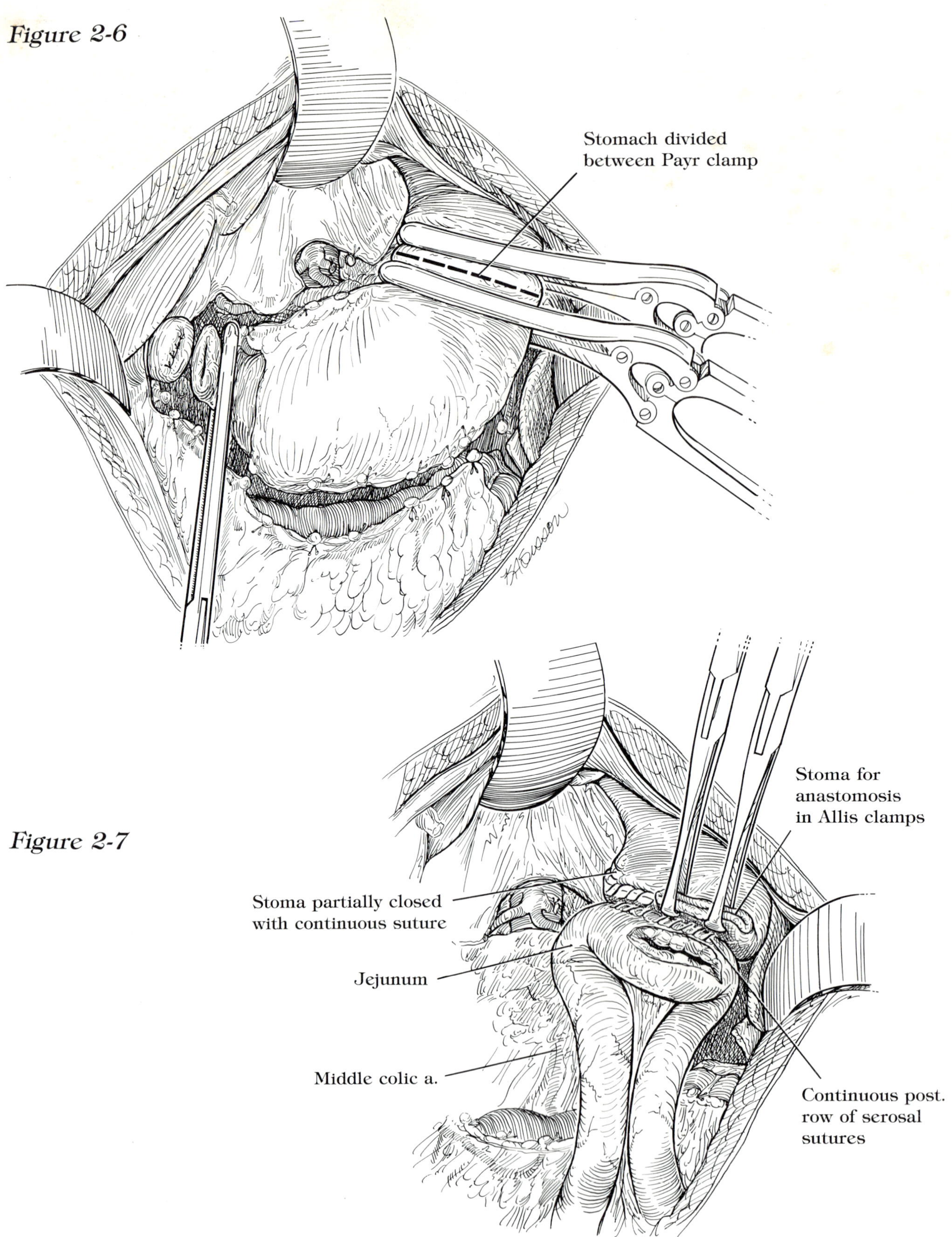

Figure 2-6
Stomach divided
between Payr clamp
Figure 2-7
Stoma for
anastomosis
in Allis clamps
Stoma partially closed
with continuous suture
Jejunum
Middle colic a.
Continuous post.
row of serosal
sutures

Figure 2-8

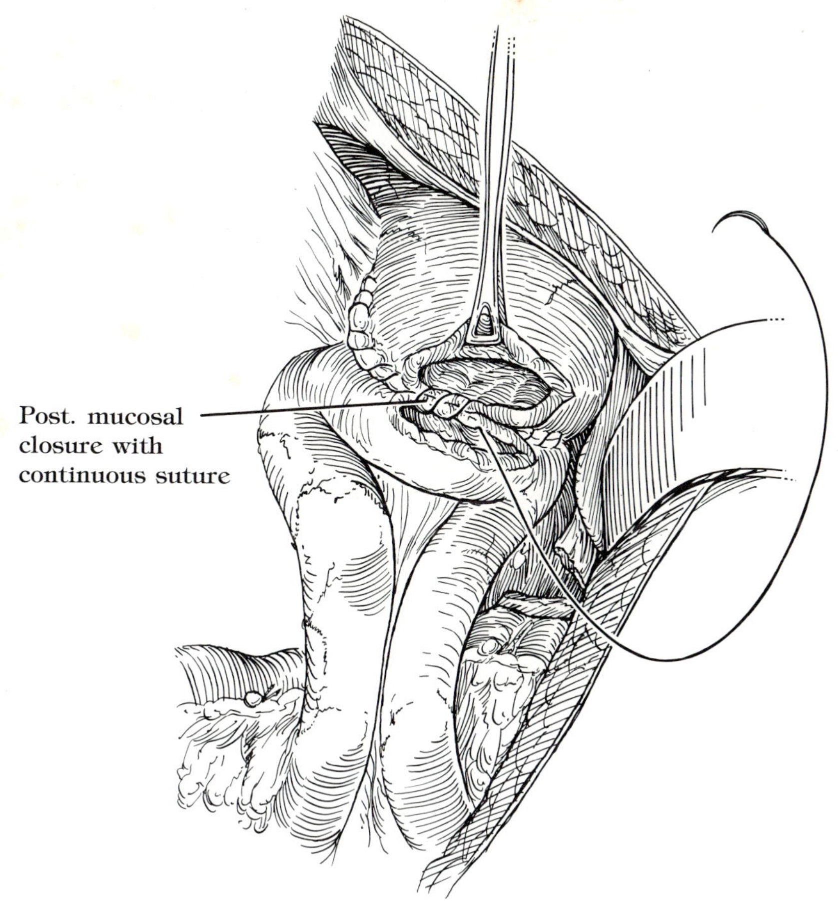

Post. mucosal
closure with
continuous suture

Figure 2-9

Figure 2-10

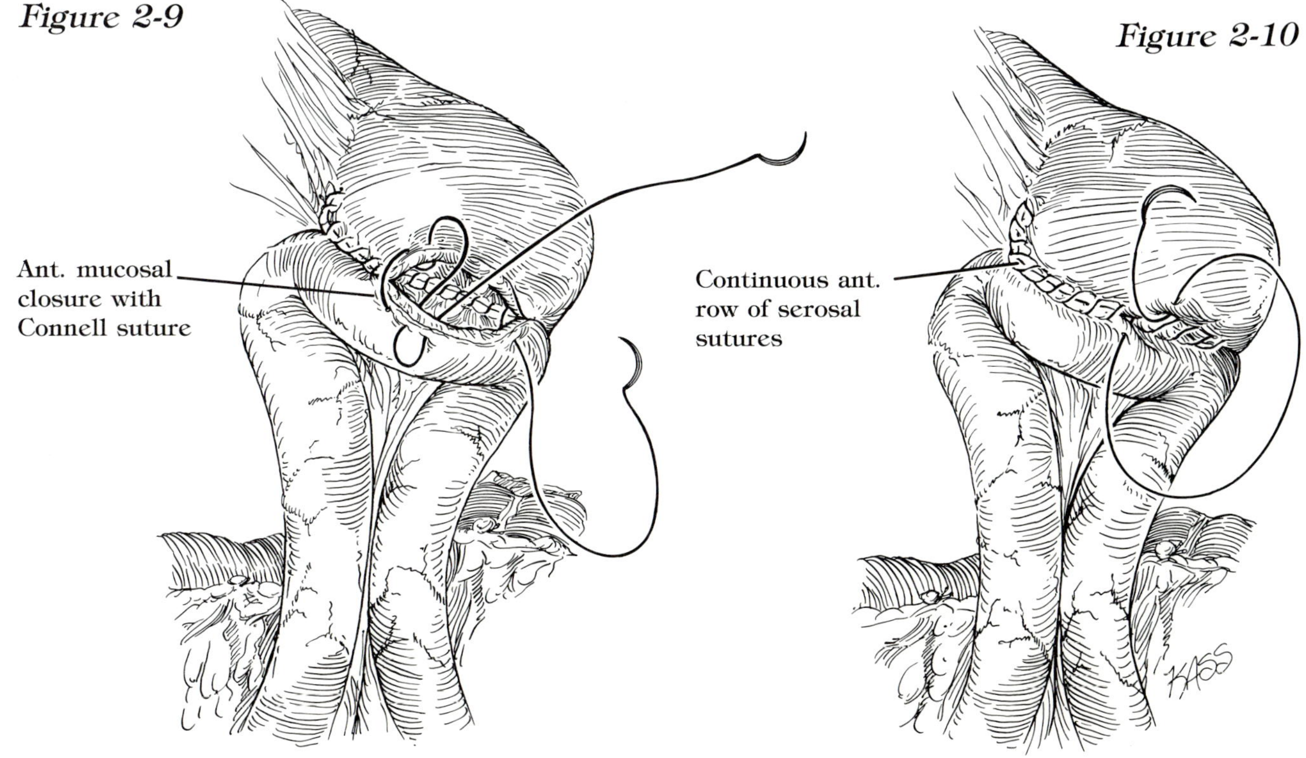

Ant. mucosal
closure with
Connell suture

Continuous ant.
row of serosal
sutures

Mapped Antrectomy

A modification of the distal gastrectomy is often preferred as an acid-reducing operation for patients with peptic ulcer disease and is described here as a mapped antrectomy with truncal vagotomy. Some surgeons may feel secure in deciding by estimate the extent of the mucosa of the gastric antrum, but this is so variable that if one wishes to be precise, exact identification should be carried out as shown in the accompanying diagrams.

The initial part of the procedure is similar to the exposure of the mobilization of the greater curvature as carried out for distal gastrectomy. A 10-cm incision is then made in the anterior wall of the stomach above and parallel to the mobilized greater curvature, careful hemostasis is secured in the cut edges by application of small hemostats (Fig. 2-11), and then Babcock clamps are placed appropriately on the upper edge of the incision to expose the posterior gastric mucosa as well as the greater and lesser curvatures. Nitrazine papers, or any other chosen form of acid identification material, are then placed in a row along the posterior wall and up on the lesser and greater curvatures as shown in Figure 2-12. Absolute hemostasis is essential to obtain an accurate recording. A temporary occluding spring clamp is placed on the gastric side of the pylorus in the mobilized distal stomach to prevent reflux of alkaline secretions from the duodenum. Betazole hydrochloride (Histalog) is then administered intravenously, resulting in an outpouring of gastric acid from the parietal cells. The difference in color of the paper (orange-red over the acid-secreting fundus and green over the alkaline-secreting antrum) (see Fig. 2-12) accurately identifies these physiologic segments of the stomach and permits accurate resection. The line of division between the antrum and the parietal cells can be marked with interrupted sutures and the gastrotomy incision closed (Fig. 2-13). Resection of the antrum can then be carried out along the line of the marking sutures, thus

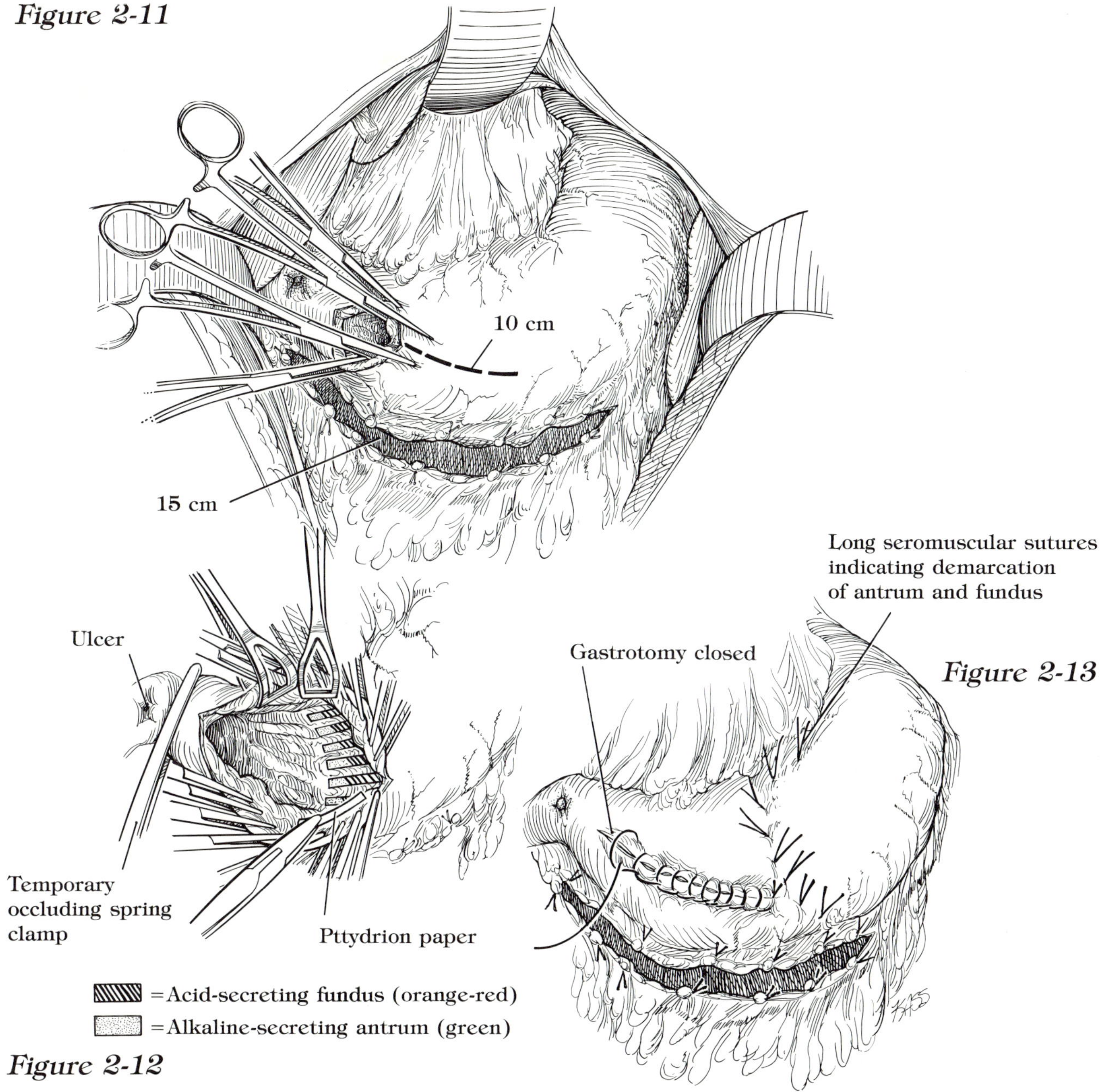

assuring a total removal of the gastrin-producing antrum mucosa. Truncal vagotomy (to be described later) is then added.

Resection of the proximal portion of the stomach (which may include varying lengths of distal esophagus) is applicable particularly to malignant lesions of the proximal stomach or lower esophagus. It is best accomplished through a left transthoracic or thoracoabdominal incision in which the diaphragm is divided along the incision down to the esophageal hiatus. The anatomic features of this approach are shown in Figure 2-14.

Proximal Gastrectomy

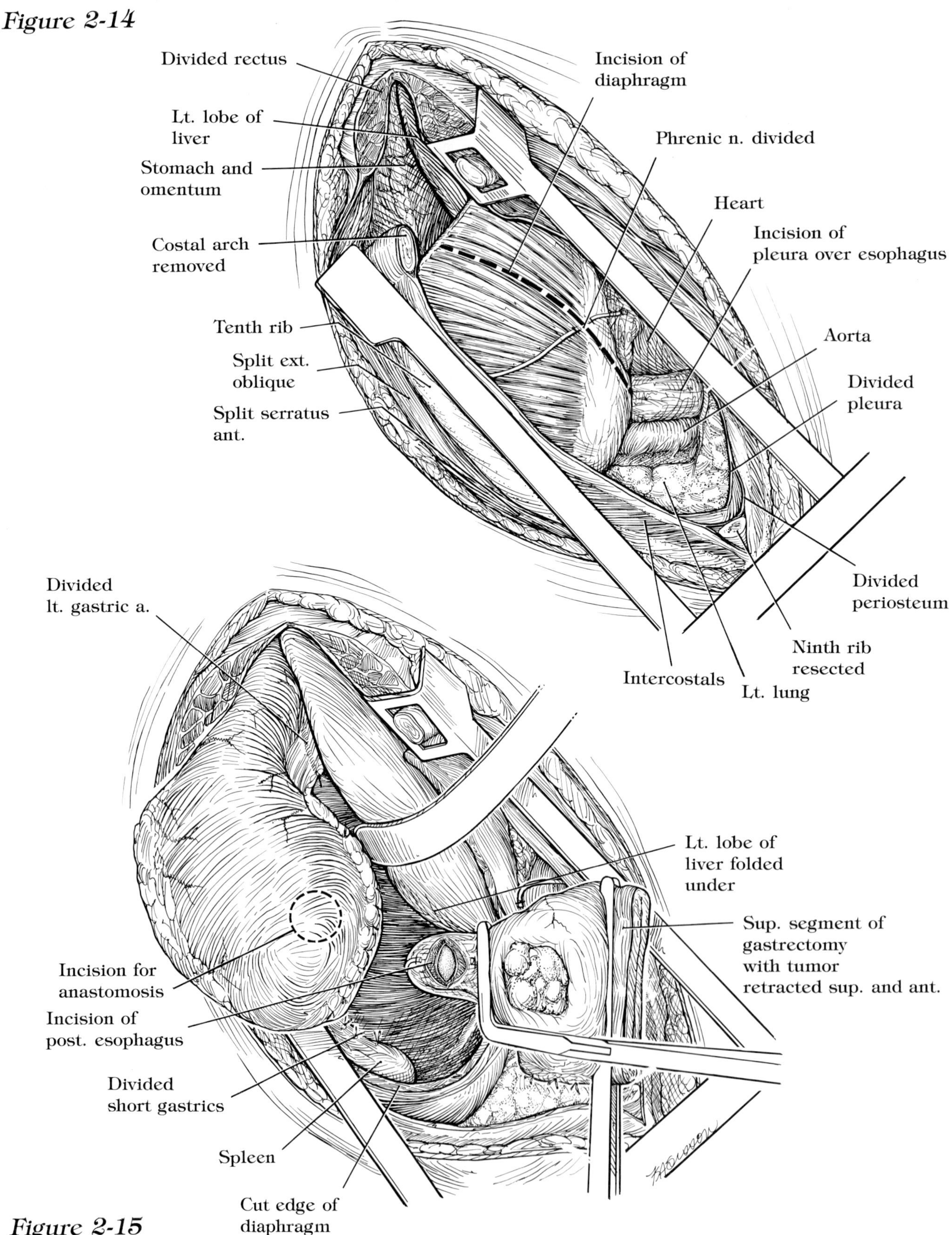

Figure 2-14

Figure 2-15

The proximal stomach may then be mobilized by dividing the branches of the left gastric and left gastroepiploic vessels as well as the vasa brevia from the spleen. (In some instances, the splenectomy may be included as a part of the operative procedure.) The lower esophagus is also mobilized and the stomach transected between clamps at a point determined by the judgment of the surgeon, depending on the disease for which the procedure has been chosen. The stomach is then closed in two layers with continuous chromic catgut, occasionally reinforced by an outer layer of interrupted silk. The specimen to be resected, which may contain a tumor in either the upper stomach or lower esophagus, is reflected upward and the point where the esophagus is to be transected is then selected. The point on the anterior wall of the stomach distal to the gastric turn-in which is chosen for the point of esophagogastric anastomosis is then identified by circular incision carried through the serosa (Fig. 2-15). The posterior wall of the esophagus, reflected upward and anteriorly, is then opened and the first posterior row of sutures is placed between the outer muscular layer of the esophagus and the serosa of the stomach (Fig. 2-16). The button of stomach is then removed and a second row of interrupted fine sutures is placed between the inner muscular layer of the esophagus and the muscular wall of the stomach (Figs. 2-17, 2-18). When these two rows have been completed, a third layer of interrupted silk then approximates the firm esophageal mucosa with the posterior wall of the anastomotic site and the gastric mucosa in the stomach. At this point, the esophagus is transected (Fig. 2-19) and the specimen removed. The esophagus and stomach are then held firmly together without undue tension by the three posterior rows of sutures, and the anastomosis is completed by similar approximation of the three anterior layers. Some surgeons prefer to include a pyloroplasty as part of the operative procedure because the vagal nerves have been transected. The completed procedure is shown in Figure 2-20.

The incision is then closed in layers using interrupted heavy silk sutures on the diaphragm and interrupted heavy silk sutures on each side of the transected costal arch to bring the arch together without sutures in the cartilage itself. It is often wise to resect a portion of the cartilage to prevent overriding. A row of interrupted silk sutures is then placed at the intercostal bundles left after the rib has been removed in the incision. The adjacent ribs are brought together with a Bailey approximator, permitting sutures to be tied without tension. Closure of the chest wall completes the operative procedure.

Total Gastrectomy

For a total removal of the stomach, an approach similar to that described for proximal gastrectomy may be used or, in thin individuals, a midline abdominal incision may give sufficient exposure. When the stomach is completely removed as a combina-

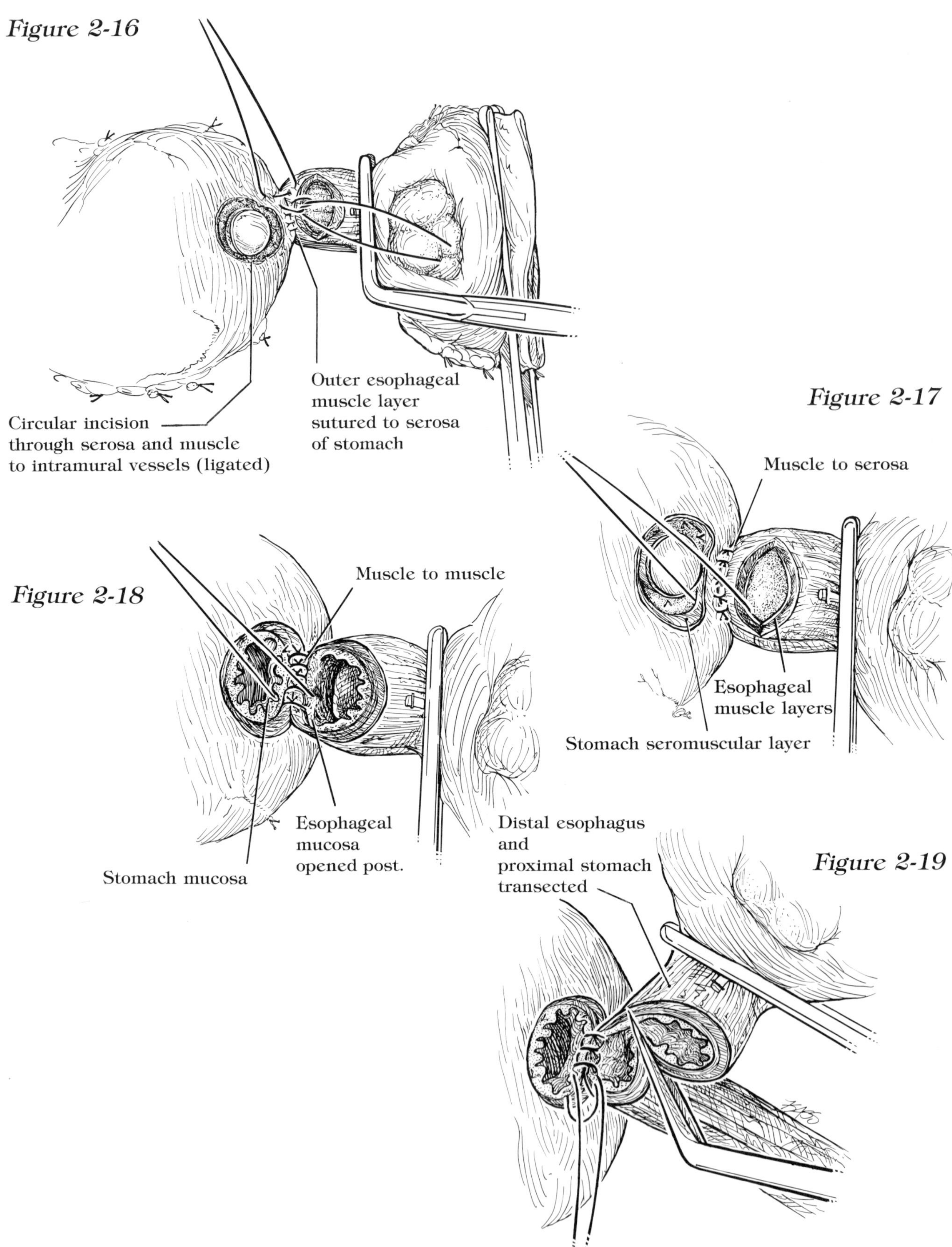

Figure 2-16
Circular incision through serosa and muscle to intramural vessels (ligated)
Outer esophageal muscle layer sutured to serosa of stomach
Figure 2-17
Muscle to serosa
Esophageal muscle layers
Stomach seromuscular layer
Figure 2-18
Muscle to muscle
Esophageal mucosa opened post.
Stomach mucosa
Distal esophagus and proximal stomach transected
Figure 2-19

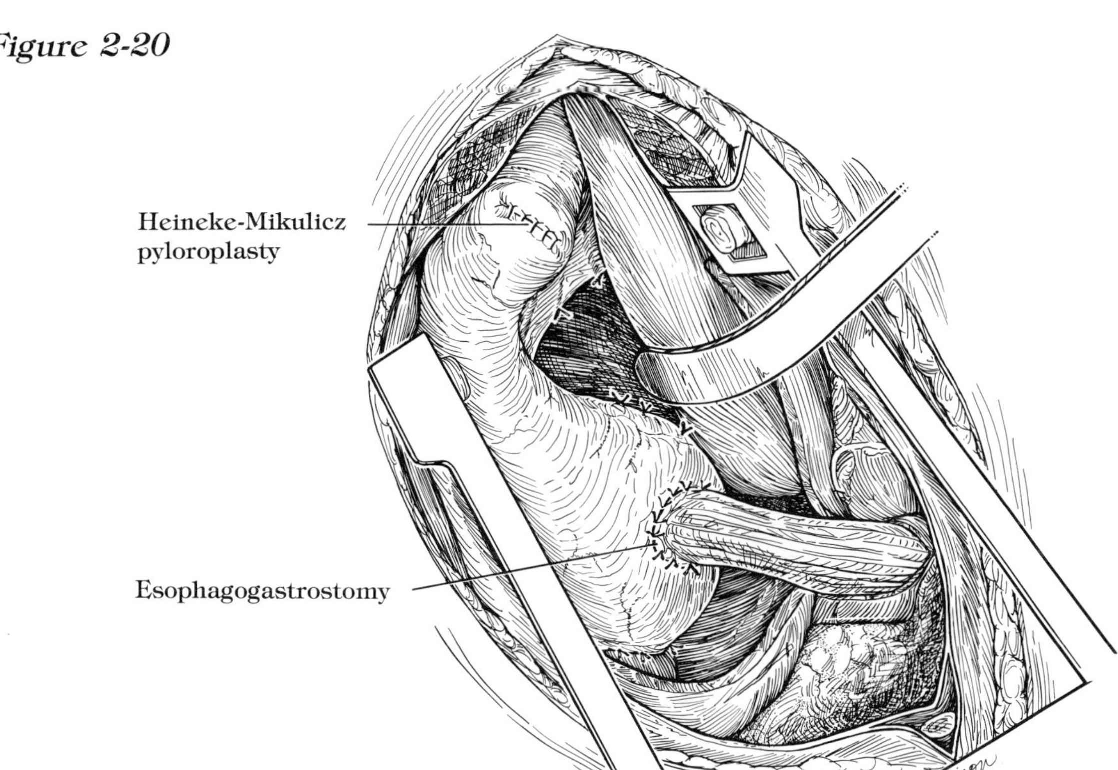

tion of what has already been described for proximal and distal gastrectomy, the duodenum is turned in by a method similar to that described after distal gastrectomy. Gastrointestinal continuity is then reconstructed by an anastomosis between the esophagus and a loop of small intestine in a manner similar to that described for the esophagogastrostomy following proximal gastrectomy.

CAUTION

The recognized risk of anastomotic leakage in any surgically established connection between the esophagus and the other portions of the gastrointestinal tract, which may occur even in the most experienced hands and after utilization of the most meticulous technique, has led surgeons to suggest that a rim of stomach may be preserved just distal to the esophagogastric junction in order to provide a safer gastrointestinal reconstruction. This is a satisfactory modification providing it does not limit the potential curability of a malignant lesion in the stomach and provided that careful attention is given to preserving blood supply to the small gastric remnant.

After the completion of the anastomosis, a long side-to-side enteroenterostomy between the limbs of the loop is usually constructed to provide a type of pouch and also to divert alkaline duodenal secretions away from the lower esophagus.

The recognition of the importance of the vagus nerve in control of gastric acid secretion, as emphasized by Dragsted, led to the introduction of a series of technical operations designed to control peptic ulcer disease while avoiding some of the recognized complications of partial gastrectomy. The advantages and disadvantages of the vagotomy procedure are not reviewed in detail here, but some generalizations can be made as an introduction to the description of the purely technical aspects.

Transthoracic vagotomy alone was early recognized as an unsatisfactory procedure because of the high incidence of recurrent gastric ulcers. The addition of pyloroplasty or posterior gastroenterostomy to the truncal vagotomy eliminated this particular disadvantage which had been caused by delayed gastric emptying, increased antral secretion of gastrin, and resulting peptic gastric ulceration. The procedure is attended, however, by occasional unpleasant complications such as persistent diarrhea, but it was also shown in long-term follow-ups to have a significantly higher incidence of recurrence of peptic ulceration than the radical distal subtotal gastrectomy.

In an effort to avoid unpleasant postoperative gastrointestinal sequelae and still achieve a high degree of ulcer control, surgeons have introduced more recent variations of selective or highly selective (parietal cell) vagotomies. The former is seldom used because the recurrence rate has been high, despite a lower incidence of gastrointestinal dysfunctions secondary to interruption of hepatic and splanchnic vagal branches. The high recurrence rate has occurred for reasons similar to those relating to truncal vagotomy as the sole operative procedure.

The highly selective (parietal cell) vagotomy supposedly corrected or protected against all previous deficits of peptic ulcer surgery by preserving hepatic and splanchnic innervation and, in addition, by preserving innervation to the antrum and pylorus. In theory the selective denervation of the parietal cell area of the stomach should protect against peptic ulceration while preserving normal gastrointestinal function and physiology. It is too soon to offer a final analysis of long-term results, but it would appear that this procedure also is attended by a high recurrence rate of peptic ulcer disease, possibly because of technical difficulties of total denervation of the parietal cell mass. Certainly, a high degree of skill and experience is required to perform the operation successfully.

The surgical techniques of these various vagotomy procedures are described separately in the following section.

This procedure is usually accomplished through an upper abdominal midline incision. The left triangular ligament of the liver is divided and the edge of the left lobe is folded back on itself and held with a retractor in order to expose the esophageal hiatus. With traction downward on the stomach, the anterior reflection of peritoneum from the stomach on to the undersurface of the diaphragm is then divided in semicircular fashion. A finger can then be introduced around the esophagus. Using the dissection plane of the finger as a guide, one can place a tape or rubber drain around the esophagus, ascertaining that the posterior vagus nerve is included. The traction on this tape or drain then brings the esophagus down into the abdominal cavity and permits identification and dissection of the right and left vagus nerves (Fig. 2-21). The left vagus nerve lies anterior to the esophagus and is the more easily identified, but the right (posterior) vagus trunk can be identified by palpation and drawn into view with a nerve hook so that transection between applied dura clips can be carried out well above the point where the nerve begins to divide on the posterior wall of the stomach (Fig. 2-22). The anterior nerve is treated in a similar fashion (Fig. 2-23) and the truncal vagotomy is completed. Attention is then directed toward the pylorus. An incision is made through the pylorus and carried 4 cm proximally and distally through the gastric and duodenal walls (Fig. 2-24). The longitudinal incision is then closed transversely (Fig. 2-25), thus insuring a widely patent outflow for the stomach as well as interrupting the function of the pyloric muscle.

The Finney pyloroplasty is another variant in which the distal stomach and posterior duodenum are brought together with an interrupted row of sutures. A U-shaped incision, as shown in Figure 2-26, is made between spring clamps. This is closed with an inner layer of continuous chromic catgut and an outer layer of interrupted silk sutures as depicted in Figures 2-27 and 2-28. The completed anastomosis (Fig. 2-29) provides the type of outflow from the stomach as shown in the type of standard pyloroplasty in Figures 2-24 and 2-25.

An extension of the vagotomy principle has resulted in the introduction more recently of two variations referred to as selective vagotomy or parietal cell (highly selective) vagotomy. Diagrammatic representations of the three variants of vagus nerve interruption are set forth in Figures 2-30, 2-31, and 2-32. The initial exposure and anatomic identification of the vagus nerves are similar to those described in the initial phases of the truncal vagotomy. For the *selective vagotomy,* dissection of the trunks of the vagus nerves is more precise to the extent that the branches diverging to the right and posteriorly near the esophagogastric junction are carefully preserved, branches from the vagus to the anterior and posterior walls of the stomach are di-

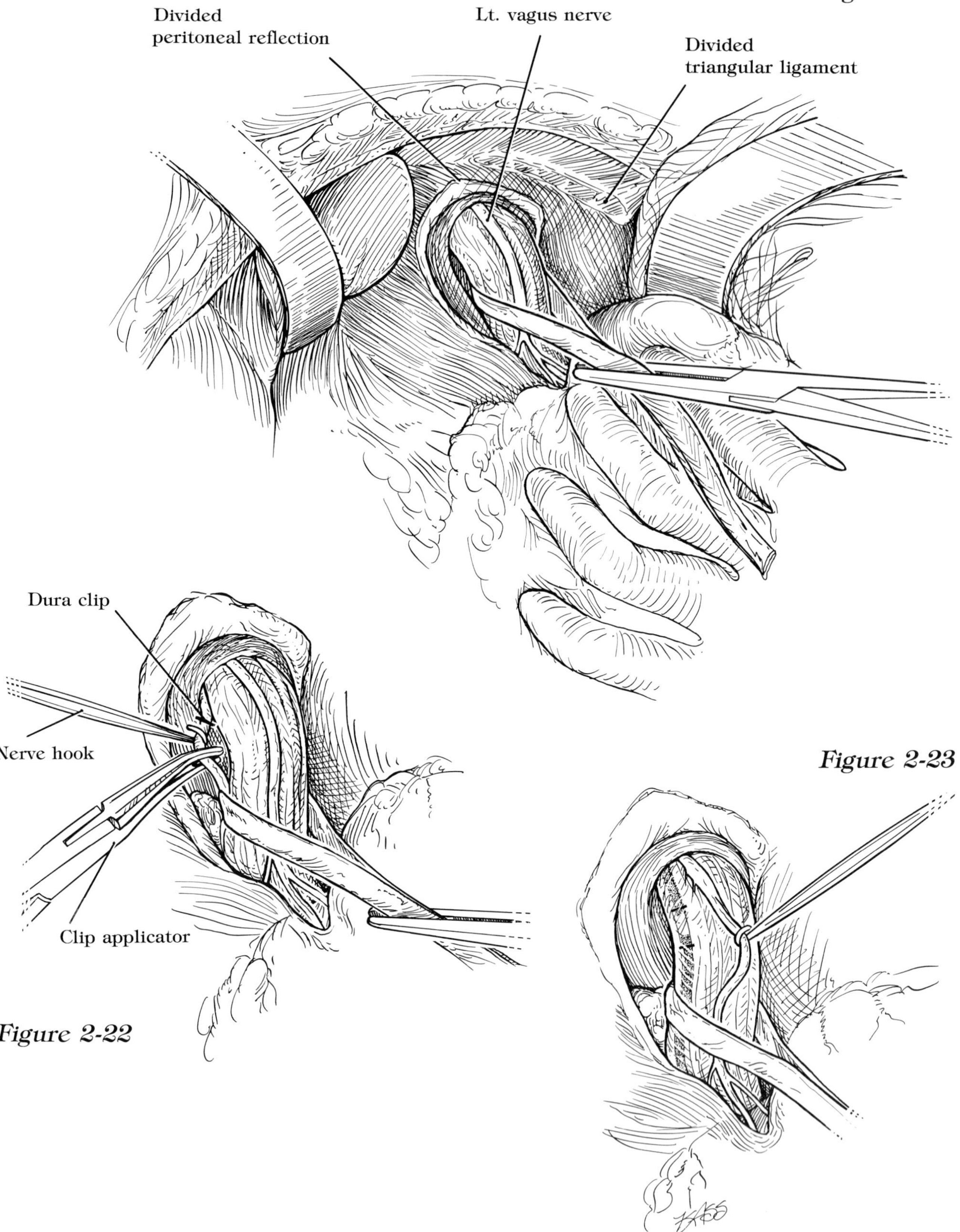

Divided
peritoneal reflection
Lt. vagus nerve
Divided
triangular ligament
Dura clip
Nerve hook
Clip applicator
Figure 2-22
Figure 2-23

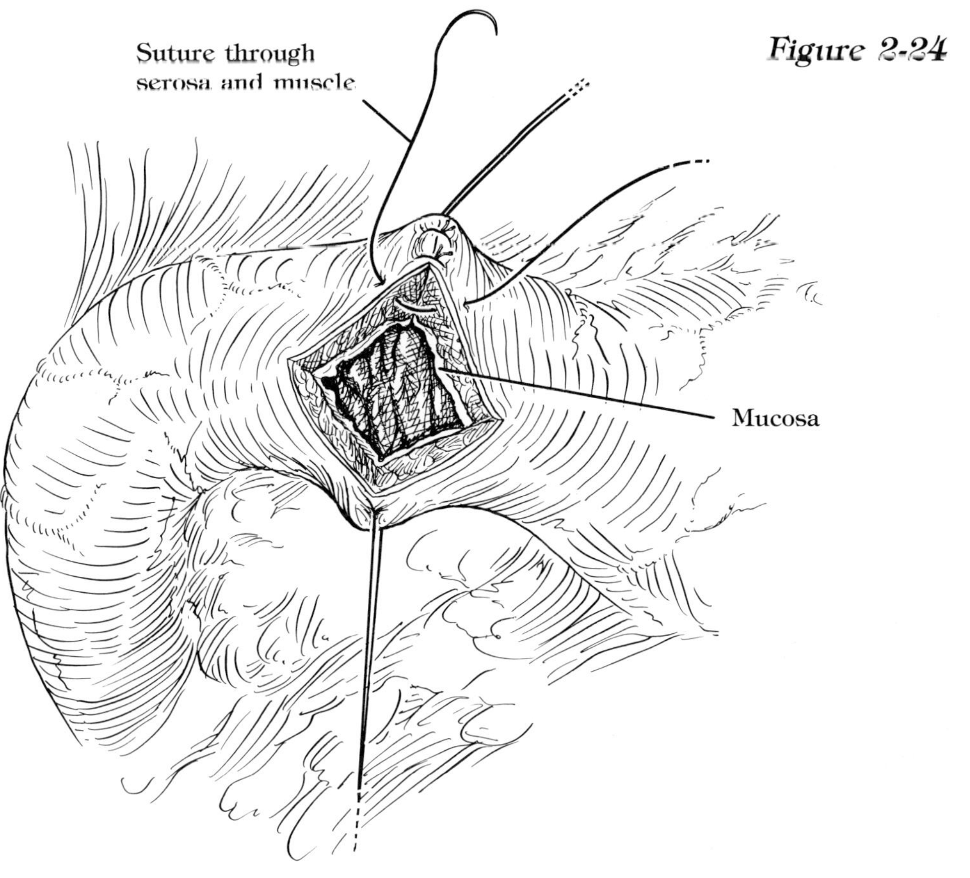

Suture through
serosa and muscle
Mucosa
Figure 2-24

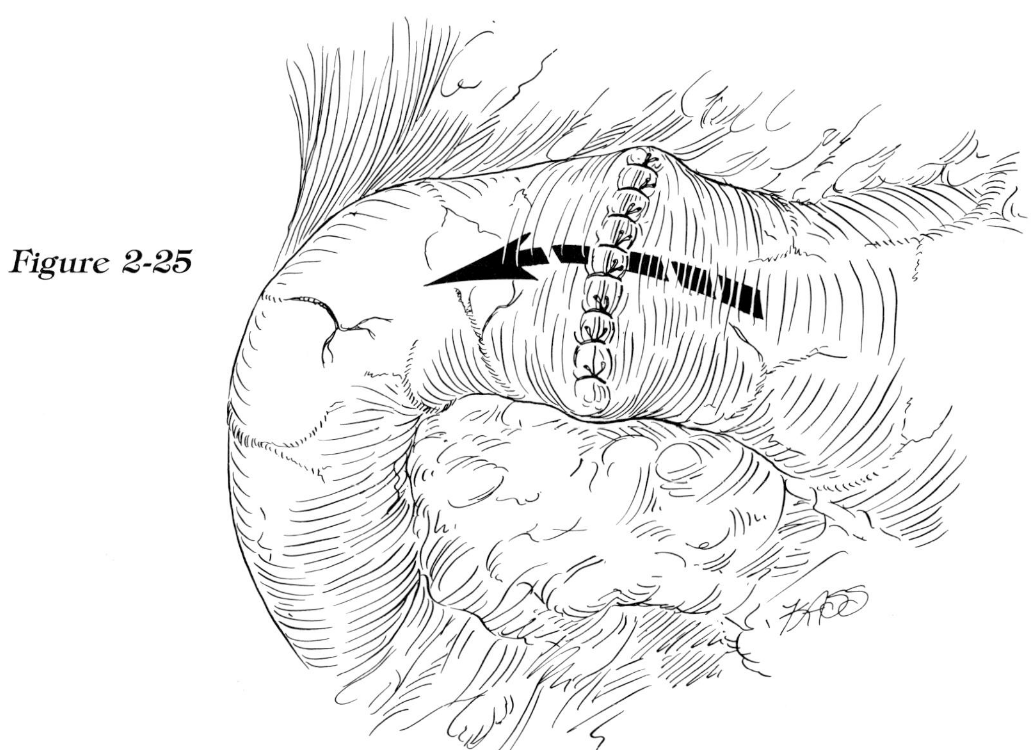

Figure 2-25

Figure 2-26

Figure 2-27

Figure 2-28

Flow through
completed anastomosis

Figure 2-29

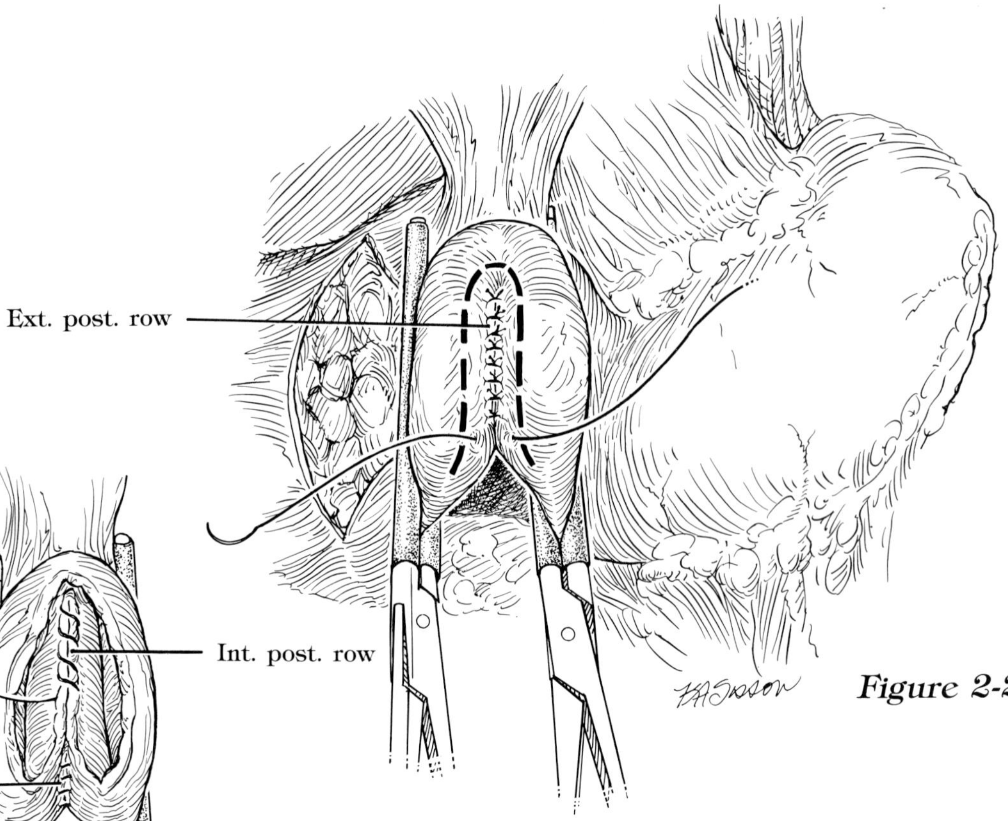

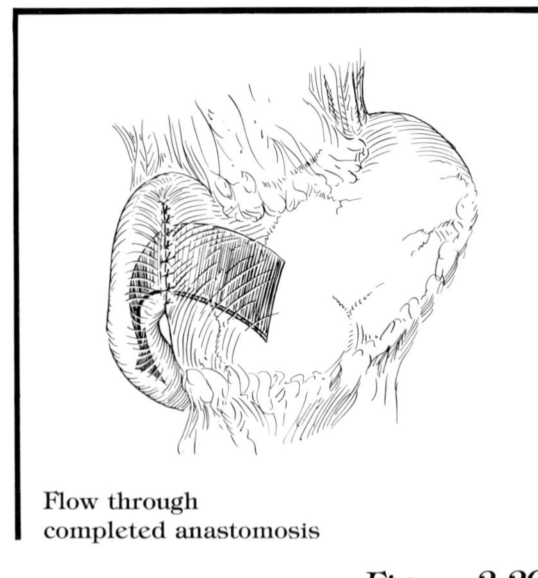

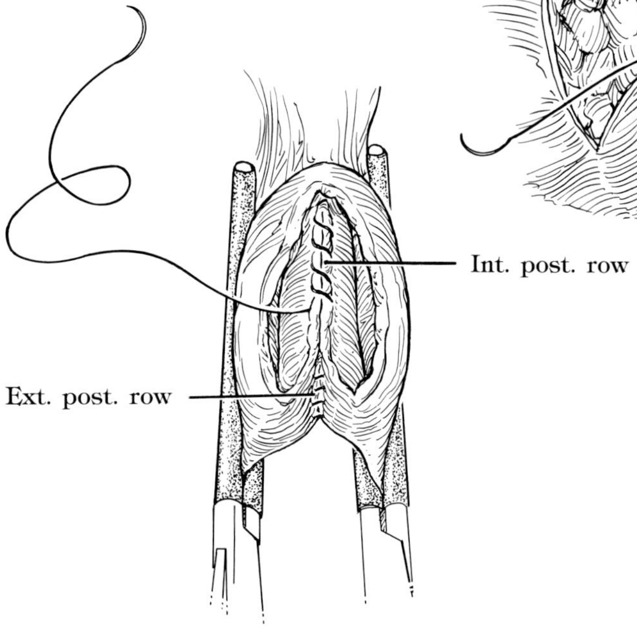

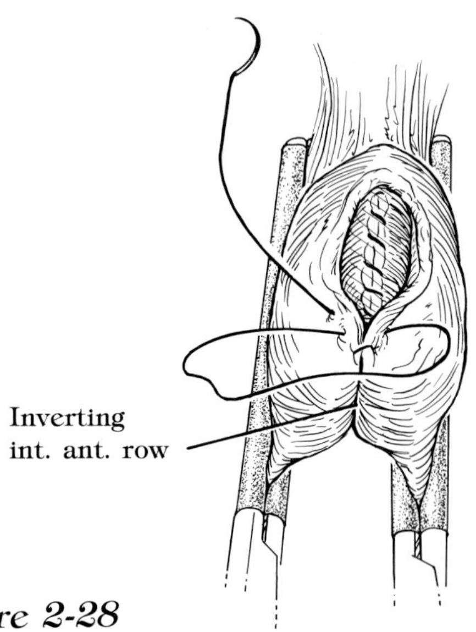

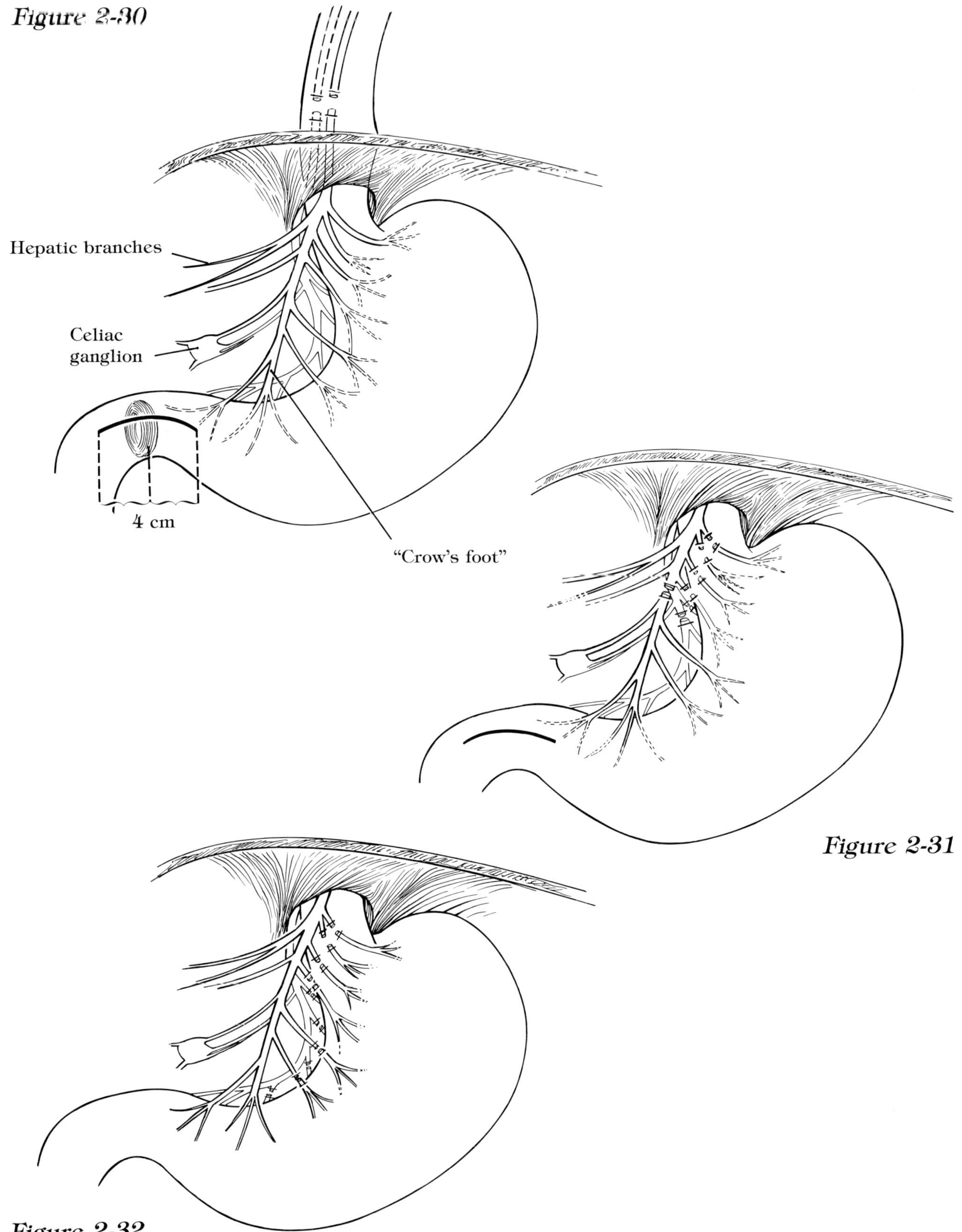

Figure 2-30
Hepatic branches
Celiac ganglion
4 cm
"Crow's foot"
Figure 2-31
Figure 2-32

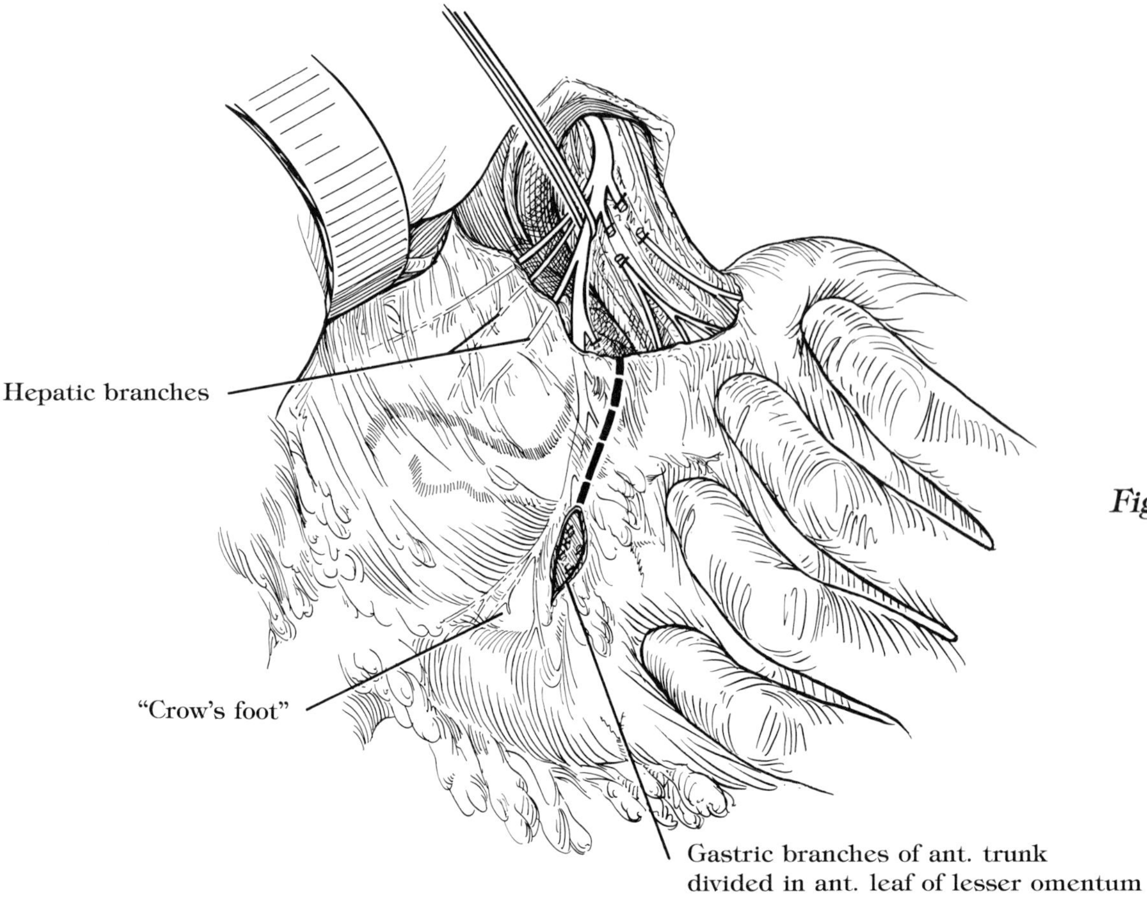

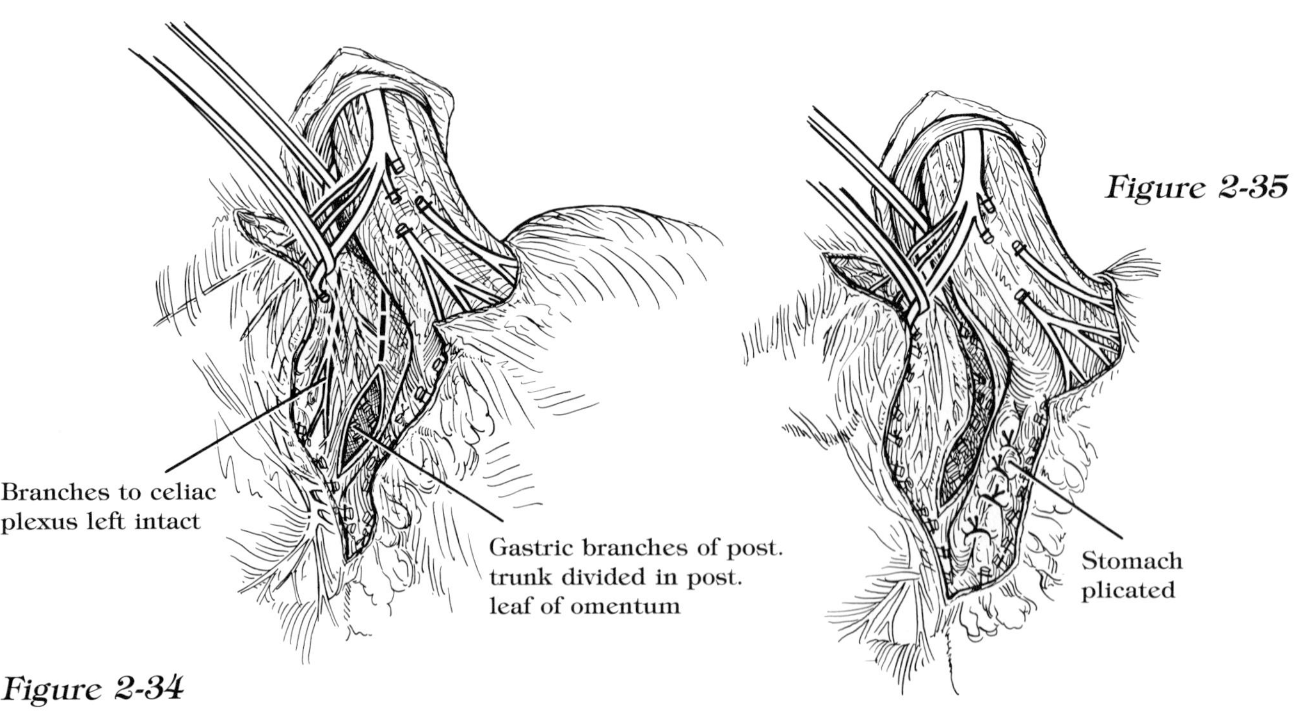

Hepatic branches
"Crow's foot"
Gastric branches of ant. trunk
divided in ant. leaf of lesser omentum
Figure 2-33
Branches to celiac
plexus left intact
Gastric branches of post.
trunk divided in post.
leaf of omentum
Figure 2-34
Figure 2-35
Stomach
plicated

vided between dura clips, and then finally the trunks of the vagus distal to the hepatic branches are completely divided (see Fig. 2-31). Anatomic details can be inferred from the text, and drawings that follow in the later modifications are referred to as *parietal cell* (or *highly selective*) *vagotomy.*

After the initial dissection of the anterior vagus nerve and division of the branches diverging onto the stomach wall, a finger is inserted through the avascular part of the lesser omentum and passed behind the omentum to the lesser curvature of the stomach. The serosa is divided along the lesser curvature, the vessels are dissected free against the finger, and the blood vessels to the lesser curvature are carefully divided between ligatures. As the dissection is carried either proximally or distally (preferably the former) along the lesser curvature, small branches of the anterior vagal trunk are identified and divided until the entire omentum has been dissected free from the lesser curvature (Fig. 2-33). When the dissection is complete along the anterior wall of the lesser curvature, a similar dissection is made of the posterior or right vagal trunk (Fig. 2-34). An essential part of the operation is identification of the "crow's foot" where the vagus nerves end in a decussation of fibers along the antrum and provide innovation to the pylorus and distal stomach. At the conclusion of the procedure, the lesser curvature of the stomach is oversewn with interrupted silk sutures to prevent any possible perforation and leak from the extensive devascularization (Fig. 2-35).

It is generally accepted that the most common condition that predisposes to gastroesophageal reflux is the existence of a sliding esophageal hiatus hernia. Given the differences of opinion as to whether the incompetent sphincter precedes the development of the hernia or whether the hernia results in the loss of the sphincter mechanism, it is accepted that reconstruction of a normal sphincter mechanism is essential to correct the characteristic symptoms of substernal burning, regurgitation, and eructations with endoscopic findings of esophagitis.

Repair of Esophageal Hiatus Hernia

Figure 2-36 is a diagrammatic representation of a sliding hernia, showing the zones of elevated pressure at the hiatus and at the sphincter. It may be that esophageal manometry based on this concept will provide better indications as to whether a symptom complex is or is not related to an incompetent sphincter mechanism and, therefore, whether or not a surgical repair is indicated.

The number of surgical approaches that have been designed and reported over the past three decades in order to accomplish the restoration of a normal sphincteric mechanism give testimony to the ultimate lack of satisfaction with any one of these various procedures. These approaches are not described in de-

Figure 2-36

Pressure
Esophagus
Sphincter
Hernia
Hiatus
Fundus

Lt. lobe of liver
folded back on itself
Divided peritoneum
Divided triangular
ligament
Esophageal Hernia
Closed
Divided lt. gastric a.
and gastrohepatic ligament
Divided
short gastric
vessels

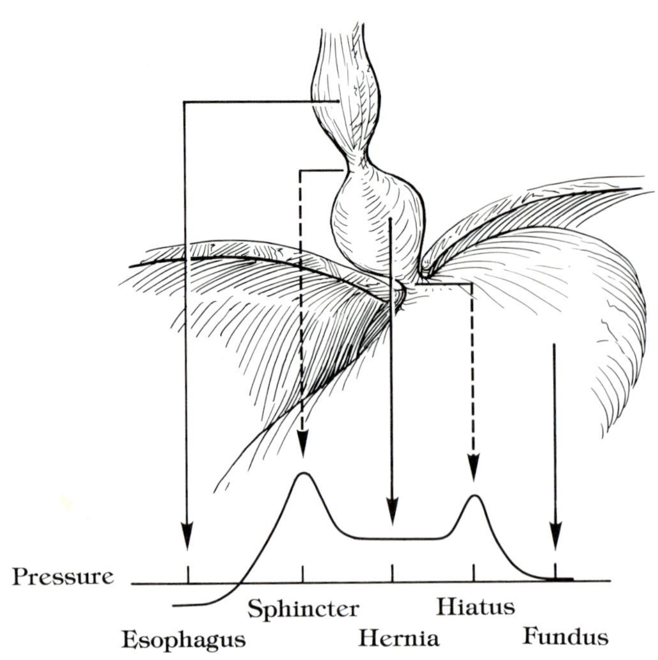

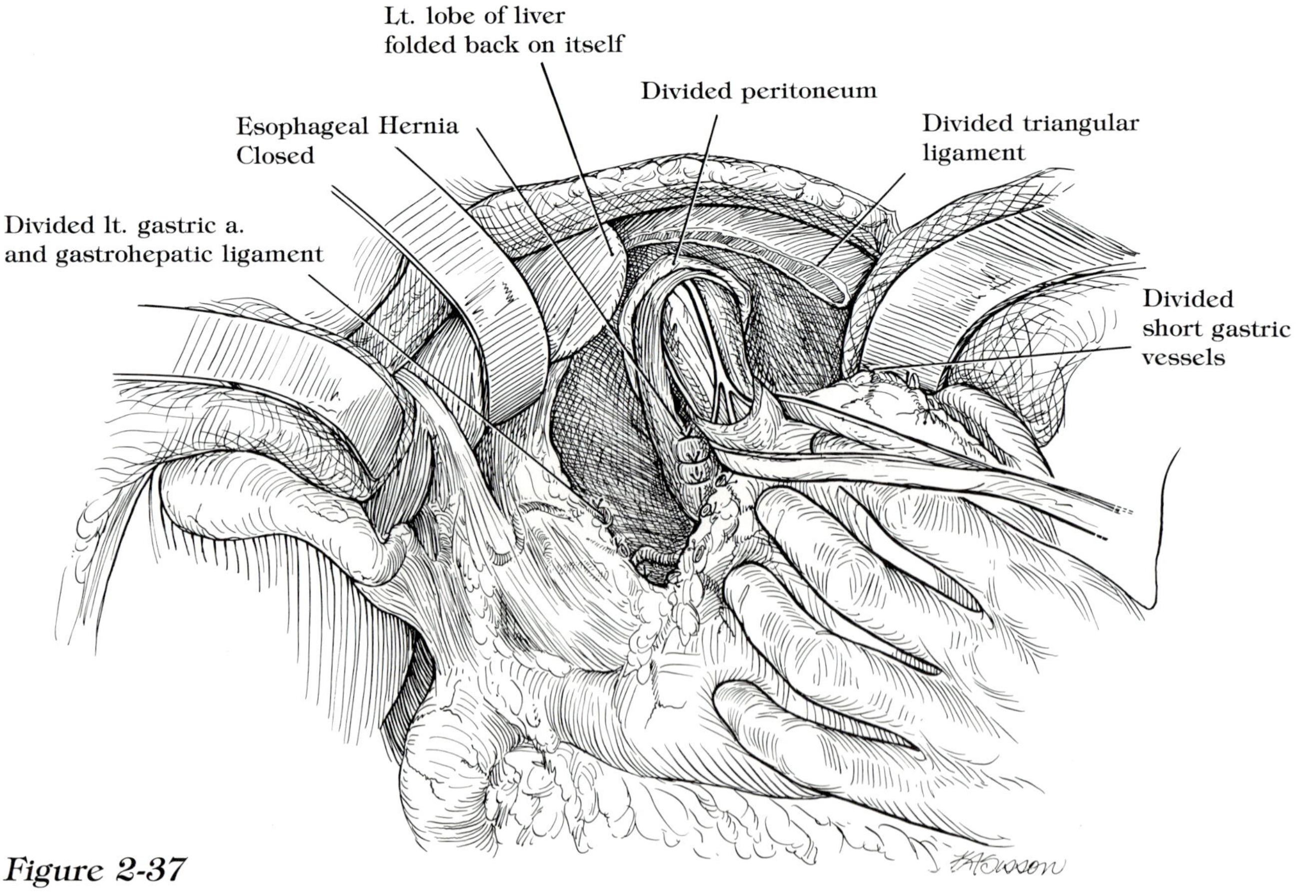

Figure 2-37

tail, but the most generally accepted surgical approach at present, called fundoplication, is described in the following section.

Exposure of the gastroesophageal junction is usually satisfactory through a midline upper abdominal incision. An anatomic view of the area is obtained as in the truncal vagotomy, by dividing the left triangular ligament of the liver and folding the left lobe on itself for exposure to the hiatus. The peritoneal reflection from the stomach to the undersurface of the diaphragm is divided and the dissecting finger is passed around the distal esophagus. Mobilization is carried out as previously described in the procedure of truncal vagotomy. Again, the use of an encircling tape or rubber drain permits continuous downward traction on the esophagogastric junction. The upper stomach is also fully mobilized, including division of some of the vasa brevia, and the wall of the stomach should be freed up posteriorly. With the esophagogastric junction drawn downward with the Penrose drain and pulled somewhat to the left, the widened esophageal hiatus can be visualized and is then narrowed by approximating the crura posteriorly with several heavy silk sutures tied to form a snug hiatus that easily admits the index finger (Fig. 2-37). In order to avoid narrowing of the distal esophagus by this and subsequent maneuvers to be described, a large gastric tube should be placed by the anesthesiologist transorally into the stomach during the fundoplication. The mobilized gastric fundus is then displaced posteriorly to the right in such a way that, when sutured, it encircles the area of the gastroesophageal junction (Fig. 2-38). Interrupted silk sutures are then used to approximate the adjacent margins of the encircling fundus (Figs. 2-39, 2-40). When the sutures are placed and the surgeon is satisfied that the plication has not unduly narrowed the esophagus, the gastric tube may be withdrawn and the incision closed.

Small Bowel Resection

Because of the easy mobilization of the small intestine, this is usually a simple technical procedure provided the anatomy of the arcades is visualized either directly or by transillumination, and the V excision of the mesentery is performed so that the proximal and distal ends of transected bowel are well vascularized. The anastomosis is one of the safest of all gastrointestinal reconstructions and may be achieved either with a single layer of interrupted silk sutures, bringing serosa to serosa, similar to what has been described in pyloroplasty or, by surgeon's preference, with a continuous inner layer of catgut with an outer reinforcing serosa layer of interrupted silk. Anastomosis can be tested by thumb and forefinger evaginated through the suture lines to determine the patency of the stoma. Then the leaves of the mesentery are carefully closed with interrupted silk sutures or continuous fine catgut, with care taken not to damage any of the preserved blood supply to the anastomotic area.

Figure 2-38

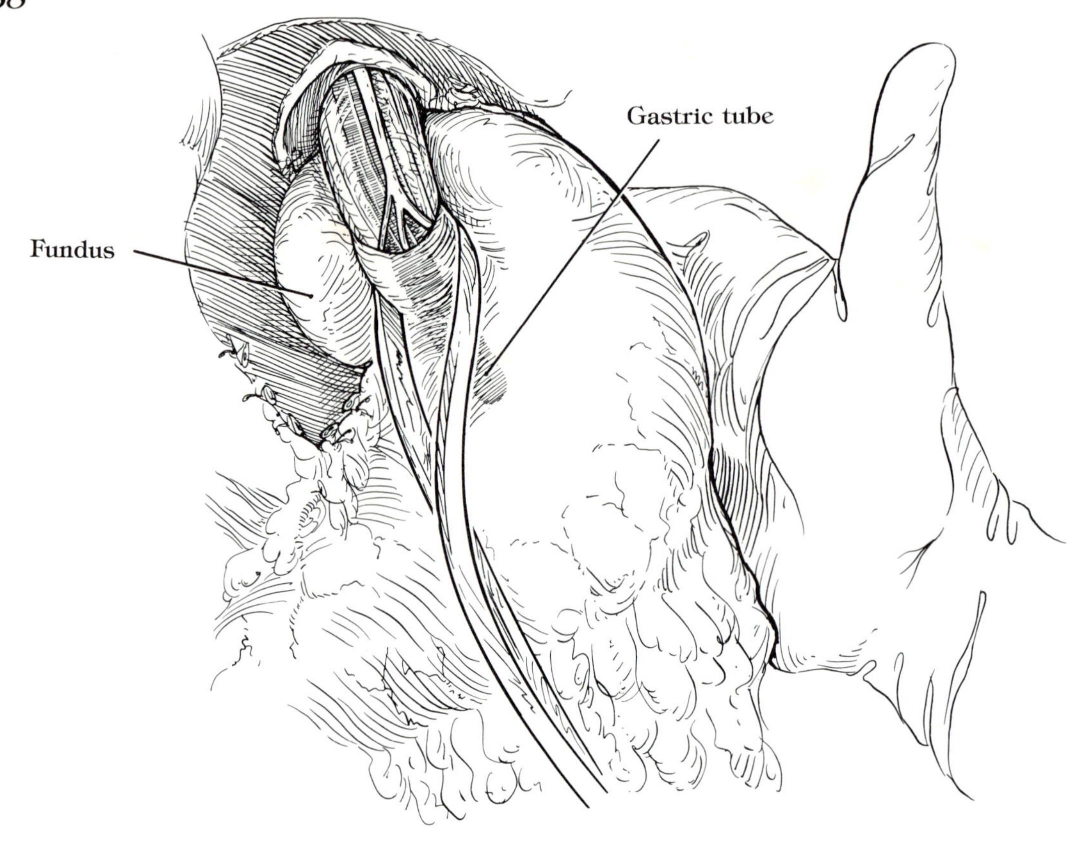
Gastric tube
Fundus

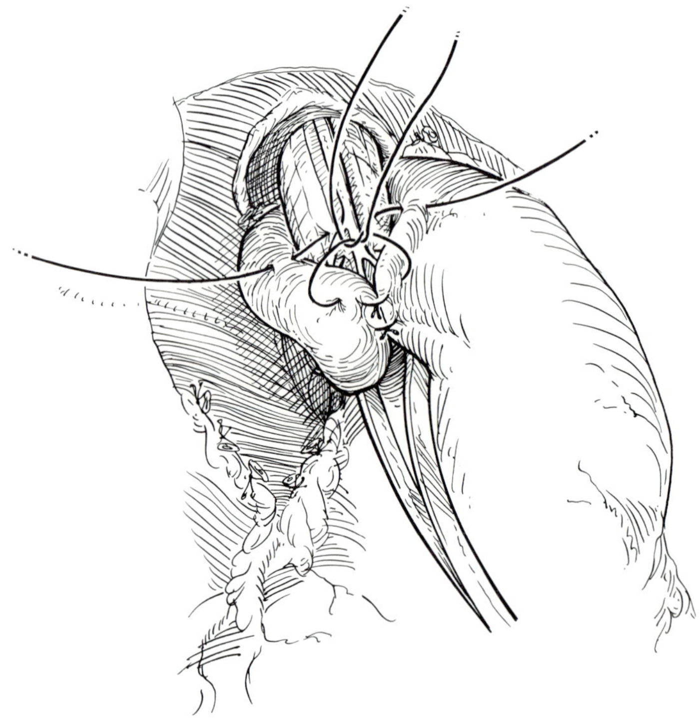
Figure 2-39

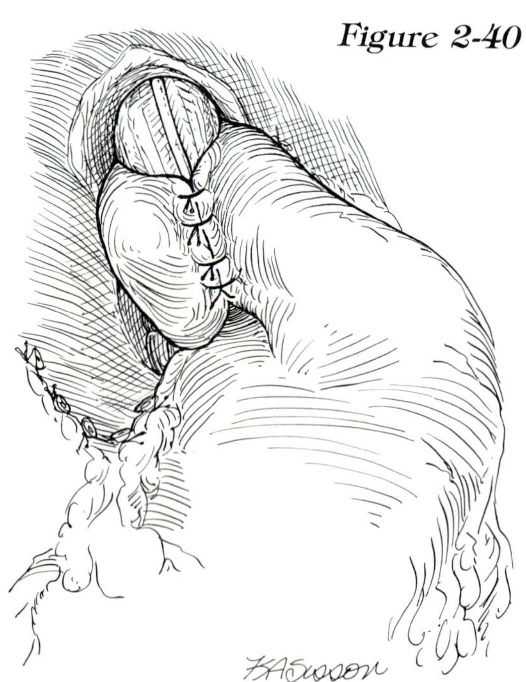
Figure 2-40

CHAPTER THREE

COLON
AND
RECTUM

The success of any colon resection depends on a knowledge of the vascular anatomy and lymphatic drainage, as shown in Figure 3-1. The points at which vessels are divided depends on the location of the lesion and the extent of the appropriate resection as indicated in Figures 3-2 through 3-8.

Colonic Resections

Two decades ago the concept was still held valid that the wider the lymphatic node dissection, the better the chance of cure. With better realization of the biological behavior of cancer, procedures such as left colectomy with high dissection of the inferior mesenteric nodes are no longer considered appropriate. The extent of resection, as shown by the dotted lines in Figures 3-2 through 3-8, is considered adequate for each of the locations indicated. It is important, either before or at the time of operation, to be certain that no metachronous lesion is coexisting. Colonoscopy or barium enema, when feasible, may be indicated preoperatively and certainly careful inspection of the colon is a necessary part of the procedure. Subsequent specific text and drawings emphasize the operative details.

The preferable incision is a right paramedian, centered at the level of the umbilicus. The attachments of the cecum are then interrupted at the lateral peritoneal reflection divided with the scissors using fingers as a guide along the entire right gutter up to the hepatic flexure. This permits mobilization of the cecum and terminal ileum which has been drawn medially up into the

RIGHT COLECTOMY

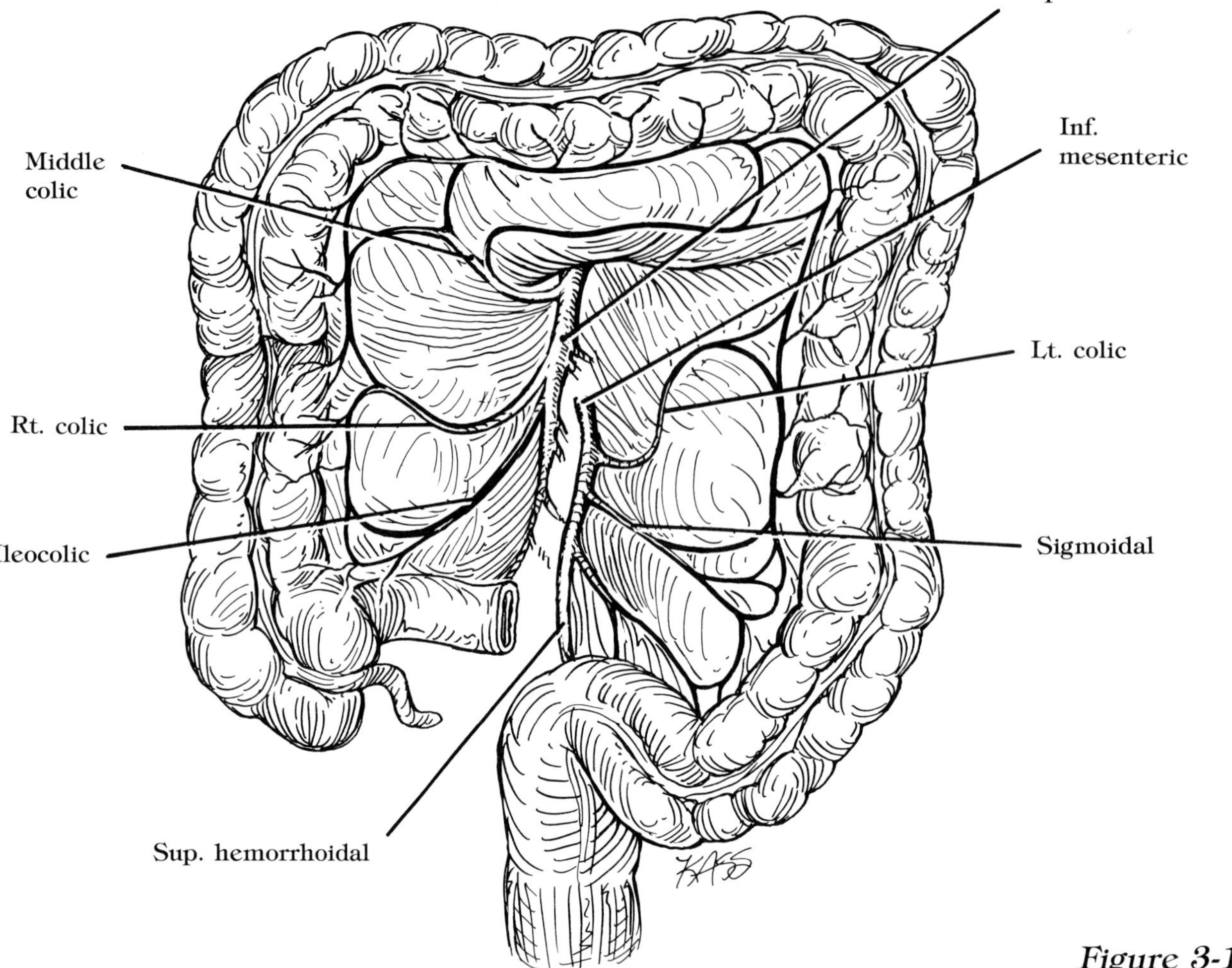

Figure 3-1

operative incision. As division of the peritoneum is then carried around the hepatic flexure, the duodenum should come into view. The attachments of the greater omentum to the hepatic flexure and transverse colon can be freed up entering the plane between the transverse mesocolon and the gastrocolic omentum (Fig. 3-9).

When the entire area to be resected has been mobilized, the appropriate branches of the superior mesenteric vessels are li-

CAUTION

During mobilization of the right colon, it is imperative to identify the course of the right ureter in the retroperitoneal retrocolic space since this could be easily drawn up with the mesentery of the bowel by blunt dissection and inadvertently injured.

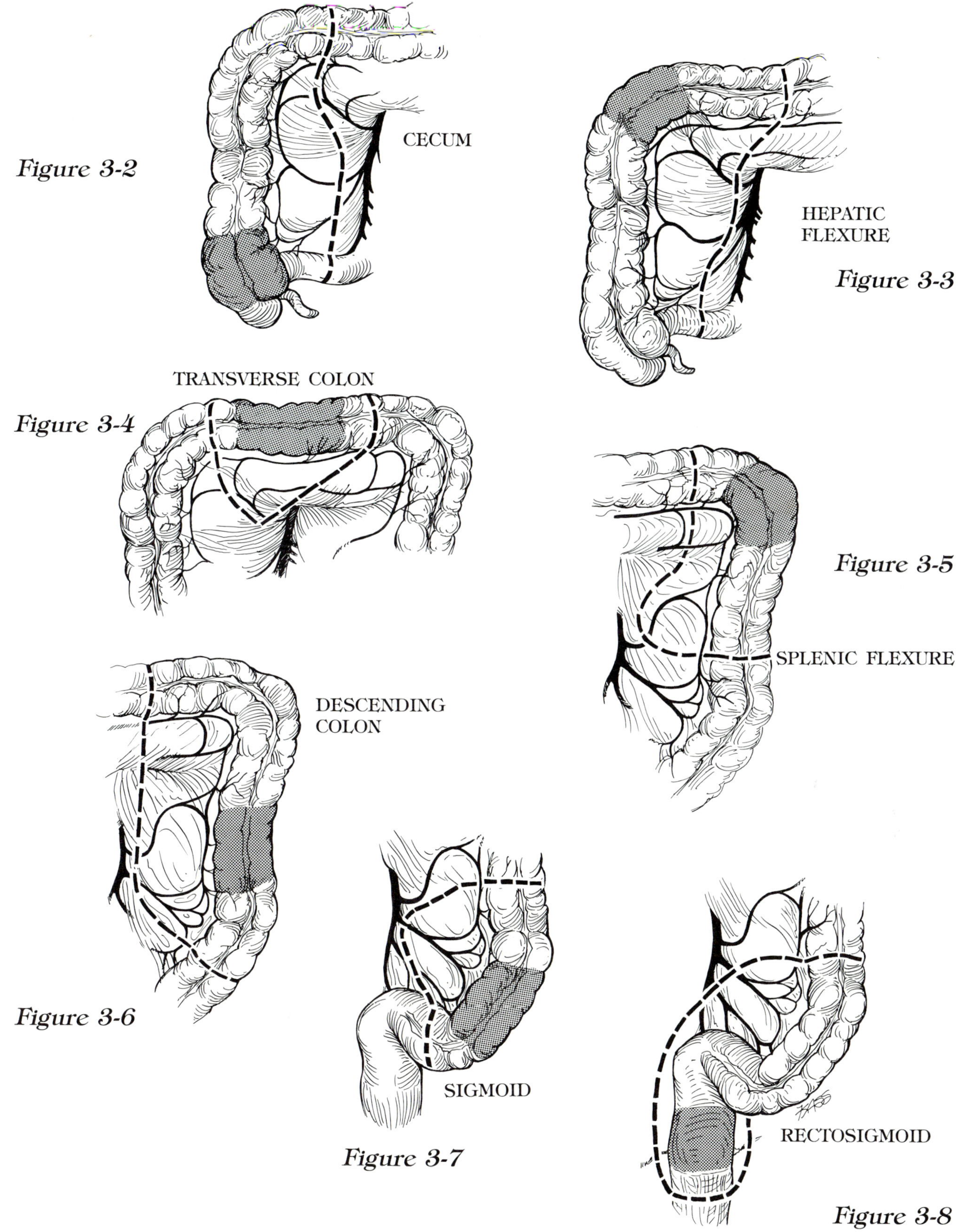

Figure 3-2
CECUM
HEPATIC
FLEXURE
Figure 3-3
TRANSVERSE COLON
Figure 3-4
Figure 3-5
SPLENIC FLEXURE
DESCENDING
COLON
Figure 3-6
SIGMOID
Figure 3-7
RECTOSIGMOID
Figure 3-8

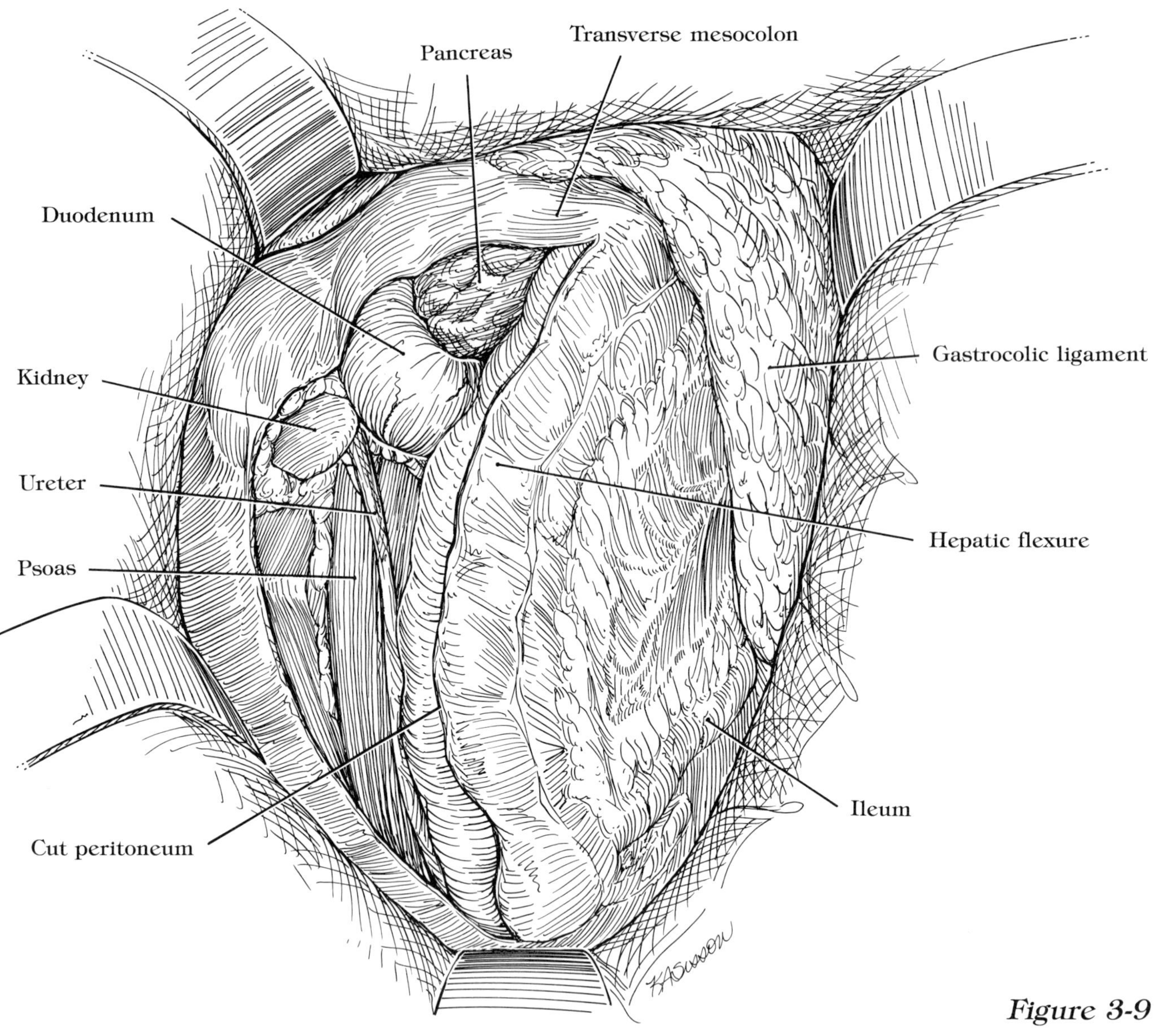

Figure 3-9

gated, with the point of division determined by the location of the lesion (see Figs. 3-2, 3-3). It is particularly important to preserve the left branch of the midcolic artery or to carry the resection far enough toward the splenic flexure to assure adequate blood supply from the left colic. A branch of the ileocolic should be identified in order to provide adequate blood supply to the terminal ileum. Once this has been accomplished, the bowel is divided between clamps, rubber-shod clamps are placed proximally and distally, and the edges of the mesenteric borders are approximated with a continuous 2-0 chromic catgut stitch. The Allen-Kocher clamps are then removed and an end-to-end anastomosis is constructed with a single layer of interrupted, nonabsorbable suture material.

CAUTION

The entire success of colon resection and anastomosis is dependent on adequate blood supply to the margins. Therefore, certain maneuvers and sequences are considered important. First, the edges of the mesentery are approximated in the event that some of the blood vessels coursing beneath the leaf of peritoneum are injured. Resulting observed or suspected ischemia can then be managed by further resection of a bowel segment without repeating that entire step. Second, the curved needle holding the continuous catgut suture should be placed parallel to the edge of the peritoneum, which provides less likelihood of vascular injury. Third, prior to the actual anastomosis, the bowel margins should be carefully inspected to ascertain the presence of pulsations in the small vessels and the existence of a healthy, pink mucosal surface at the cut edges. Fourth, a single-layer anastomosis of interrupted sutures is believed to be less likely to interfere with vascular supply at the anastomotic edge. In the hands of surgeons utilizing this technique, it has proved at least as safe and satisfactory as a two-layer closure.

TRANSVERSE COLECTOMY

Through a transverse upper-abdominal incision, the gastrocolic omentum is opened and a plane is identified between the gastrocolic omentum and the transverse mesocolon. A portion of the greater omentum with the area to be resected is left on the bowel. After ligation of the appropriate vessels (see Fig. 3-4), end-to-end anastomosis is carried out as described. The same precautions and sequence of technical maneuvers are followed as in right colectomy.

LEFT COLECTOMY

This procedure is approached through a left paramedian incision centered at the umbilicus, but perhaps carried farther up toward the costal margin than is usually necessary on the right side. The lateral attachments of the sigmoid colon are divided. The peritoneal reflection into the left gutter is divided with scissors, using two fingers as a dissecting and identifying maneuver (Fig. 3-10). As the bowel is mobilized and drawn medially, the left ureter should be identified as it crosses the bifurcation of the common iliac artery and vein and followed superiorly in order to assure its preservation. The left spermatic or ovarian vessels also can be visualized at this point and preserved. Perhaps the most difficult part of this procedure is the mobilization of the splenic flexure. With retraction by an assistant on the

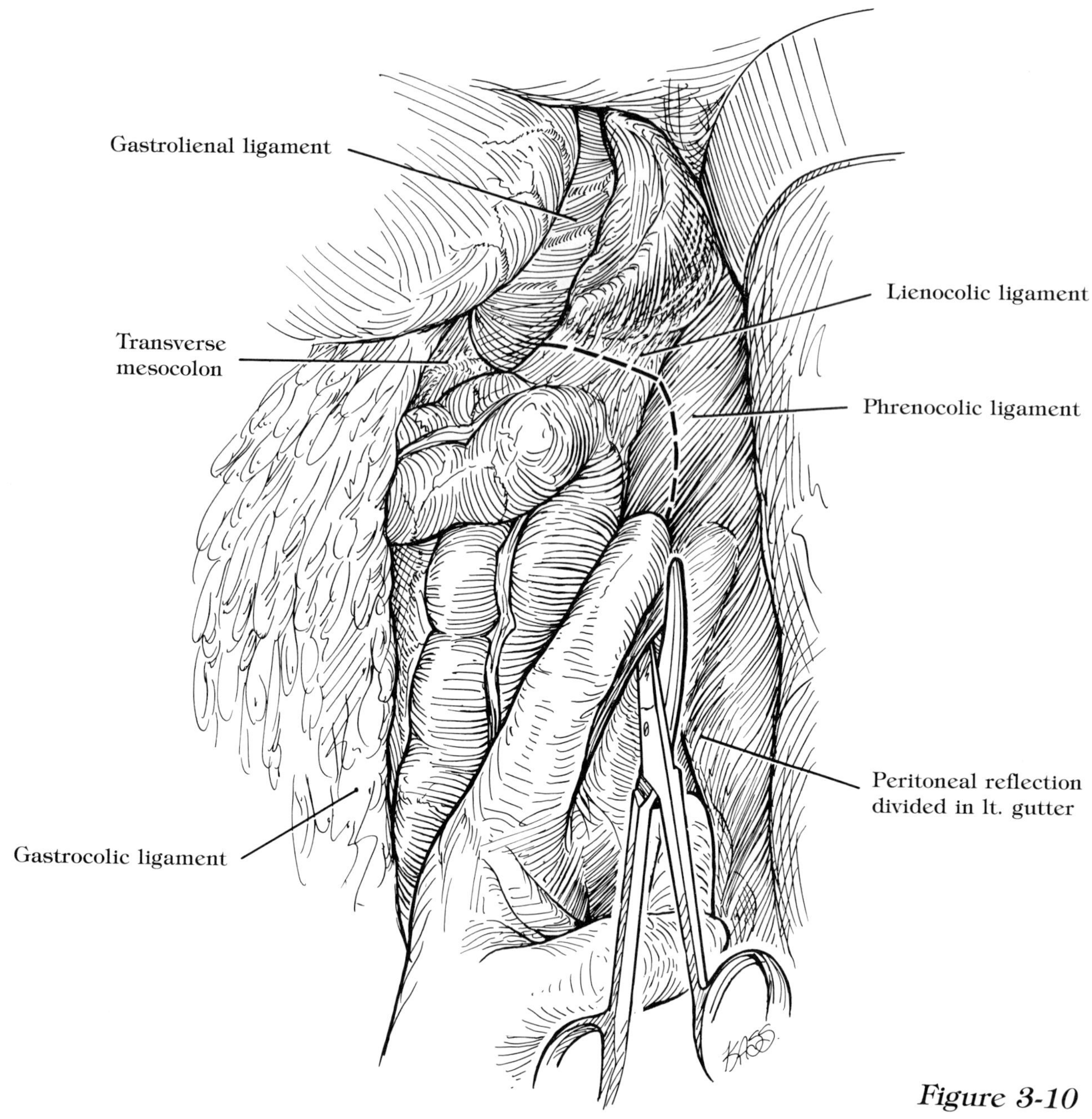

Figure 3-10

upper end of the incision and traction downward of the mobilized descending colon, one can cautiously proceed to divide the lienocolic ligaments. At this point, mobilization of the greater omentum off the splenic flexure and transverse colon makes dissection easier, although any segment of the greater omentum near a malignant lesion should be left attached to the bowel and removed with it. As one then draws the splenic flexure downward, the transverse colon is mobilized and dissection is performed according to the pattern shown for the location of the lesion (see Figs. 3-5, 3-6). Anastomosis between the transverse colon and distal sigmoid is then accomplished in the manner already described. See cautionary notes under the section on right colectomy.

For a lesion of the midportion of the sigmoid loop, a left paramedian incision centered below the umbilicus is made. The operation is begun as described for a left colectomy by mobilization of the sigmoid, again carefully identifying and preserving the ureter and spermatic or ovarian vessels. Once the bowel is mobilized, clamps are placed, the vascular supply is identified and ligated, and the bowel is divided (see Fig. 3-7). Often it is necessary to mobilize the splenic flexure in order to obtain sufficient length of bowel to bring down to the distal sigmoid. The left colic artery must be identified and preserved. In terms of the distal blood supply, inferior mesenteric artery must be identified and a terminal sigmoid branch preserved if an anastomosis is to be constructed above the pelvic floor. See cautionary notes under the section on right colectomy.

This operation is designed for lesions at or just below the pelvic floor where it is estimated that an adequate resection from malignant disease can be carried out and still preserve a section of rectum for anastomosis (see Fig. 3-8). Again the sigmoid colon and entire left colon and splenic flexure are mobilized unless there is sufficient length of bowel to reach well down into the pelvis without tension. An incision is made in the pelvic reflection from the rectosigmoid to the posterior wall of either the uterus or the bladder, dissection is carried down anteriorly, and then the peritoneal incision is carried upward along the mesentery. Lateral peritoneal flaps are raised for later reconstruction of the pelvic floor (Fig. 3-11). Adequate visualization of both ureters is essential, and they can be retracted laterally with the peritoneal flaps. Dissection is then carried down on each side of the rectosigmoid to the levator ani muscles, dividing and ligating the middle hemorrhoidal vessels (see Fig. 3-11). A right-angled Wertheim clamp is then placed well below the pelvic floor at a distance of at least 10 cm below the gross extension of the lesion. Holding ligatures are placed on each side of the rectum, and the bowel is divided and brought up out of the pelvis (Fig. 3-12). The bowel is transected superiorly between clamps. One must again make certain that blood supply is adequate from the branches of the left colic artery since the superior hemorrhoidal and sigmoidal vessels are ligated. An open single-layer anastomosis is then formed well below the pelvic floor, which can then be closed with a continuous 2-0 chromic catgut stitch above the area of anastomosis (Figs. 3-13, 3-14). In such a low anastomosis, it is advisable to bring a drain or suction catheter out between the coccyx and the anus so that it lies in the hollow of the sacrum but does not abut the actual

Bladder retracted
Middle hemorrhoidal vessels divided
Levator ani m.
Ureter in peritoneal flap
Lesion
Sigmoid colon

Mesentery
Rectum divided
Sup. hemorrhoidal vessels
Sigmoid branches
Inf. mesenteric vessels

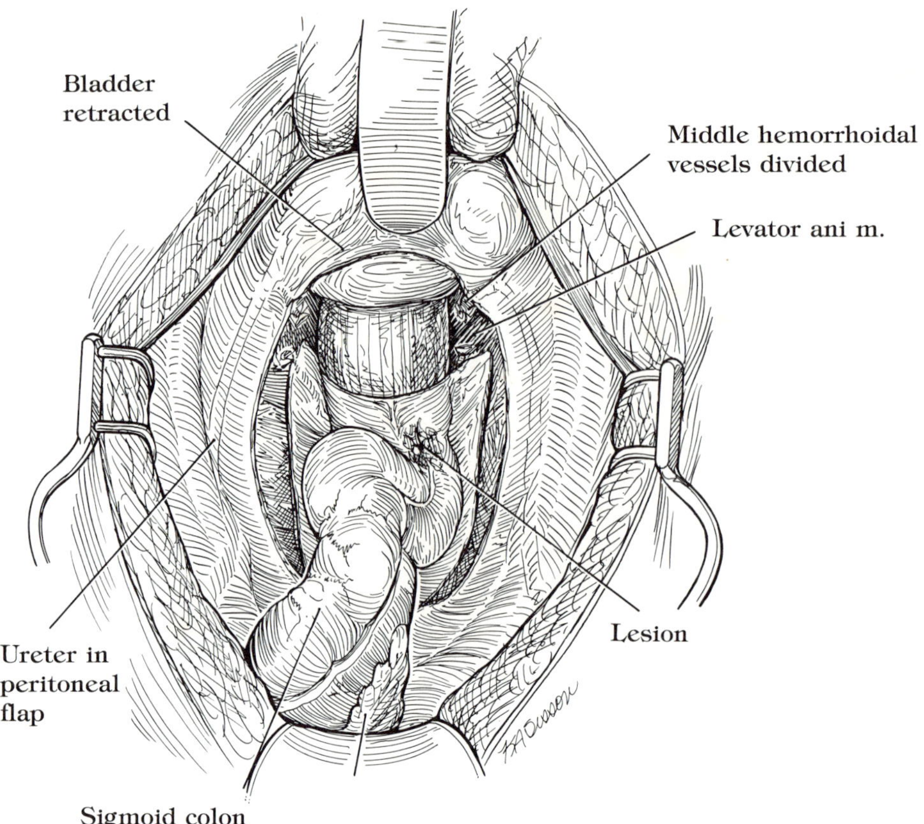

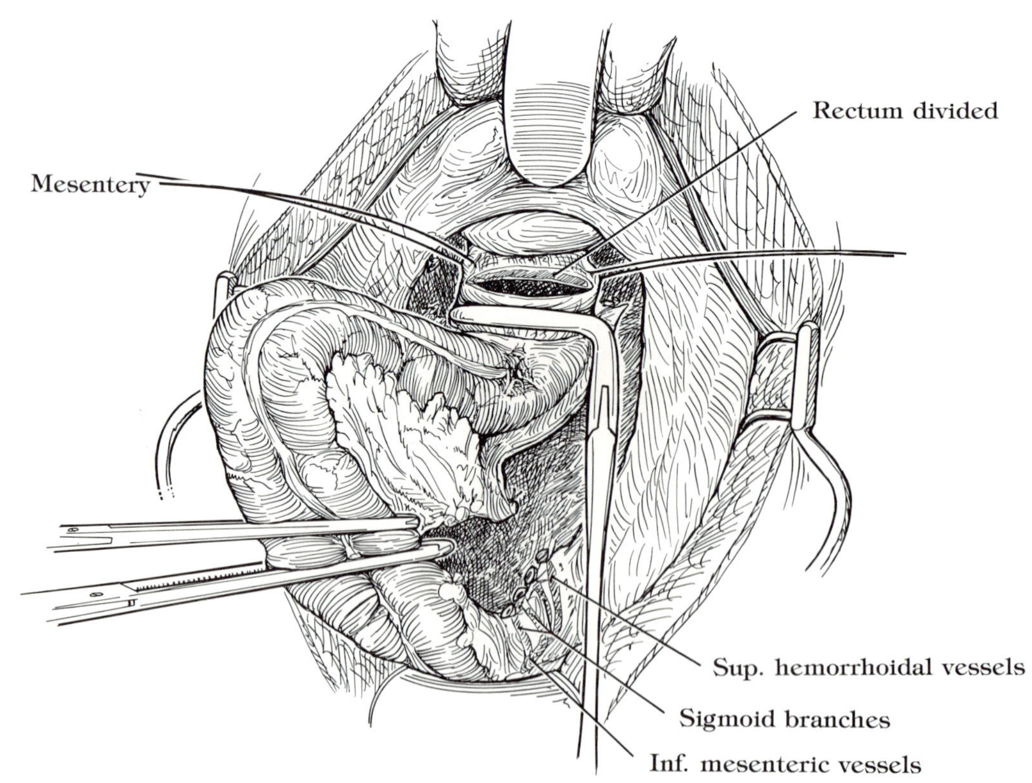

Figure 3-12

anastomotic site. Because of the dubious blood supply to the distal bowel from the inferior hemorrhoidal system, a complementary transverse colostomy is considered mandatory as part of the operative procedure.

CAUTION

Surgeons have long noted the surprisingly high incidence of clinically obvious or radiologically demonstrable anastomotic leaks after this procedure. For this reason, a complementary transverse colostomy should be used, except in circumstances where the anastomosis is very simple, the blood supply to the distal segment excellent, and no reservations exist about either the vascularity of the bowel edges or the construction of the anastomosis itself. The time for closure of the transverse colostomy is extremely variable and again depends on these various factors. It is occasionally possible to close the colostomy within two weeks of the initial resection and prior to the patient's departure from the hospital. On the other hand, when the resection has been performed for extensive diverticulitis with a severe degree of inflammation in the mesentery and the extension of the process below the pelvic floor, it may not be wise to close the colostomy for periods up to six months following the initial operation. In many instances radiologic demonstration of an intact anastomosis reassures the surgeon that the appropriate time has come for closure.

As mentioned in the Preface, stapling devices may be used in any of the anastomoses. One in particular (the EEA stapler) is designed for and is useful in the construction of bowel anastomoses low in the pelvis.

COMBINED ABDOMINAL-PERINEAL RESECTION

With a left paramedian incision extending from the pubis upward to the umbilicus, the sigmoid colon is mobilized as in the previous procedures and the peritoneal floor is opened as described for the anterior resection (see Fig. 3-11). The middle hemorrhoidal vessels are divided and ligated over Moynihan clamps. The rectum is mobilized out of the hollow of the sacrum down the levator ani muscles and the vagina or the bladder, as the case may be, is freed up anteriorly from the rectum. The superior hemorrhoidal vessels are then identified, clamped, cut, and doubly ligated. The bowel is divided at a point in the mid-sigmoid colon that leaves sufficient free length of mobile colon to bring out through the abdominal wall as a colostomy. The distal bowel is oversewn and placed down in the pelvis, and the peritoneal floor is closed with continuous 2-0 chromic cat-

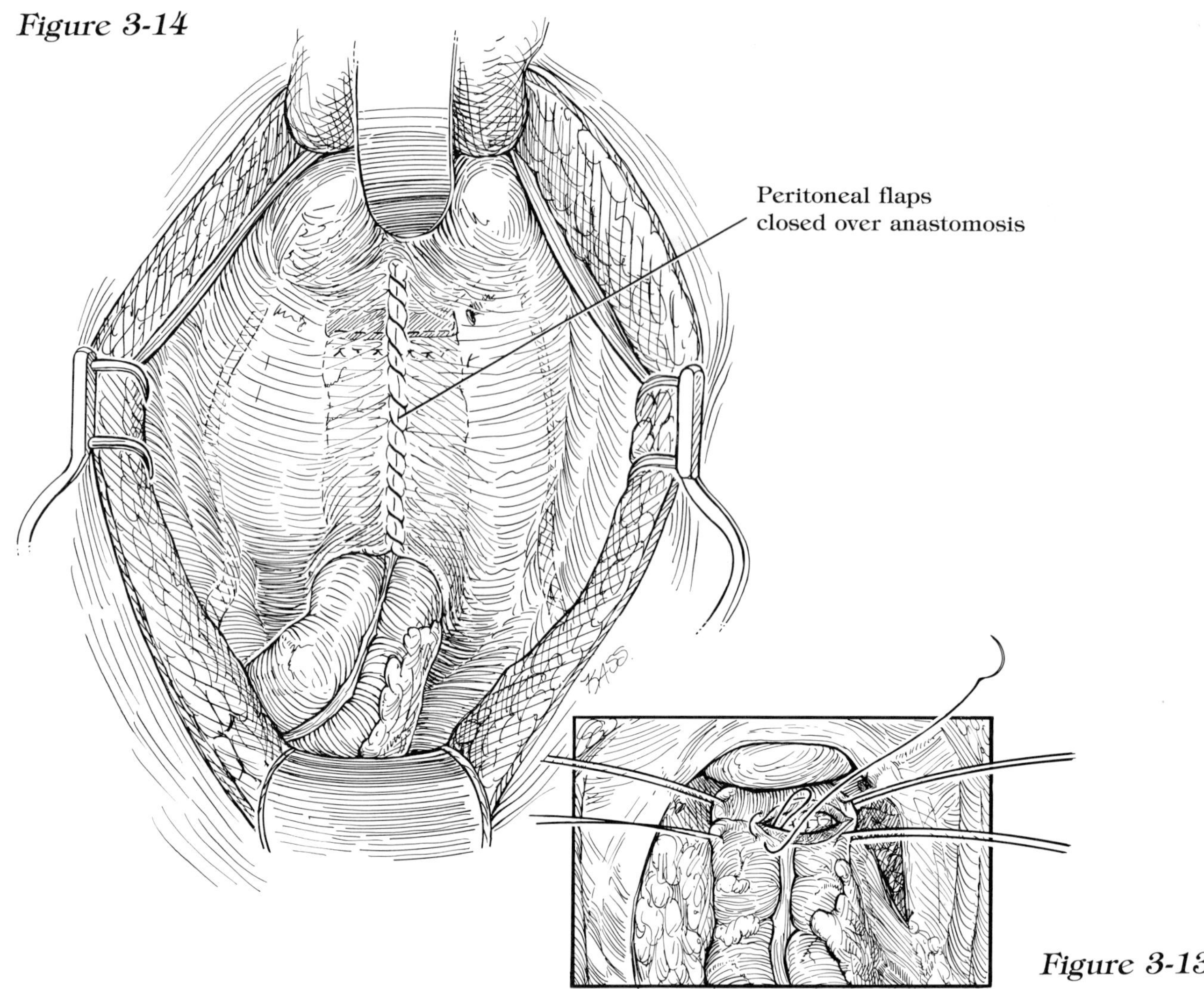

gut. An ellipse of skin is removed at a point about midway between the anterior superior iliac spine. The umbilicus, fascia, and muscle are incised and spread with scissors, and the peritoneum is divided. A Kocher clamp is placed through the stoma site and the bowel is drawn through the opening (Fig. 3-15). The left gutter is then carefully closed with continuous 2-0 chromic catgut (Fig. 3-16), the ureter is again identified and preserved, and the lateral peritoneal reflection of the mesentery is brought to the lateral abdominal peritoneal wall up to the opening for the stoma. This obliterates the space through which a loop of small bowel could potentially herniate and cause intestinal obstruction. The bowel is fixed to the anterior abdominal wall at the peritoneal level. The incision is closed, the clamp is removed from the colostomy, and maturation of the colostomy is achieved by approximating the mucosa and submucosa to the skin edges with interrupted sutures of 3-0 chromic catgut placed with a cutting needle.

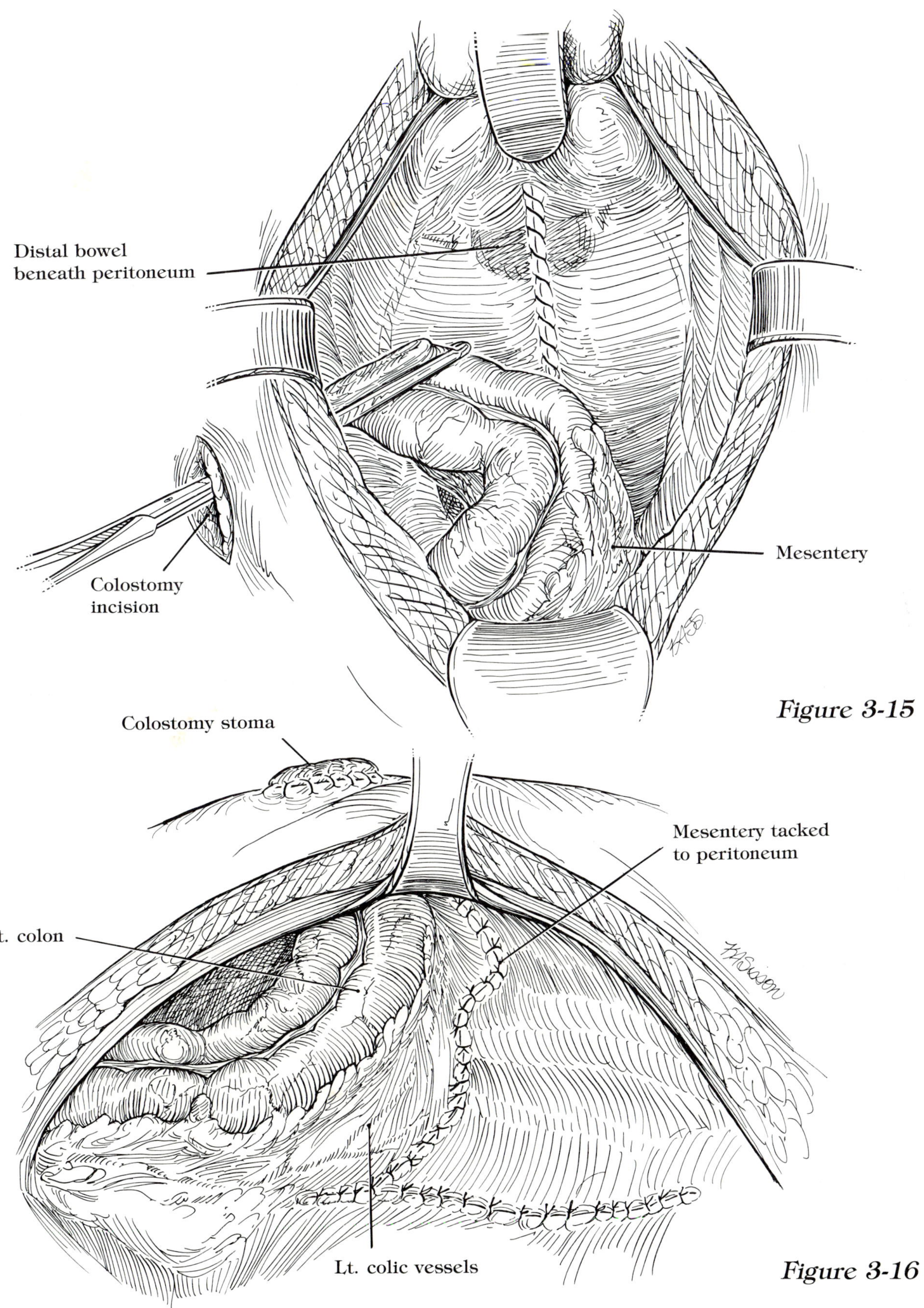

Figure 3-15

Figure 3-16

CAUTION
Viability of the colostomy must be ascertained by careful observation since it is possible for one to interfere with the blood supply by drawing the bowel through an overly narrow opening in the abdominal wall. If the surgeon suspects ischemia, either the opening through the abdominal wall may be enlarged or, if this is unsuccessful or if the bowel is clearly nonviable, a further segment should be drawn through the wall even if this requires reopening the operative incision. As often as possible, however, vascular supply and viability should be ascertained prior to closure of the laparotomy incision.

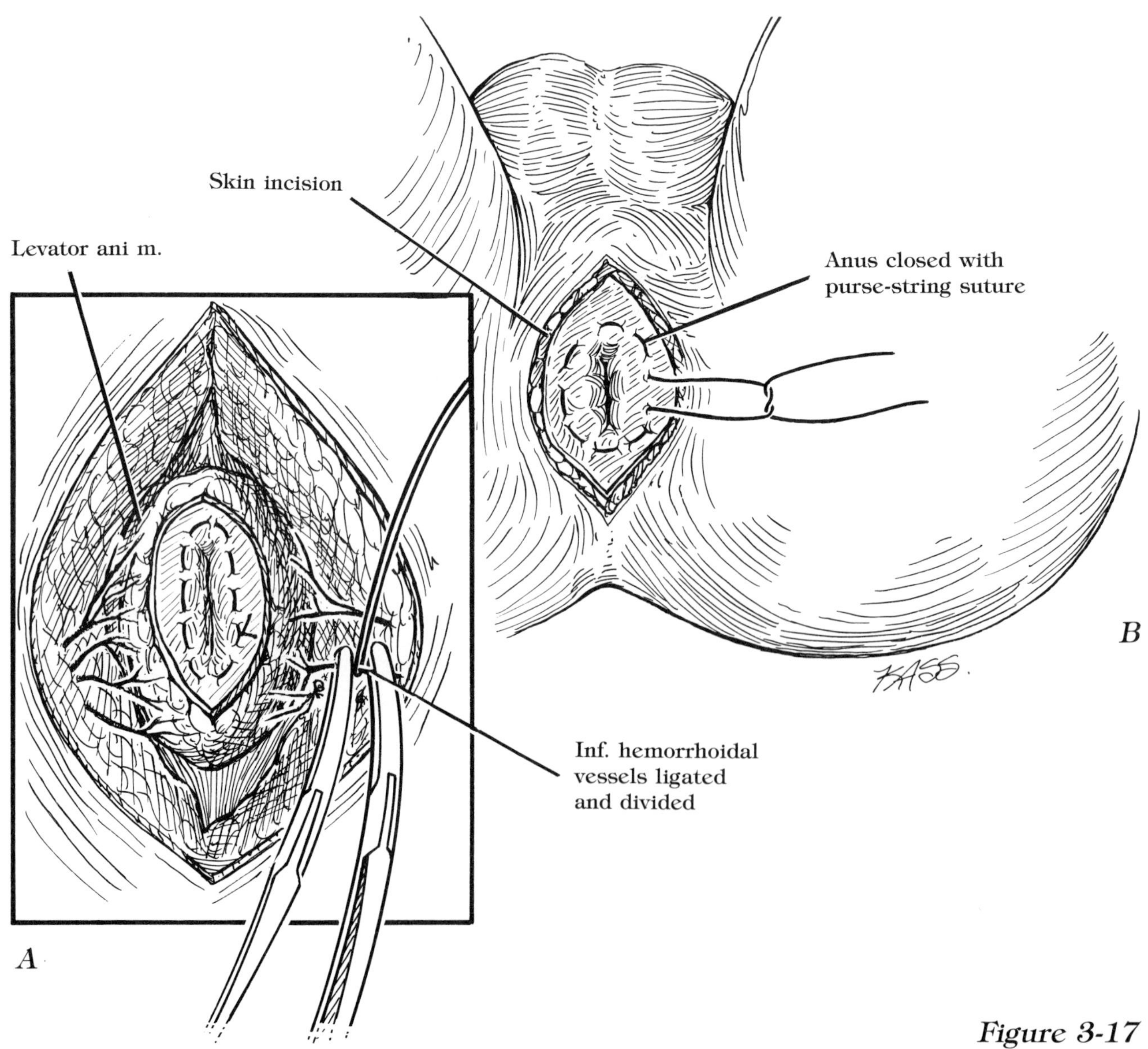
Levator ani m.
Skin incision
Anus closed with
purse-string suture
Inf. hemorrhoidal
vessels ligated
and divided
A
B

Figure 3-17

This procedure should leave a button of colon with everted mucosa fixed properly in position for adequate application of whatever type of appliance is indicated (see Fig. 3-16). The patient is then placed in lithotomy position, the perineum is prepared, and an elliptical incision is made around the anus. This is oversewn and the entire field is reprepped and draped carefully (Fig. 3-17A). A perianal incision is then carried down to the levator ani muscles, which are identified and divided. The individual branches of the inferior hemorrhoidal system are ligated as they are encountered (Fig. 3-17B). Perhaps the simplest maneuver is to enter the retrorectal space in the area between the anus and the coccyx and then, with fingers behind the levator ani muscles, to divide them with a scalpel. The bowel, which has been previously placed below the pelvic floor, is then brought out posteriorly. Under direct vision and by sharp dissection, it is mobilized off the prostatic capsule or the posterior wall of the vagina until the entire rectum is removed. The perineal incision is then closed with 2-0 chromic catgut sutures subcutaneously and interrupted silk sutures to skin; room is left posteriorly for insertion of a suction catheter.

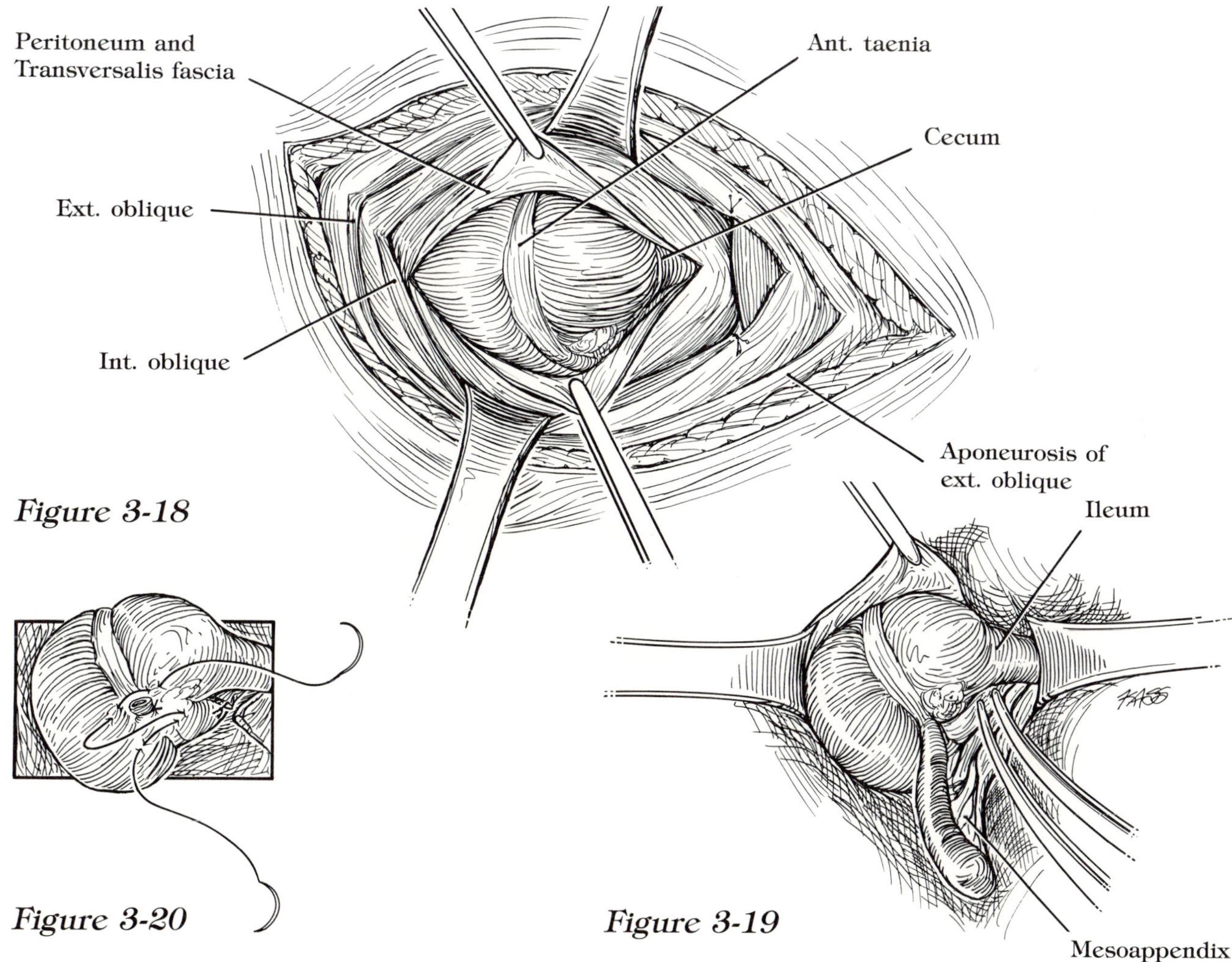

Figure 3-18

Figure 3-20

Figure 3-19

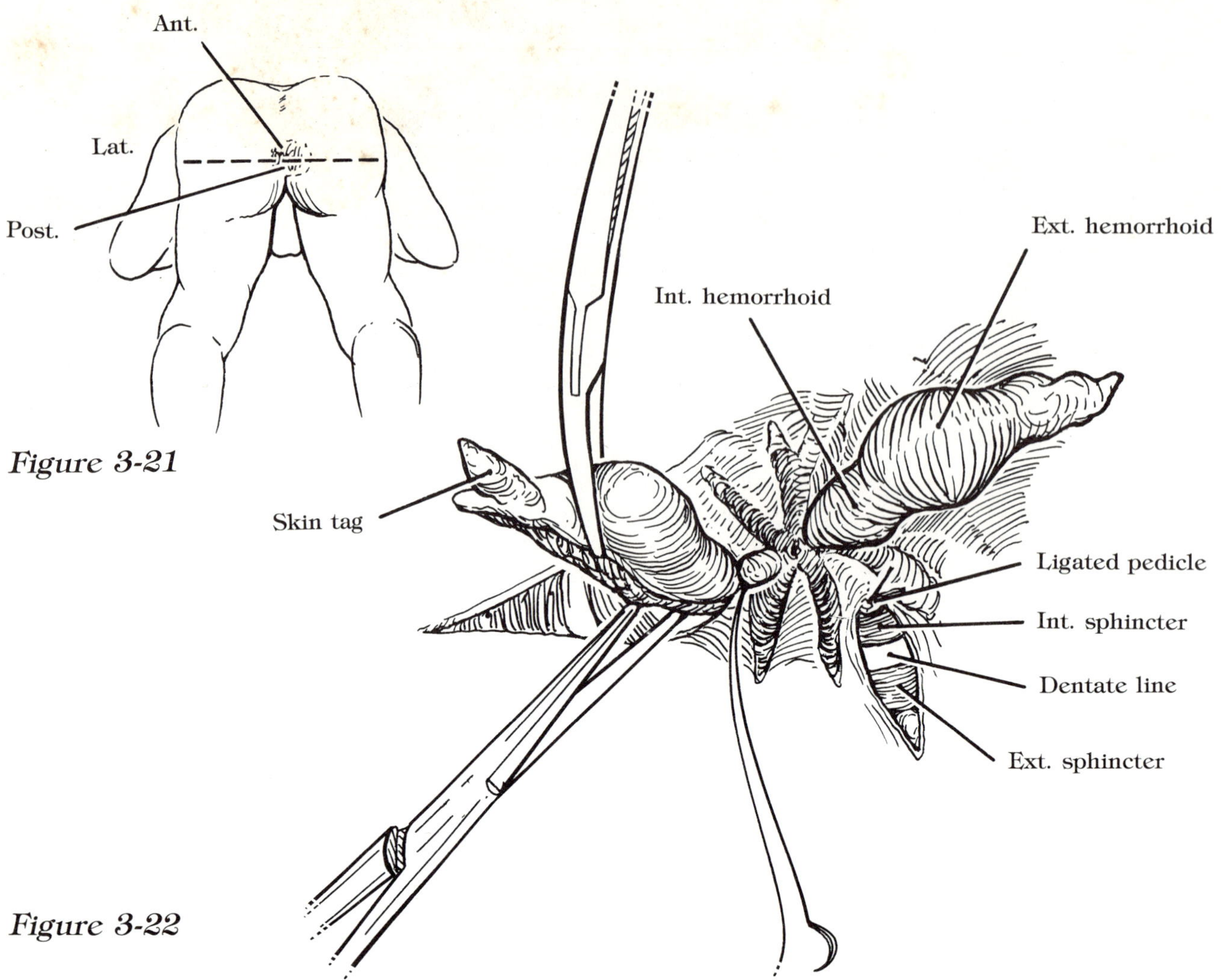

Figure 3-21

Figure 3-22

Appendectomy   The operative incision for appendectomy may be a right lower quadrant muscle-splitting (McBurney), transverse (Rocky) in which dividing the rectus sheath gives added exposure, a right paramedian, or a right pararectus.

The first (McBurney) and the paramedian incisions are most commonly used. The latter is preferred for female patients since better exposure of the pelvis is possible if right adnexal disease proves to be the cause of the symptoms.

In Figure 3-18, the cecum is exposed through a muscle-splitting incision, and the location of the appendix is identified by a taenia leading to the fat pad found at its base. The appendix is delivered through the incision, which is carefully walled off with gauze. The mesoappendix is exposed for identification and ligation of the blood supply (Fig. 3-19). After removal of the appendix with cautery, the stump is ligated with plain catgut and inverted with a Z stitch (Fig. 3-20). Use of drainage depends on the presence of extensive local infection at the time of operation.

Anal Surgery

The position of the patient on the table at the time of anal surgery may be varied to suit the needs and customs of the operating team. In Britain, it is common to perform anal surgery with the patient in stirrups in the lithotomy position. In other parts of Europe and in some parts of North America, the left lateral or Sims's position has been used widely. The Bouie or prone jack-knife position is most commonly used in this country. An advantage of this position is that the entire team can gain easy view of the operative area from any point. The lithotomy position is not well suited for anterior anal problems because visualization is limited.

Hemorrhoidectomy

With the patient in the Bouie position, the four quadrants are infiltrated with lidocaine-epinephrine solution. A Hill-Ferguson retractor is inserted into the anal canal displaying the right anterior hemorrhoidal bundle. Countertraction of the skin in the right anterior gluteal area further shows the hemorrhoid. The hemorrhoid is grasped at the anal verge, and gentle traction is placed upon it. A 3-0 chromic catgut suture is passed around the base of the hemorrhoid at the level of the rectal ampulla, and the hemorrhoid is ligated (Figs. 3-21, 3-22).

OPEN TECHNIQUE

Traction is placed on the perianal skin, and any external skin tag is included in the excision. An ellipse of external skin tag and hemorrhoid is removed, demonstrating the most superficial portion of the external sphincter muscle. The dissection includes the mucosa, submucosa, and hemorrhoidal plexus, but spares the internal sphincter, which is recognized as a pale muscular structure lining the anal canal and occurring deep to the hemorrhoid. The dissection is carried elliptically to the ligated base, and the hemorrhoid is thus excised. Any minor bleeding points are ligated or treated with the electrocautery. The left lateral and the right posterior hemorrhoidal bundles are treated similarly. Any excess skin is excised with the scissors so that the skin edges lie flat. A one-quarter-inch Penrose drain is placed within the rectum to signal the presence of postoperative bleeding. The size of the open wound may be decreased by suturing the ligated pedicle to the anal wall at the level of the internal sphincter.

CLOSED TECHNIQUE

After excision of the hemorrhoidal bundle, the cut edges of the mucosa of the anal canal may be approximated by carrying the ligating suture out to the outer limits of the excision in a continuous over-and-over fashion. The drain is inserted at the conclusion of the closed technique in a manner similar to that used in the open technique.

Anal Fissure

Superficial fissures, if they require operative treatment, are usually easily managed by simple sphincter dilatation to a diameter of three fingers maintained for a period of two minutes. Operative treatment of the more chronic anal fissure involves the local infiltration of epinephrine and lidocaine and the placement of a suture at the top of the fissure above the hypertrophied anal papilla (Fig. 3-23). The area so included in the suture is then ligated. The external skin tag, fissure, and hypertrophied anal papilla are excised elliptically down to the floor of the fissure, which is usually the internal sphincter muscle. Anal sphincterotomy may be performed through the floor of the incision and should include the internal sphincter muscle for a distance of about 1.5 cm. Healing of the wound after excision of deep anterior or posterior fissures may be delayed, and lateral sphincterotomy is often preferable in such instances. After excision of the anal fissure, the wound may be left open or may be closed by continuing the ligating suture to the anal verge, approximating the edges of cut anal canal mucosa. A one-quarter-inch Penrose drain is inserted into the anal canal (Fig. 3-24).

The anal fissure need not always be excised. In the presence of deeply indurating midline fissures, attempted total excision of the fissure is inadvisable. In such instances, simple excision of the hypertrophied anal papilla and enlarged external skin tag aids in healing the fissure after *lateral sphincterotomy*. This is usually best performed in the *right lateral region* with the left index finger inserted into the anal canal. A size-11 scalpel blade is inserted into the intermuscular groove and is passed outside the internal sphincter muscle to 1.5 cm (Fig. 3-25). The blade is then turned to face the mucosa of the anal canal, and the internal sphincter muscle is divided by pressure toward the finger

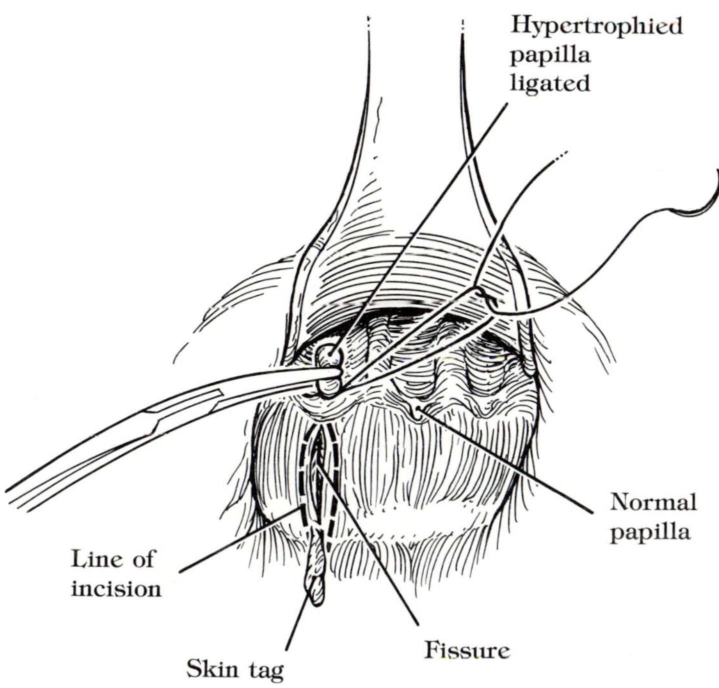

Figure 3-23

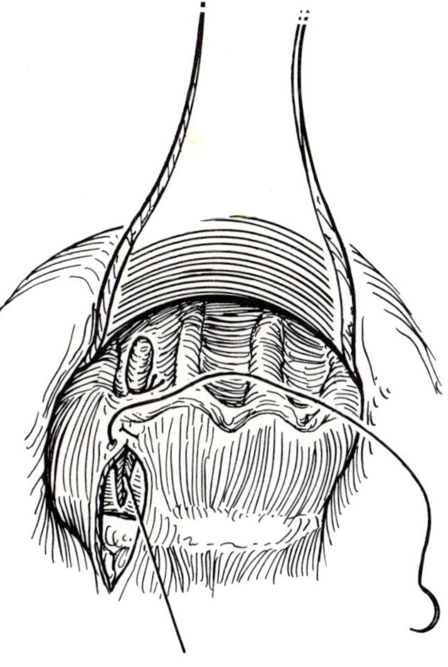

Figure 3-24

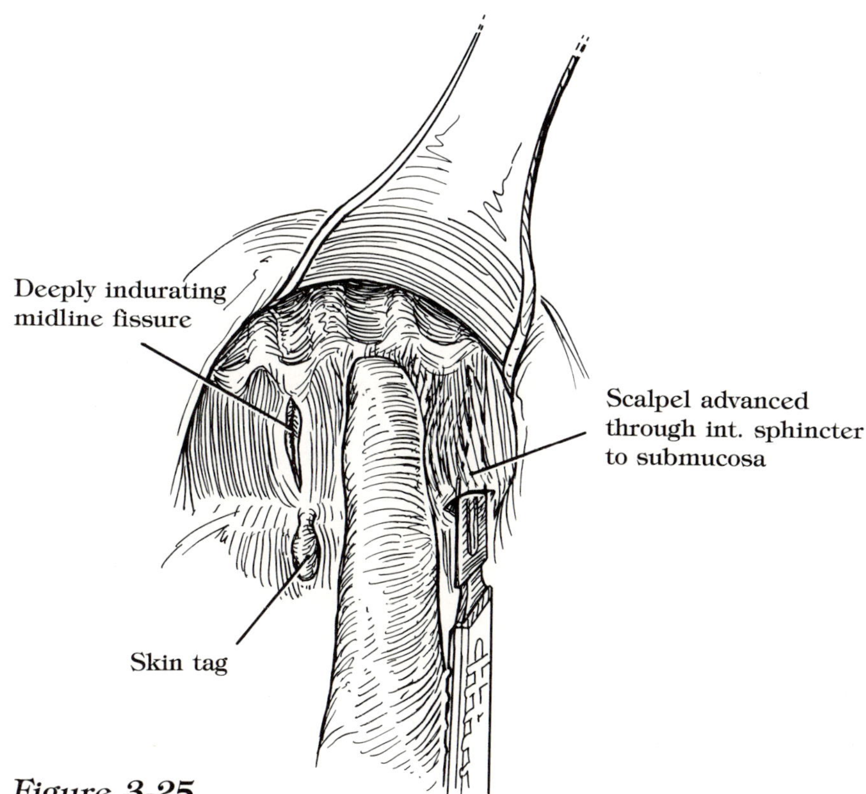

Figure 3-25

that has been inserted into the anus. The muscle fibers are felt to divide before the advancing scalpel so that mucosa and submucosa only separate the knife blade and the inserted finger. The defect in the internal sphincter muscle is readily palpable with the examining finger. Pressure from the inserted finger is maintained on the divided area for five minutes following completion of the sphincterotomy and withdrawal of the knife to insure adequate hemostasis. No suture is necessary to close the puncture wound through which the knife blade has been inserted.

<table>
<tr><td>Anal Fistula</td><td>The patient is placed on the operating table in the Bouie position, and the perineal region and perianal area are prepared as for hemorrhoidectomy and excision of fissure. The region of the fistula is examined digitally and, thus, the tract is often palpable. A probe is gently inserted into the external orifice and passed down the tract to its point of entry into the anal rectum (Fig. 3-26). Fine, malleable, silver probes are often useful in this situation. Entry into the anal canal must not be forcible; otherwise, the site of the internal orifice will not be definitely established. Fistulous tracts with orifices anterior to a line bisecting the anus usually are radial to the internal opening at the crypt level. Tracts having their orifice posterior to the line bisecting the anal canal tend to be circumferential to the posterior aspect of the anal canal and enter the canal in the posterior midline at the crypt level. External orifices that lie any distance from the anal canal tend to represent fistulous tracts that travel circumferentially and have a posterior, internal orifice. Fistulas having their internal opening above the level of the levator muscles are usually inoperable since division of the entire tract and the involved musculature may result in incontinence. All other fistulas may be excised by passing the probe through the tract from the external to the internal orifice and then cutting down upon the tract to convert the fistula into a ditch open to the anal canal (Fig. 3-27). Portions of the external and internal sphincter muscles are divided during this incision. Overhanging edges of anal skin and anal canal mucosa should be excised to flatten the ditch as broadly as possible in order to permit healing from the base upward. The floor of the fistula may or may not be excised. All granulation tissue, however, should be curetted away from the floor of the saucerized wound. The incision of the fistulous tract and the excision of the overhanging edges of tissue and base of the tract are often best performed using the electrocautery knife to achieve maximal hemostasis. Large wounds should be packed gently with iodoform gauze. Shallower wounds need no packing. The packing should be removed the day after operation. If no packing is used, a one-quarter-inch Penrose drain is inserted into the anal canal.</td></tr>
</table>

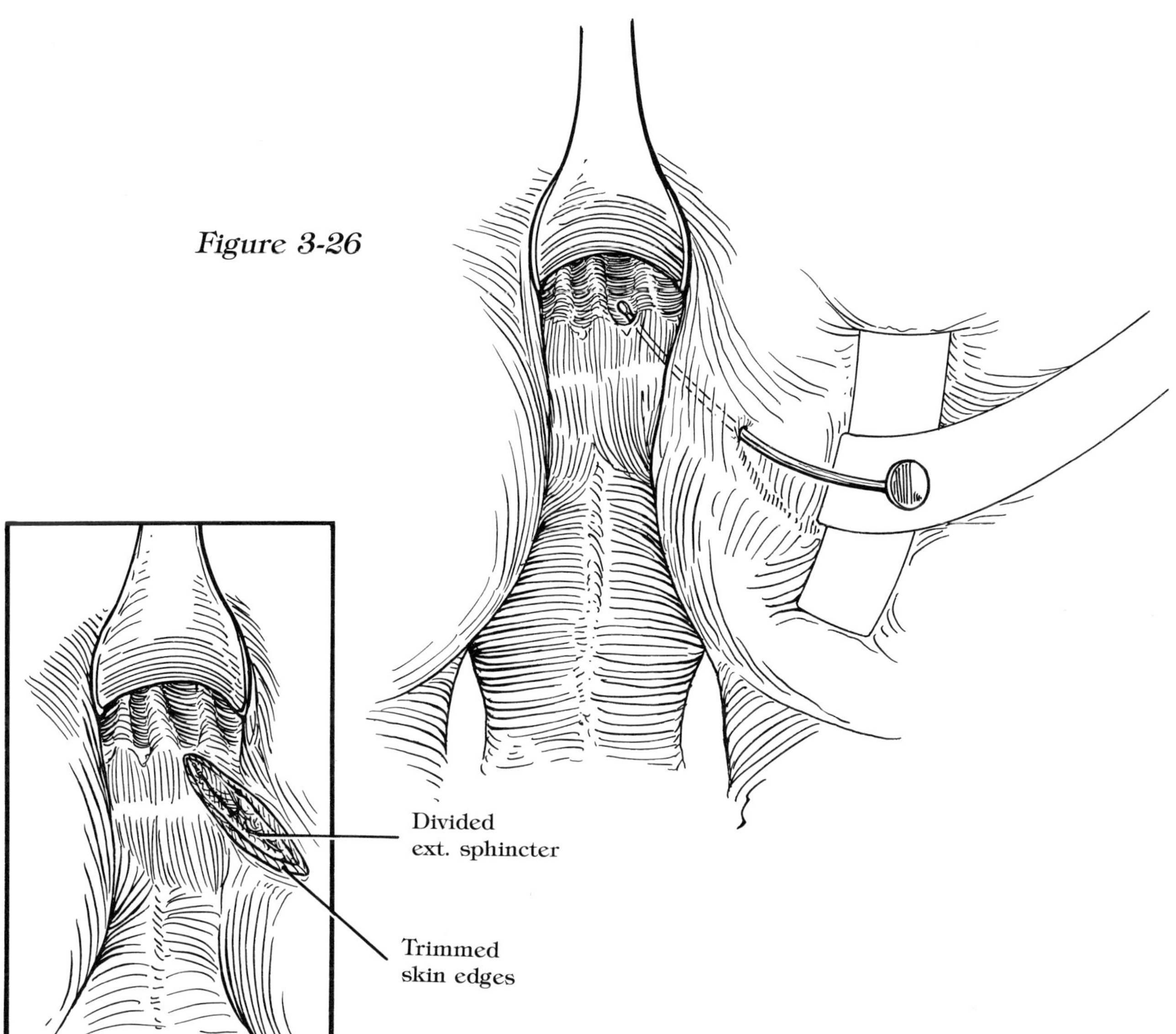

Figure 3-26

Figure 3-27

CHAPTER FOUR

PANCREATICOBILIARY SYSTEM

The simplest major operation on the pancreaticobiliary tree is the cholecystostomy. It is used rarely today, but there is still the occasional elderly or poor-risk patient with cholecystitis that is not subsiding and requires operative drainage.

Cholecystostomy

In this instance, one would choose a procedure that could be performed under local anesthesia. The operative approach is through a short subcostal incision directly over the gallbladder which is, under these circumstances, often palpable. When the peritoneum is opened and the inflamed necrotic gallbladder visualized, a trocar is inserted through the wall and the liquid, purulent material evacuated. The gallbladder can then be drawn up into the wound with Babcock forceps, the stone or stones evacuated through a combination of maneuvers including digital expression of stones from deep in the gallbladder, use of stone forceps, and irrigation (Fig. 4-1). A large catheter in which multiple holes have been cut is then inserted into the gallbladder and two or three purse-string sutures in two layers are closed about the tube. The incision is then closed, leaving the tube coming through the incision after being fixed to the skin (Fig. 4-2).

Acute cholecystitis or recurring bouts of subacute cholecystitis are the ordinary indications for removal of the gallbladder. Since cholecystitis is almost invariably related to the presence of gallstones and a calculus cholecystitis is rare, the definition of stones by ultrasonic examination is strong confirmatory evidence that the clinical diagnosis of acute cholecystitis is probably correct. If further validation is needed, a HIDA scan can be used as a measure of function of the gallbladder and of the presence or absence of obstruction of the cystic duct. Because these

Cholecystectomy

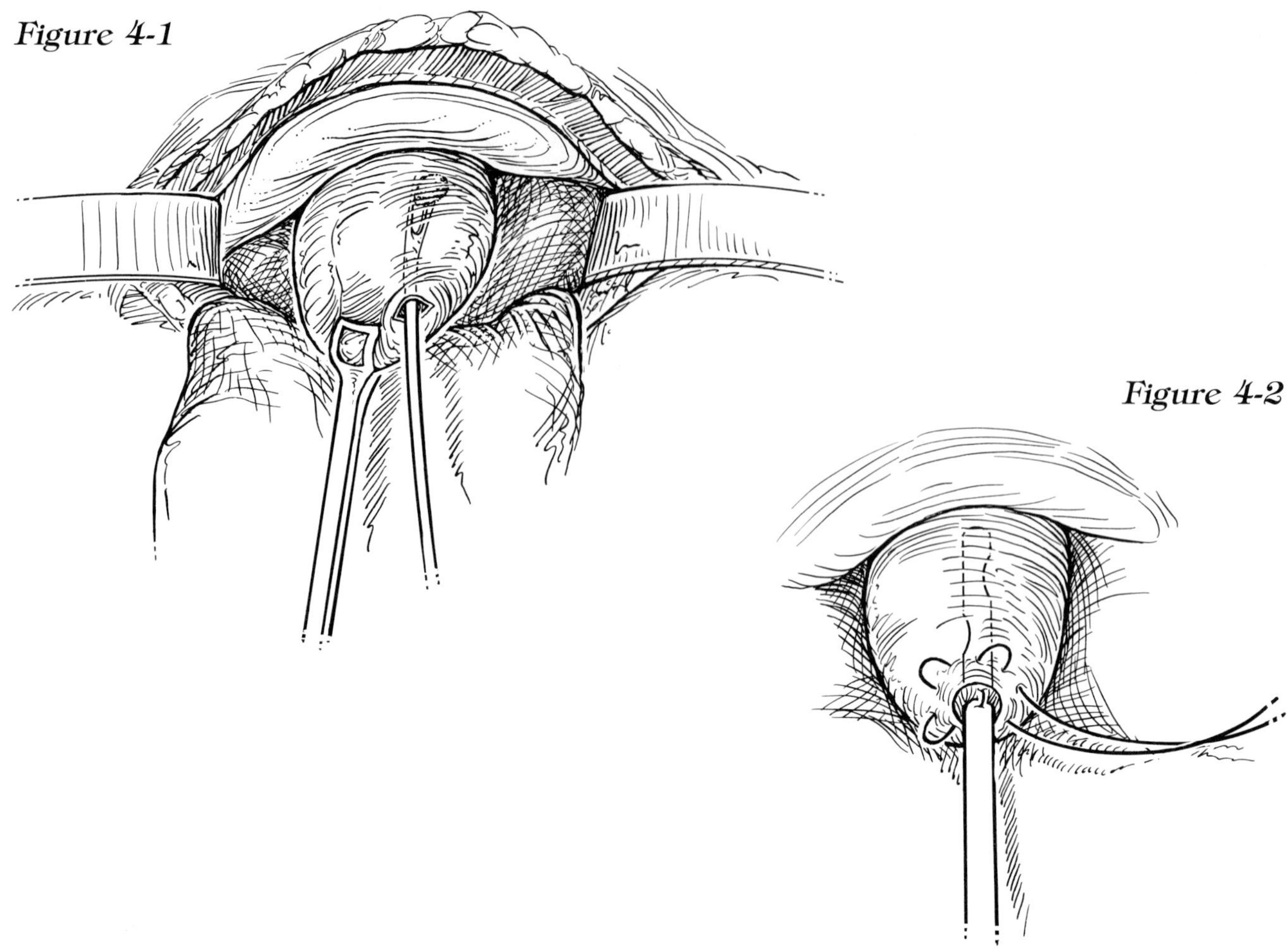

recently introduced techniques have sharpened the accuracy of diagnosis of cholelithiasis and cholecystitis, errors in evaluating the nature of the problem should be rare.

A different operative approach is used for cholecystectomy because one is never certain prior to operation whether or not choledochotomy is indicated. A paramedian incision is more satisfactory for choledochotomy and is, therefore, usually recommended for cholecystectomy in which exploration of the bile duct may be indicated. After general exploration (which is carried out unless purulent material or pericholecystic abscess is present), a hand is inserted above the liver mobilizing the right lobe of the liver downward for better exposure of the gallbladder and gastrohepatic ligament. The hepatic flexure is then packed inferiorly away from the operative field. The assistant's left hand is inserted over a wet gauze pack with the middle finger inserted into the foramen of Winslow and the index finger lying above the gastrohepatic ligament in such a way that it retracts the duodenum medially. Not only does this provide excellent exposure, but it permits the assistant to occlude completely the hepatic inflow if sudden hemorrhage from one of the major vessels occurs during the operation (Fig. 4-3). A ring forceps is then applied to the dome of the gallbladder, evacuating it first through a trocar if it is so tense that it cannot be held with an instrument. The decision is then made whether to remove the gallbladder from above downward or below upward. Unless the anatomy is thoroughly obliterated by a diffuse cellulitic process, it is probably better to define the anatomy and remove the gallbladder from below upward. The ampulla of the gallbladder is then grasped with a Moynihan clamp after it has been dissected free from the gastrohepatic ligament, and traction upward then puts the cystic artery and the cystic duct on tension. Using sharp and blunt dissection, the surgeon identifies and isolates both the duct and artery (see Fig. 4-3). The ligation of the cystic artery is a crucial part of the operation. It is imperative that one does not mistake a curving right hepatic artery for the cystic artery; therefore, all the anatomy in this area must be thoroughly identified before any clamps are applied. A right-angle instrument is then passed around the cystic artery and a 0 chromic catgut ligature placed near the gallbladder. A similar tie is passed around the cystic artery as it begins to bifurcate over the surface of the gallbladder and then tied down snugly. A right-angle clamp is placed on the cystic artery, which is then tied down snugly, and the artery is divided. A second tie can then be placed around the right-angle clamp; this procedure serves as a precaution against a single tie breaking or slipping during the course of securing the ligature. Once the cystic artery is divided, the cystic duct is then dissected free to its junction with the common bile duct. Here, a right-angle clamp is placed across it, with care taken that the side of the common duct has not been tented up. Another clamp is placed up near the Hartman's pouch, and the duct is divided and ligated. With traction upward on the gallbladder, removal of the gallbladder is begun by dividing peritoneal reflections on both sides of the gallbladder fossa (Fig. 4-4). This is carried upward with sharp and blunt dissection. The operation should leave sufficient leaf of peritoneum on each side to permit a satisfactory closure. When about half of this dissection has been completed, it is simpler to begin the closing suture of 3-0 chromic catgut at the depths of the gallbladder fossa before the gallbladder is finally removed (Fig. 4-5). The surgeon carries this suture upward, obliterating the gallbladder fossa and reperitonealizing the area from which the gallbladder has been removed. A cigarette drain is placed in the hepatorenal fossa and Morison's pouch and is brought out through the abdominal wall via a small muscle-splitting incision.

Choledochotomy

The surgeon undertaking an operation for calculus disease in the gallbladder should maintain a high index of suspicion that stones may have passed through the cystic duct and lodged in

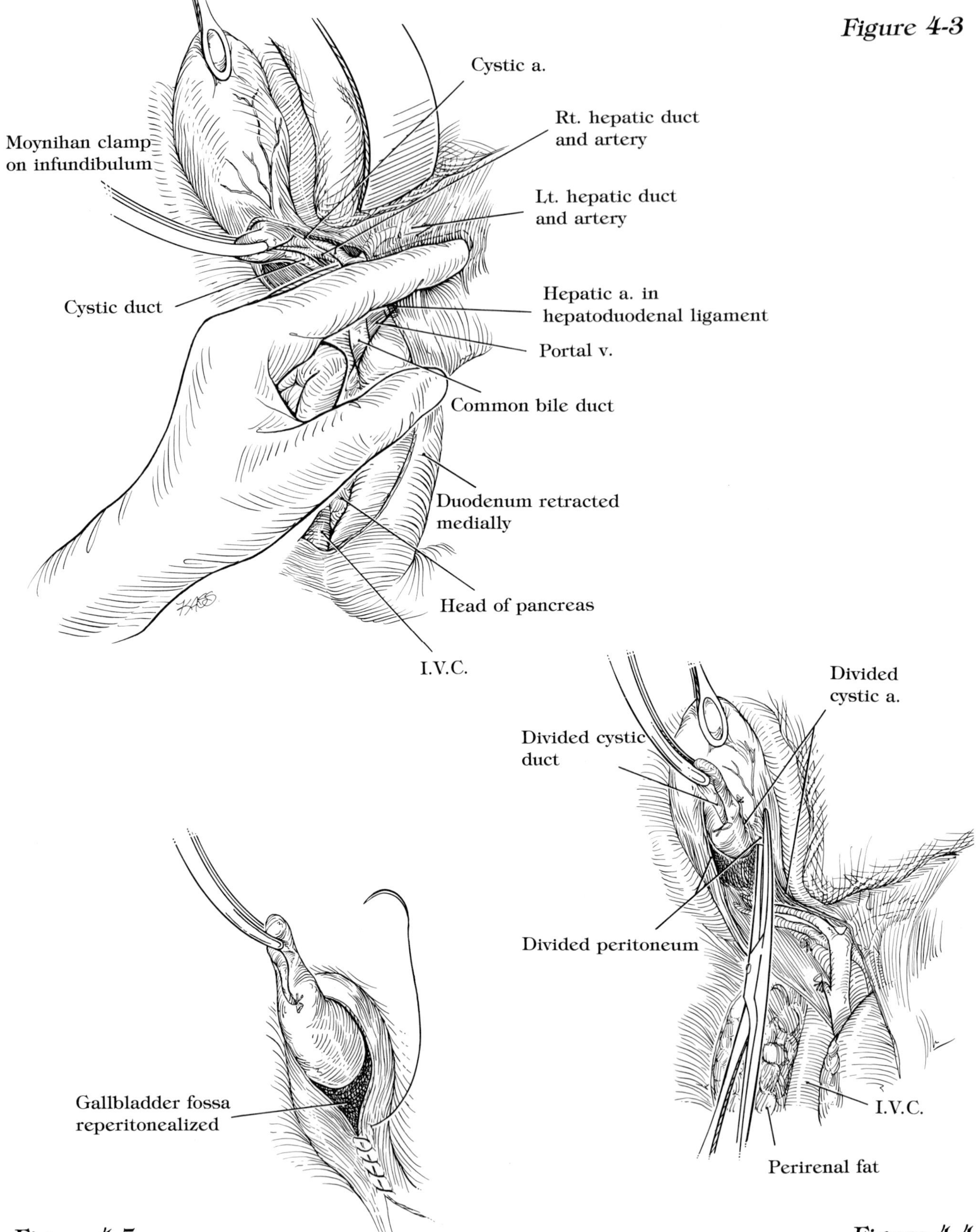

Figure 4-3

Figure 4-5

Figure 4-4

the biliary tract itself. The usual indications given for exploration of the common bile duct include bouts of colicky pain, jaundice, dark urine, shaking chills, and pancreatitis. To these clinical signs and symptoms can be added bilirubinemia and bilirubinuria with elevation of the liver enzymes and normal hepatocellular function. A radiologic examination of the biliary tract at the time of cholecystectomy should be performed in any instance where common duct disease is suspected. The technical aspects of this procedure are described in this section. In addition to calculus disease of the biliary tract, the surgeon may encounter noncalculus, malignant or benign obstructions causing dilatation of the biliary tract and clinical and chemical findings consistent with obstructive jaundice. Often a percutaneous transhepatic cholangiogram should be done preoperatively both to establish drainage of the biliary tract and to define the nature and location of the obstructing lesion.

If opening the common bile duct is indicated, the duct is aspirated with a fine needle and syringe in order to be certain that it is not a blood vessel. Often a preliminary cholangiogram is taken by inserting a fine catheter into the bile duct through the gallbladder or through the wall of the cystic duct directly. Fine sutures are placed on each side of the wall of the common bile duct. By holding these on traction, the surgeon can make an opening in the anterior wall of the duct. The duct is then explored using a number of maneuvers such as the introduction of stone forceps, irrigation of the duct with an irrigating syringe and fine catheter, and the introduction of Bake's dilators to stretch the sphincter of Oddi and to ascertain that a free passage exists into the duodenum (Figs. 4-6, 4-7). These maneuvers, as well as external digital exploration of the duct, are continued until the surgeon is thoroughly satisfied that the common bile duct and its major tributaries in the liver are completely patent and free of calculi. From the instruments available at present, it would appear that the use of a choledochoscope will soon be a part of the standard procedure for exploration of the bile duct. When patency has been assured as a result of these maneuvers, a T tube is then placed in the duct and fixed there with a suture of 5-0 chromic catgut placed through the superficial layer of the wall of the T tube and the duct itself. The duct is then closed about the T tube using 5-0 chromic catgut (Fig. 4-8). The duct is aspirated to remove all air bubbles and then a postoperative cholangiogram is obtained with the patient on the operating table. The drain is then placed down in Morison's pouch, and the drain and T tube are brought out through a small subcostal muscle-splitting incision and sutured in position.

Most cases of chronic recurrent, fibrosing, or calcereous pancreatitis are related to calculus biliary tract disease or to the heavy persistent ingestion of alcohol. In addition, however, there are

Chronic Pancreatitis

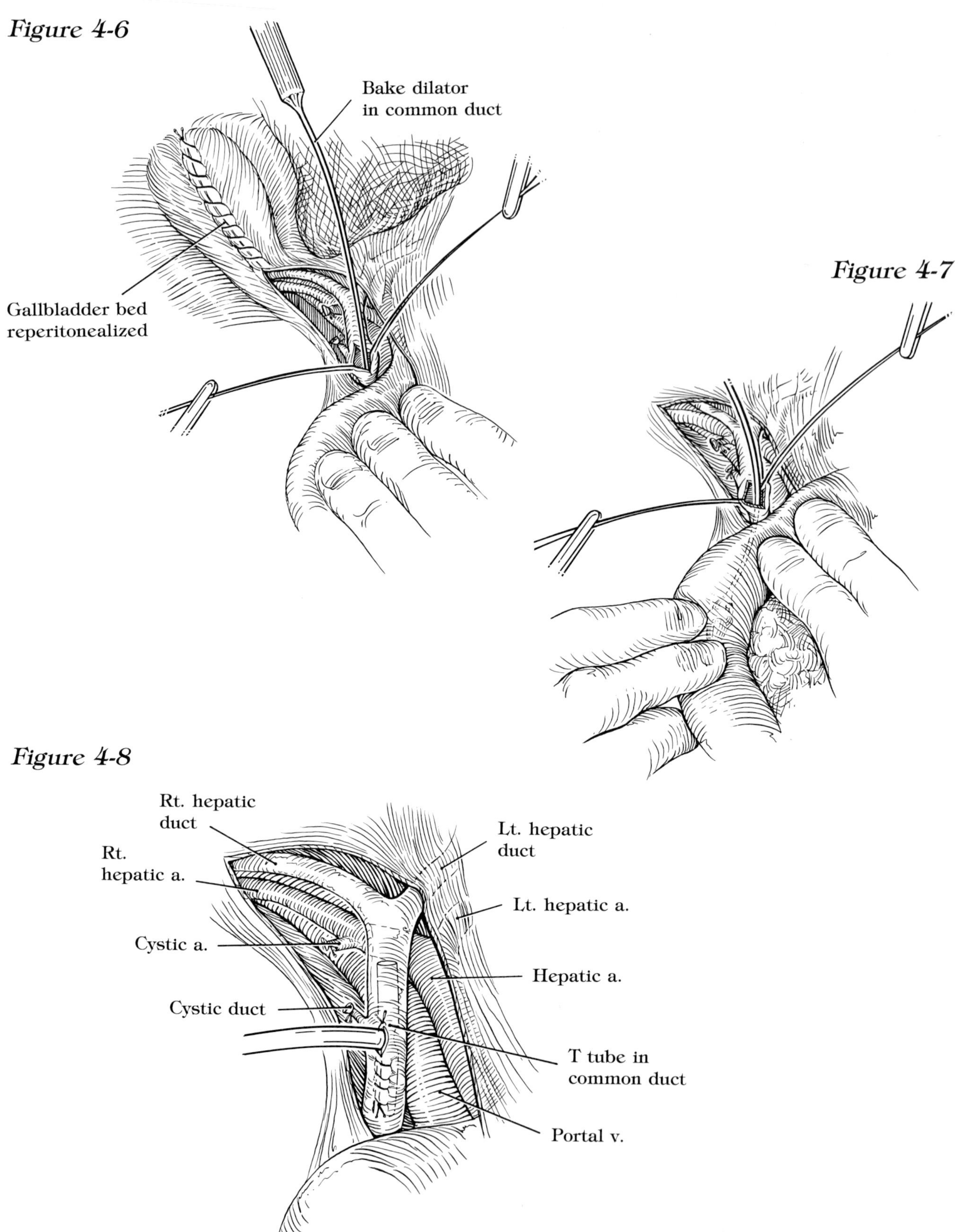

Figure 4-6

Bake dilator
in common duct

Gallbladder bed
reperitonealized

Figure 4-7

Figure 4-8

Rt. hepatic
duct

Rt.
hepatic a.

Cystic a.

Cystic duct

Lt. hepatic
duct

Lt. hepatic a.

Hepatic a.

T tube in
common duct

Portal v.

congenital and metabolic problems associated with pancreatic disease. The advent of duodenoscopy and retrograde catheterization of the common bile duct and the pancreatic duct have led to a more rational and ordered approach to surgery for chronic pancreatic disease. If biliary calculi exist, it is imperative that the gallbladder be removed and the biliary tract thoroughly exonerated as a potential factor in the evolution of chronic pancreatitis. Therefore, this section begins with a description of transduodenal exploration of the ampulla of Vater. Even in the absence of biliary calculi, stenosis of the ampulla or orifice of the duct of Wirsung may be related to bouts of pain, although in the absence of dilation of the pancreatic or biliary ductal systems, the surgeon should be wary of concluding that these apparent stenoses are necessarily related to bouts of abdominal pain.

In order to identify and approach the ampulla of Vater, a choledochotomy is first performed and a dilator is introduced through the common duct to the opening of the duct through the papilla into the duodenum (Fig. 4-9). By digital palpation of the tip of the dilator, the exact location of the sphincter can be ascertained and a short longitudinal incision made in the duodenum (Fig. 4-9). With holding stitches placed through the opening of the sphincter, a right-angled scissors is then introduced and the sphincter divided for a distance between 10 and 15 mm (Fig. 4-10).

TRANSDUODENAL
SPHINCTEROPLASTY

> CAUTION
>
> An incision longer than this introduces the possibility of a lateral duodenal fistula, since the division may extend beyond the intrapancreatic portion of the common bile duct. This is a disastrous complication; great care should be taken with this particular maneuver.

With ampulla and sphincter thus divided, usually one can identify the ostium of the pancreatic duct. The usual location is approximately where it is shown in Figure 4-11, although there are numerous anomalies in terms of the exact location at or near the opening of the sphincter. It is sometimes necessary to administer intravenous secretin or to stimulate a flow of pancreatic juice and further identify the sphincter. Once the pancreatic ductal orifice has been identified and any appropriate abnormalities corrected, a plastic closure of the sphincterotomy is effected approximating the mucosa of the duodenum and the epithelial lining of the common duct using 4-0 chromic catgut sutures, as shown in Figure 4-12. The longitudinal opening of

Figure 4-9
Figure 4-10
Figure 4-11
Divided ampulla
retracted by sutures
Divided
sphincter of Oddi
Ostium of
pancreatic duct
Figure 4-12

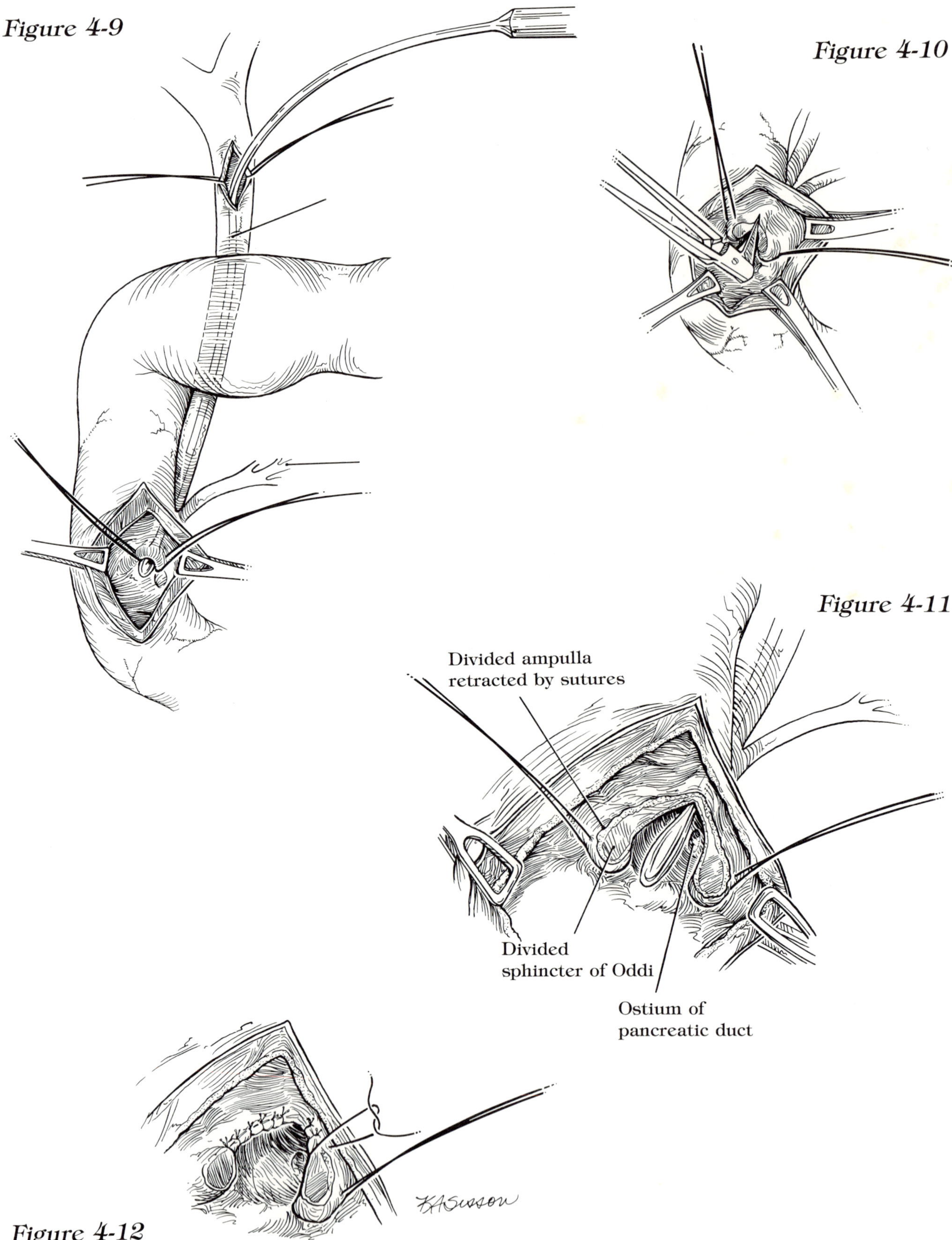

the duodenum is then closed transversely using a double layer of continuous 3-0 chromic catgut and an outer layer of interrupted silk sutures. If further operation on the pancreas is indicated, sometimes the closure of the duodenotomy is deferred so that the pancreatic duct may be explored simultaneously from the duodenal opening and from an opening farther back in the ductile system in the body or tail of the pancreas. If a preliminary pancreatogram has not been obtained by duodenoscopy and catheterization, it may be indicated to perform an operative pancreatogram by introducing a ureteral catheter through the ostium prior to any further surgical procedure.

If the results of endoscopic retrograde cholangiopancreatography and other studies suggest that an obstructed and dilated pancreatic ductal system, often containing calculi, cannot be completely drained by transduodenal sphincterotomy, then a retrograde approach is indicated to establish satisfactory drainage and to permit removal of calculi from the pancreatic duct. At times the abnormalities are such that correction requires resection as well as drainage. Therefore, a highly individualized approach can be taken utilizing the possibilities of varying degrees of partial pancreatectomy with or without concomitant retrograde drainage or a fillet procedure that evacuates and drains the duct without removal of the pancreas. These procedures are described in detail.

This procedure is begun by mobilizing the spleen and tail of the pancreas after the lesser omental sac has been entered in the midportion of the body. The pancreas is usually transected in a fishmouth fashion and the distal body and tail removed with the spleen.

CAUTION

It is possible to perform a distal pancreatectomy and preserve the spleen, but this procedure may be technically impossible in the presence of extensive pancreatitis. At any rate, because preservation of the spleen seems to be of more importance to children and young adults than to the older age group, it does not seem essential in most patients with pancreatitis.

This procedure requires ligation of the splenic vein at the time of transection. The pancreatic ductile system can then be approached and evaluated in a retrograde fashion. Retrograde drainage is established by bringing up a Roux-en-Y limb of jeju-

Retrograde Drainage Procedures and Resections

PARTIAL PANCREATECTOMY AND RETROGRADE END-TO-END PANCREATICO-ENTEROSTOMY

num for an anastomosis which is carried out using an outer row of interrupted nonabsorbable sutures and an inner row of continuous 3-0 chromic catgut. Whenever possible one attempts to achieve a mucosa-to-mucosa approximation between a dilated pancreatic duct and the mucosa of the jejunum. The anastomosis is usually constructed with a small plastic tubing as a stent. This procedure is illustrated in Fig. 4-13 and is sometimes referred to as the Duval procedure.

SIDE-TO-SIDE PANCREATICO-ENTEROSTOMY

Another method of establishing retrograde drainage of the pancreatic ductile system is by opening the irregularly dilated main pancreatic duct throughout most of its length in the body and tail of the pancreas, thus accomplishing a "fillet" of the pancreas. A Roux-en-Y limb of jejunum is then brought up and opened longitudinally so that it can be sewn in position over the widely opened pancreatic duct, as shown in Figure 4-14. Variants of this procedure are often collectively referred to as a Puestow procedure.

DRAINAGE OF PSEUDOCYST

A pseudocyst that has developed as a result of one or more attacks of pancreatitis usually requires either external drainage or, preferably, internal drainage into the gastrointestinal tract through the stomach or jejunum, depending on the presentation of the cystic mass. If the cyst displaces the stomach anteriorly and seems fixed to the posterior wall, the best approach is probably a transgastric drainage. This is accomplished by opening the anterior wall of the stomach, entering the cyst through the posterior wall, and finally placing a running stitch around the newly contructed opening between the cyst and the posterior wall of the stomach, as shown in Figure 4-15.

CAUTION

Postoperative bleeding from the suture line site has been a relatively common complication of cyst-gastrostomy and raises the question of whether polyglycolic or nonabsorbent suture material should be used in oversewing the edges of the cyst-gastrostomy.

The anterior gastrostomy is then closed with a double layer of continuous chromic catgut and an outer layer of interrupted silk sutures. Another common presentation for a pancreatic pseudocyst is an inferior bulge through the transverse mesocolon; in this instance, drainage is appropriately instituted by a defunctioned limb of jejunum, as shown in Figure 4-16.

Post. mucosal
wall sutured
to pancreas
Sup. mesenteric
vessels
Roux-
en-
Y
Proximal
jejunum
Distal
jejunum
Opened pancreas
and duct
Roux-en-Y

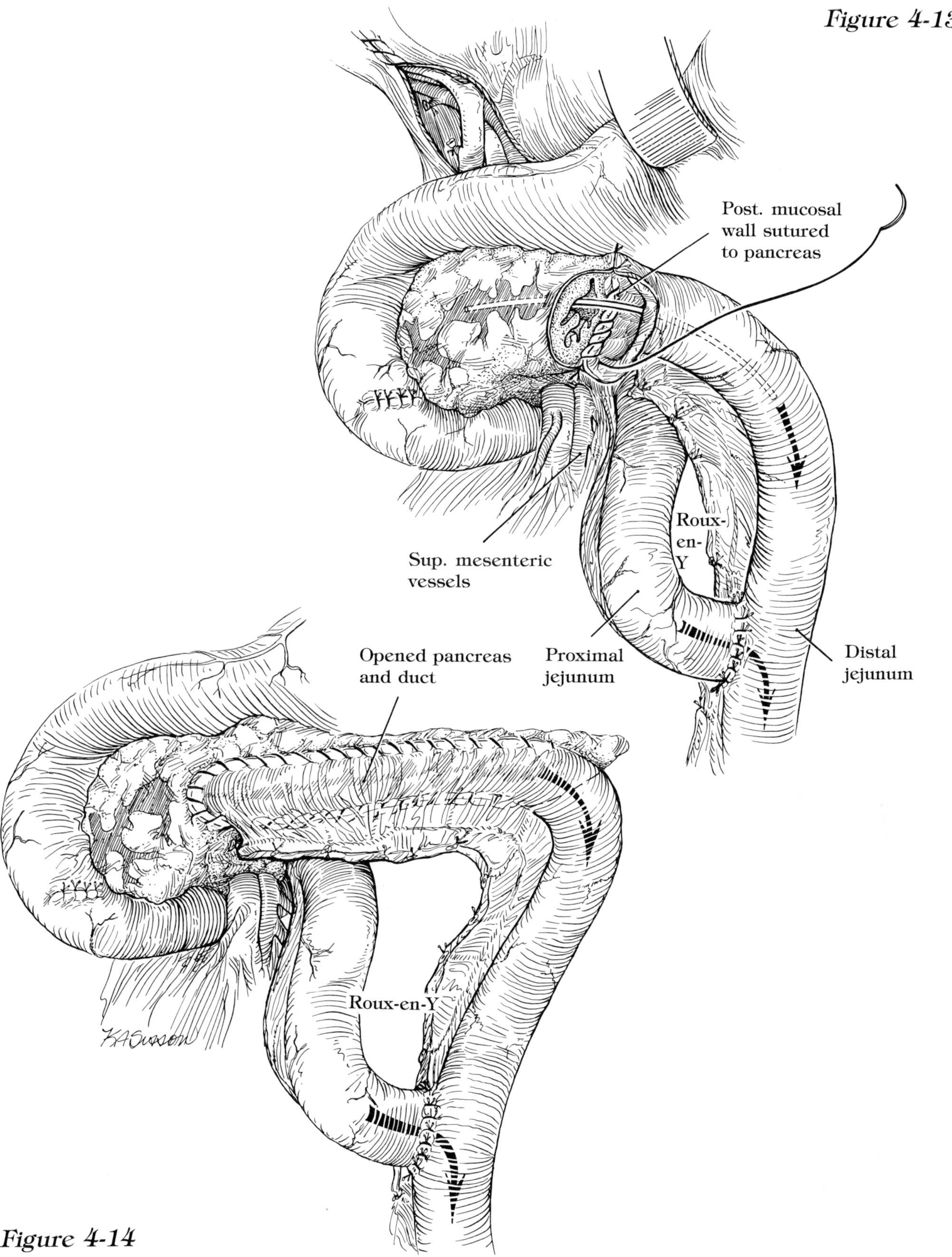

Figure 4-14

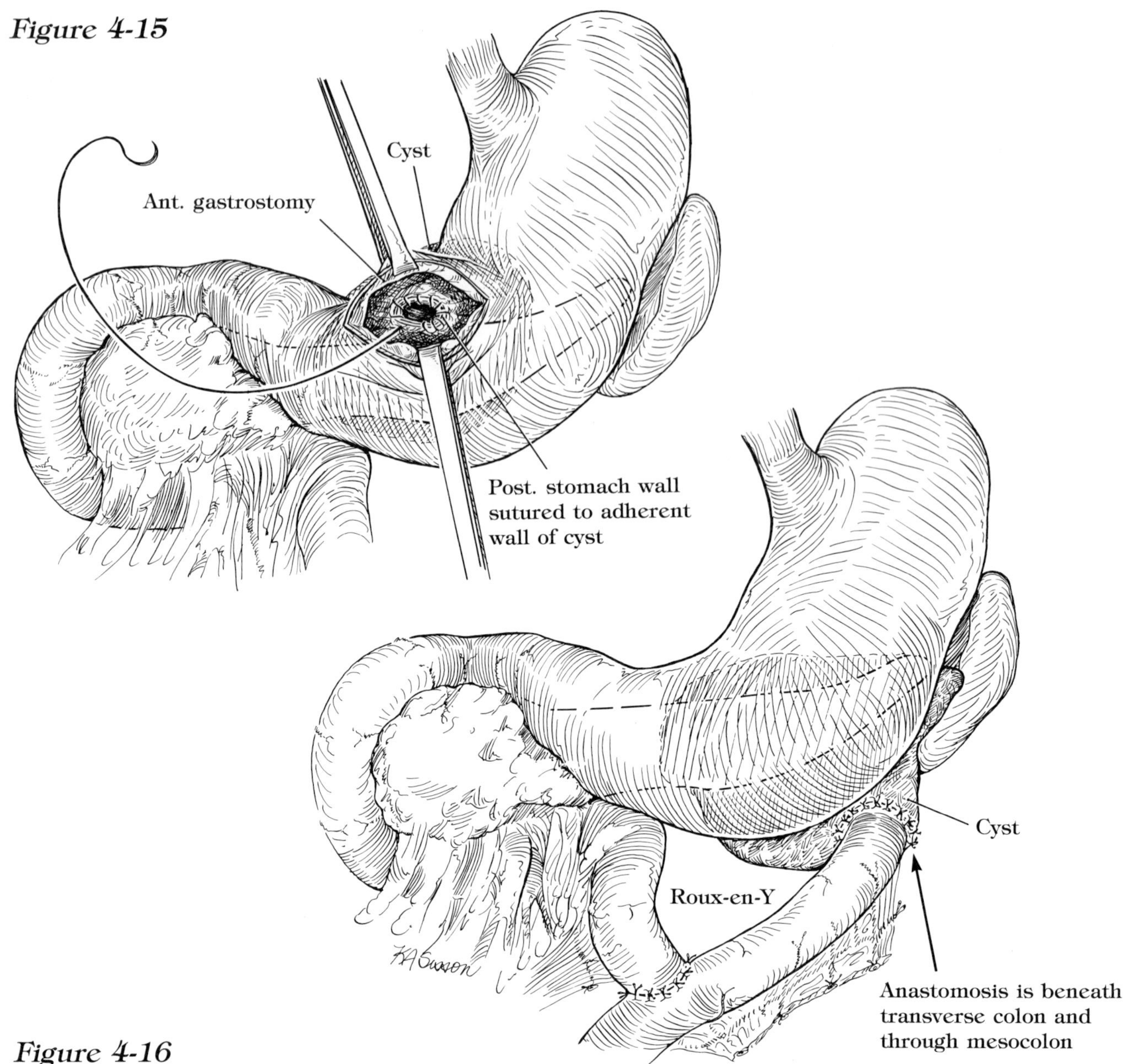

Figure 4-16

PANCREATECTOMY

Under some circumstances, a 90% pancreatic resection is advocated. This is achieved, as described previously, by mobilization of the spleen and then the body and tail of the pancreas after entering the lesser omental sac. The pancreas is elevated off the superior mesenteric and portal venous confluence where the splenic vein is ligated. Further dissection around the superior mesenteric vessels permits removal of all but a thin rim of pancreas following the curve of the duodenum (Figs. 4-17, 4-18). If a total pancreatectomy is indicated, as it may be occasionally, the initial part of the distal pancreatectomy is combined with the Whipple operation, which is described in the following section.

This procedure is indicated for certain malignant lesions arising in the head of the pancreas, ampulla of Vater, distal common bile duct, or midduodenum, although occasionally extensive intractable pancreatitis may indicate a total removal of this organ. The ideal candidates for the Whipple operation are those patients who have small obstructing lesions near the entry of the common bile duct to the duodenum which may result in early diagnosis. Ordinarily these prove to be lesions arising in the ampulla itself, the distal bile duct, or the duodenum adjacent to the ampulla. The results of resection for cancer of the head of the pancreas have been dismal. The majority of cases are inoperable at the time of the first exploration because of either the size of the lesion, the extent of local invasion, or regional or distant metastases. Even in those patients in whom the tumor is apparently favorable, less than 10% five-year survival is the ordinary figure given in most large series. As a result, most surgeons are restrained in undertaking the Whipple procedure. It is wise to limit this operation to the most favorable anatomic cases in patients in good general health without other systemic disease. These poor results have also led a number of surgeons to perform total pancreatectomy for carcinoma arising in the ductal system of the pancreas because of the relative frequency of microscopic disease at the resection margin and the occasional identification of multifocal disease. Further comments will be made on this subject under the section on total pancreatectomy.

Pancreatico-
Duodenectomy
(Whipple Operation)

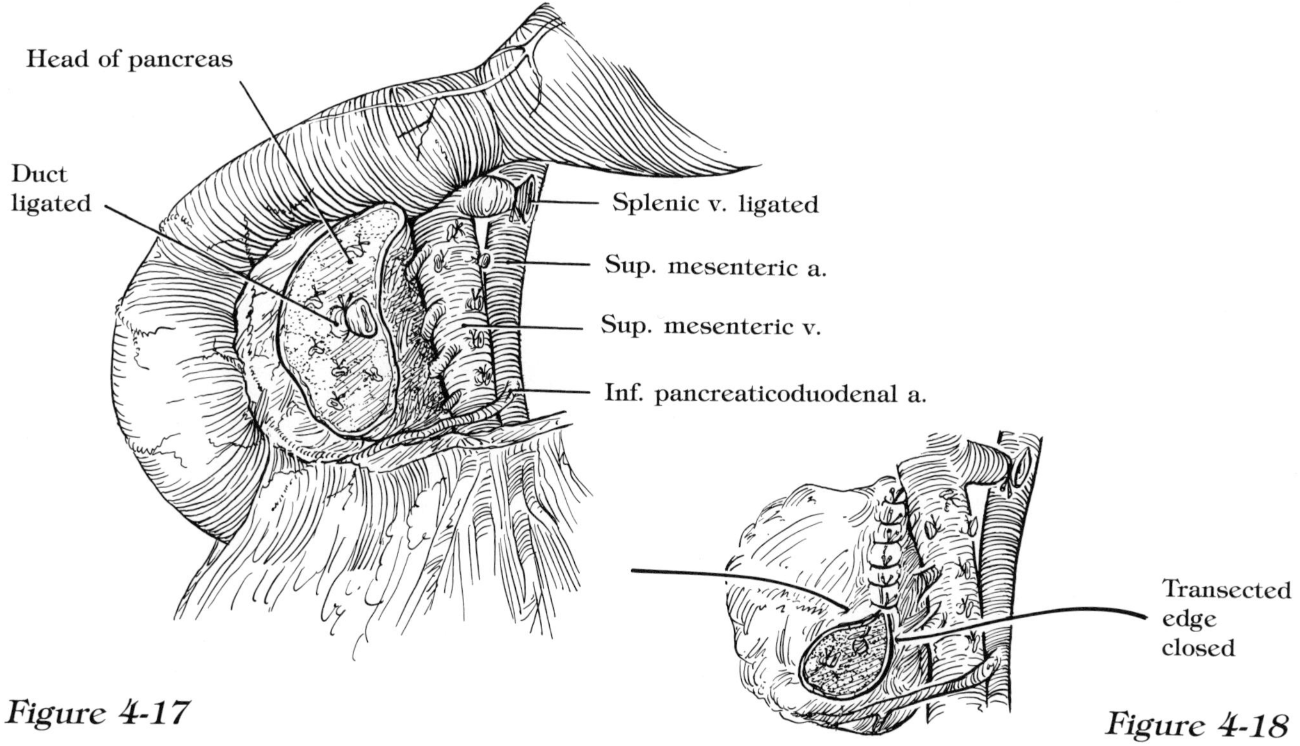

Figure 4-17

Figure 4-18

Either the midline or transverse incision curving downward at both ends gives satisfactory exposure, but if a total pancreatectomy is indicated, then a transverse ("frown" or "chevron") incision is preferable. After exploration for determination of the size, extent, and resectability of the tumor, surgical procedure is begun. Prior to this, microscopic confirmation of the diagnosis may be indicated but, as has been indicated so often in the literature, this often presents the pathologist with difficult problems. Mobilization of the head of the pancreas is begun by incising the lateral reflection of the peritoneum off the duodenum and carrying out what is classically referred to as the Kocher maneuver. This permits the surgeon to introduce his fingers retroperitoneally behind the head of the pancreas and gives further information on the extent and resectability of the tumor (Fig. 4-19). As the duodenum is mobilized and the hepatic flexure and the right transverse colon are reflected downward, the entire third and fourth portions of the duodenum can be brought into view. This maneuver is often facilitated by early division of the ligament of Treitz and partial mobilization of the first portion of the jejunum and the fourth portion of the duodenum (Fig. 4-20). As the surgeon proceeds with this mobilization of the ligament of Treitz and portions of the duodenum and jejunum, the superior mesenteric vein can be identified from below as it crosses the upper gastrointestinal tract at the ligament of Treitz. At this point, the surgeon may elect to enter the lesser omental sac to mobilize the stomach, antrum, and pylorus off the pancreas by dividing the branches of the gastroepiploic. The surgeon should now have a sufficiently clear anatomic picture to determine operability and then can proceed to transect the stomach between clamps for better exposure of the superior border of the pancreas. When this is done, the celiac axis can be visualized and the left and right gastric arteries ligated (Fig. 4-21). Dissecting down the superior border of the pancreas and following the course of the proper hepatic artery, the surgeon then encounters, divides, and ligates the gastroduodenal artery.

CAUTION

The not infrequent anomaly of a divided hepatic arterial inflow, with the left hepatic artery arising from the left gastric artery and the right hepatic artery arising directly from the superior mesenteric artery, complicates the operative procedure. However, both the hepatic arteries can be preserved by careful dissection, particularly if preliminary angiography has alerted the operating surgeon to the presence of this anomaly.

Figure 4-19

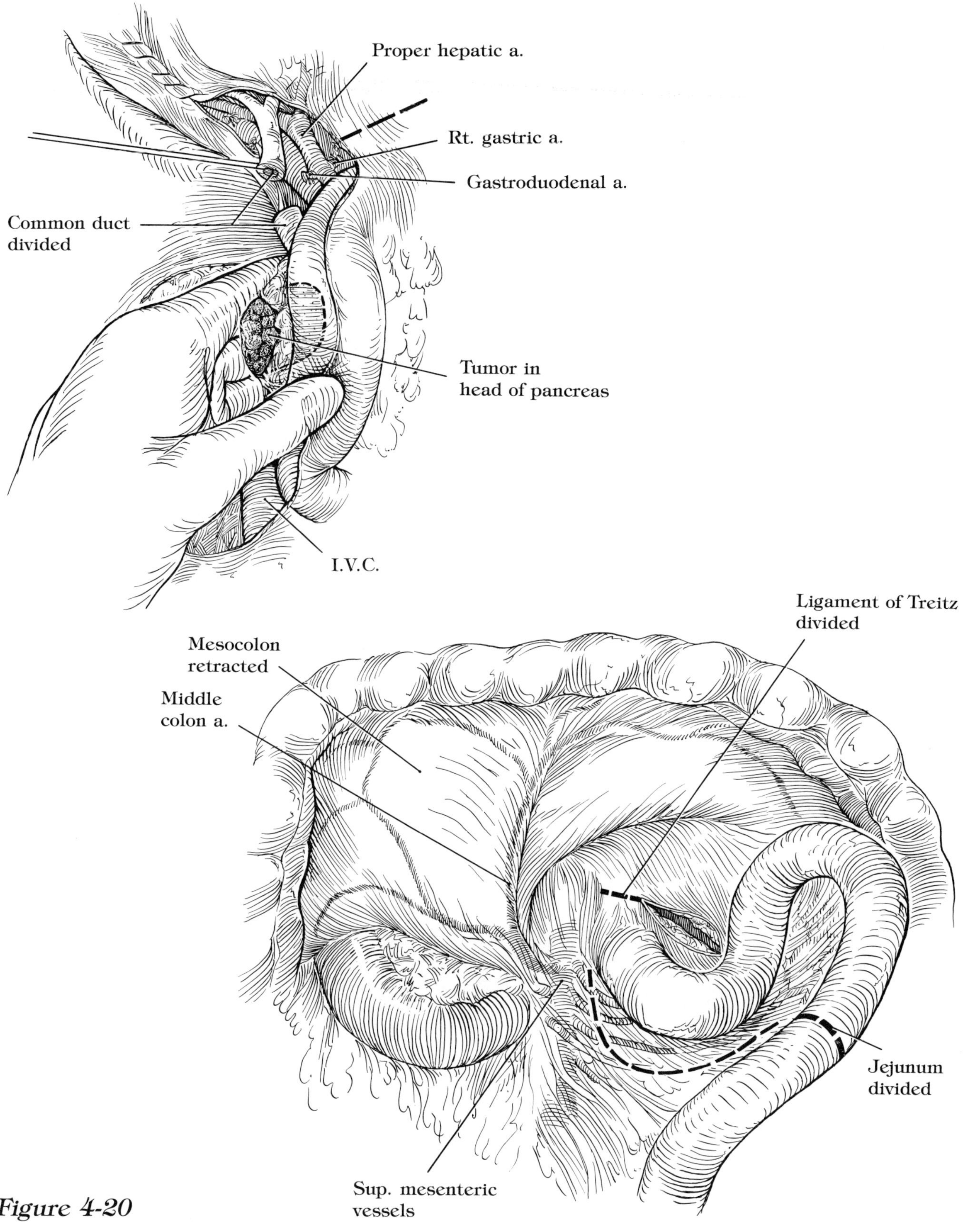

Proper hepatic a.
Rt. gastric a.
Gastroduodenal a.
Common duct
divided
Tumor in
head of pancreas
I.V.C.
Mesocolon
retracted
Middle
colon a.
Ligament of Treitz
divided
Jejunum
divided
Sup. mesenteric
vessels

Figure 4-20

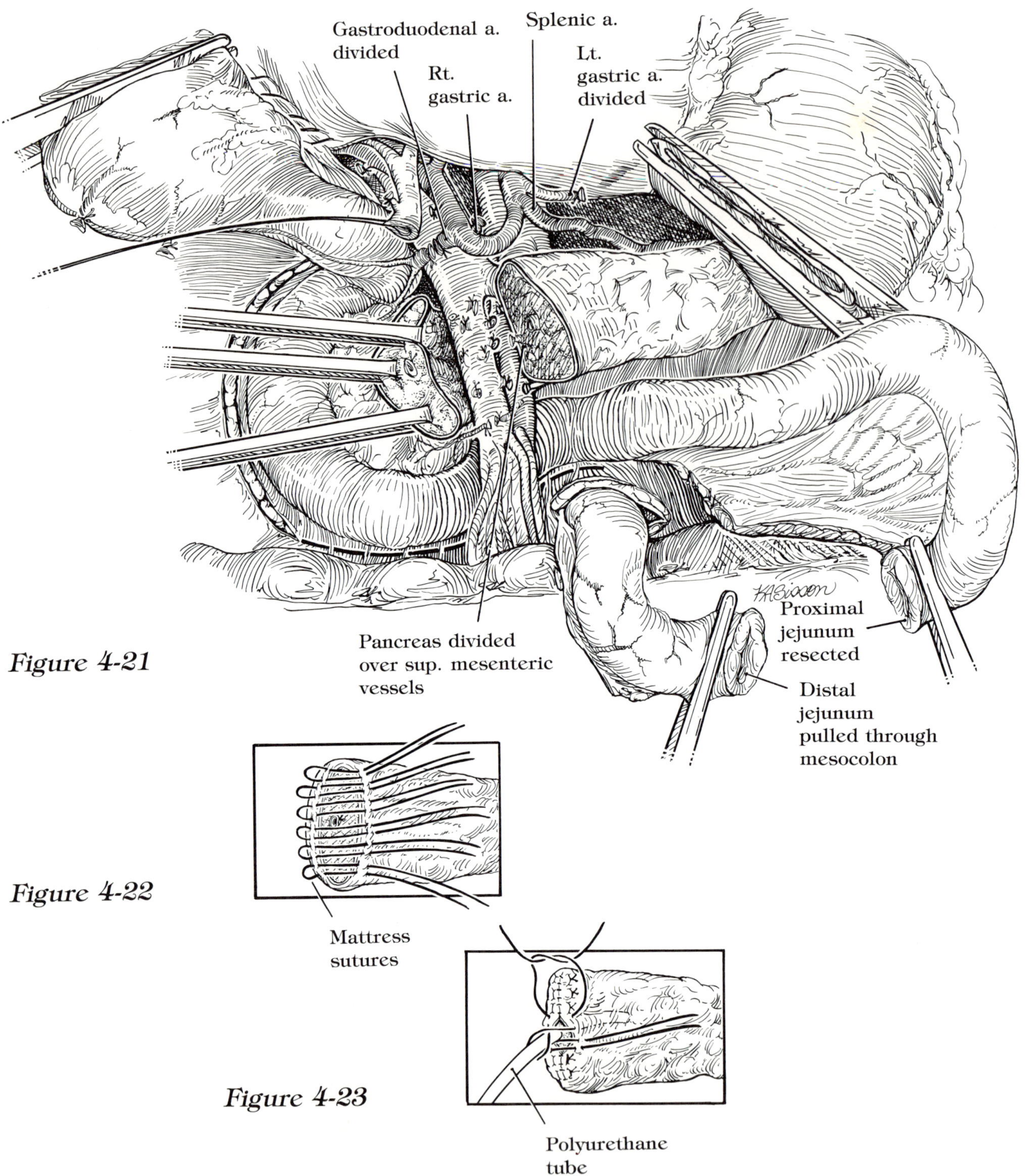

Figure 4-21

Figure 4-22

Figure 4-23

The common duct should be the next structure in the gastro-hepatic ligament that is encountered. In cases of obstruction at the outlet of the bile duct, identification is usually quite simple because of the enormous dilatation of the duct itself. When this is dissected carefully from the underlying portal vein and divided, one can then direct attention to the pancreas itself. The superior and inferior borders of the pancreas should be followed to the point where the organ crosses the superior mesenteric vein (this area may have already been partially identified by previously described dissection from below). A number of large venous tributaries enter the superior mesenteric vein, but these mostly occur laterally and posteriorly. Therefore, careful blunt dissection beneath the body of the pancreas as it crosses the superior mesenteric vein should make it possible to elevate the gland and transect it using a fishmouth incision for more satisfactory anastomosis and closure later. The only remaining attachments of the pancreas and gastrointestinal tract are below the ligament of Treitz and behind the superior mesenteric vein where the uncinate process sweeps posteriorly. The upper jejunum may then be transected at an appropriate point and drawn through the opening of the mesentery in the transverse mesocolon at the ligament of Treitz for ultimate removal with the specimen. After this, the distal portion of the upper jejunum which has been transected can be drawn up through the transverse mesocolon for ultimate anastomosis. The status of the operation at this point is shown in Figure 4-21; all that remains is dissection behind the superior mesenteric vein to mobilize the uncinate process of the pancreas and to permit complete removal of the distal stomach, duodenum, upper jejunum, head of the pancreas, and distal common bile duct.

Reconstruction may be accomplished with either an end-to-end or an end-to-side pancreaticoenterostomy.

CAUTION

This particular anastomosis is the source of the most troublesome complications and most of the deaths resulting from this operative procedure. A leak of pancreatic juice in this area induces serious morbidity and the likelihood of one or more drainage procedures; in addition, the erosive action of the proteolytic enzymes can set off massive and often lethal intra-abdominal hemorrhages. Thus, meticulous attention should be paid to a mucosa-to-mucosa approximation of the edges of the dilated pancreatic duct and the mucosa of the duodenum. Whether an end-to-end or side-to-end anastomosis is used, the serosa of the jejunum should be securely fastened to the capsule of the pancreas, inverting as much as possible of the transected end (Figs. 4-22, 4-23).

In either case, it is essential to also reestablish biliary and gastrointestinal continuity. The common duct is then anastomosed to the side of the jejunum with an inner layer of continuous 3-0 chromic catgut suture and an outer layer of interrupted silk. Gastroenterostomy is carried out ordinarily using a Hofmeister anastomosis with two layers of continuous 3-0 catgut suture. The point at which the jejunum has been brought through the mesocolon for these anastomoses is closed loosely around the bowel with interrupted silk sutures. Ordinarily, the gallbladder is removed prior to closure of the abdomen since it is functionless once the sphincter mechanism has been removed. The final reconstruction is shown in Figure 4-24A, B.

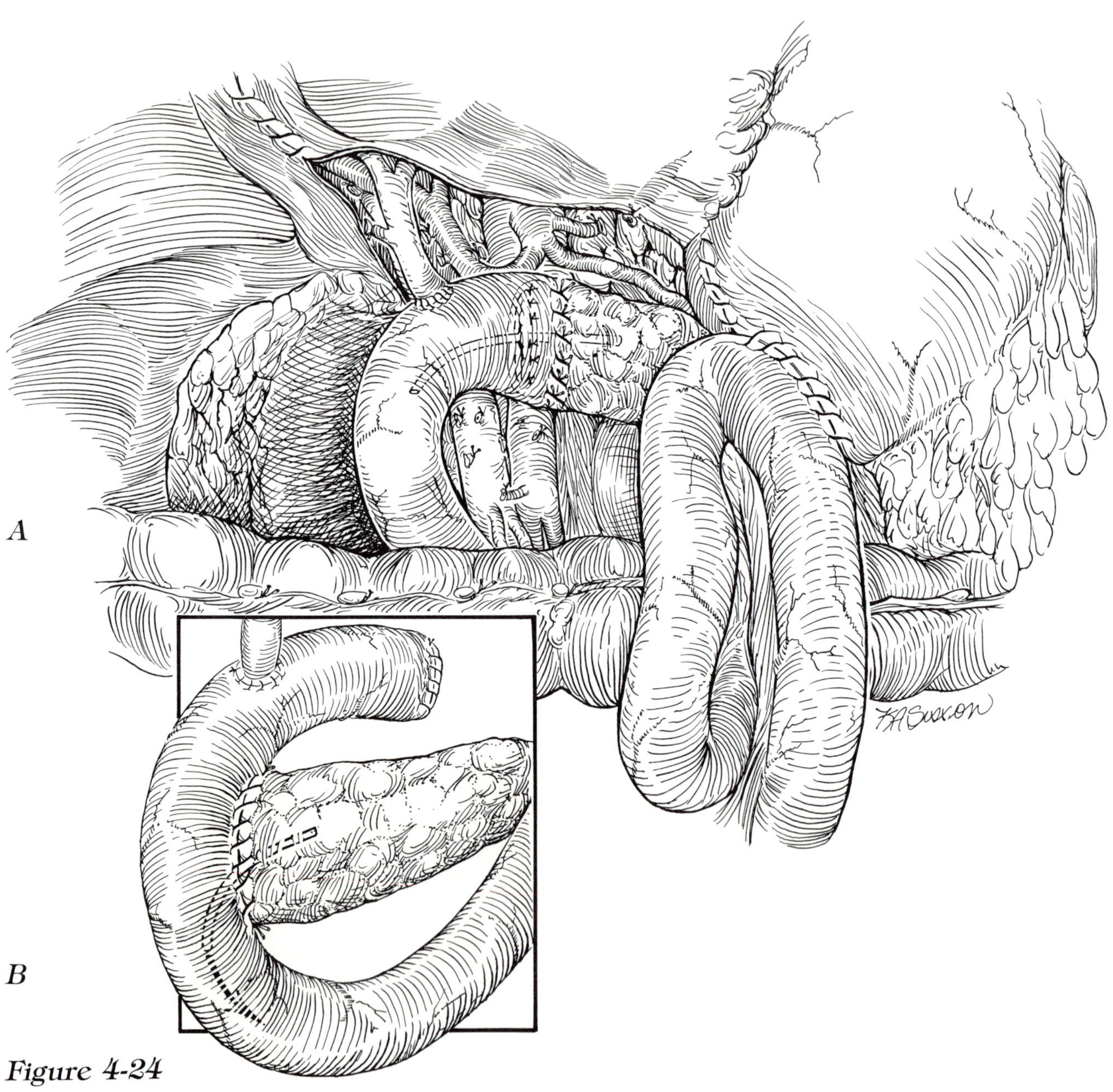

A

B

Figure 4-24

CHAPTER FIVE

LIVER AND PORTAL CIRCULATION

Major resections of the liver are a relatively recent advent in the surgical field since these extensive procedures were introduced less than 30 years ago by Lortat-Jacob in Paris and popularized in this country by Pack, Quattlebaum, and others. The main indication for major hepatic resection is the presence of primary or metastatic malignant disease. The problems of primary hepatocellular carcinoma or cholangiocarcinoma need no extensive discussion. If the tumor is resectable and the patient's condition warrants, then the operation is undertaken; if not, then considerable palliation may be achieved by a combination of dearterialization, regional infusion, and radiotherapy. The presence of apparently solitary or at least surgically resectable metastatic disease in the liver presents the surgeon with a problem that requires thoughtful appraisal. Under the most favorable circumstances a five-year cure rate of no more than 20% can be expected. One would think that a longer time interval between the removal of the primary and the appearance of the metastasis would increase survival. Although this has not been firmly established, it is one of the reasonable suppositions one can make in evaluating the feasibility of surgery. The location of the primary is, of course, of prime consideration, and one can limit hepatic resections for metastatic disease for patients whose primary arose in the colon or, on occasion, from some unusual source. Metastatic spread from cancers of the stomach, duodenum, and pancreas are almost by definition incurable. There are some benign indications for major hepatic resection, such as tumors secondary to oral contraceptives which may present with

Hepatic Resections

massive hemorrhage, symptomatic cavernous hemangiomas, bile duct cysts, or abscesses which, because of their location, are more amenable to resection than to drainage.

> ## CAUTION
>
> Most major hepatic resections may be carried out through an abdominal incision. Occasionally, however, because of the location in the posterior superior segment of the right lobe, it may be necessary to extend the incision into the chest in order to obtain appropriate visualization of the suprahepatic vena cava in the entrance of the right and left hepatic vein.

RIGHT HEPATIC LOBECTOMY

Although limited wedge resections and closure with mattress sutures may be carried out for peripheral small tumors or for trauma, the most difficult standardized operative procedure on the liver is referred to as *right hepatic lobectomy*. It actually consists of the anatomic removal of the right, caudate, and quadrate lobes. The operation is begun through a right upper quadrant paramedian or a subcostal incision. Once a pathologic condition has been defined and resectability ascertained, the incision is then extended if necessary across the costal margin into the chest through the sixth interspace or by removal of the sixth rib. Dissection is begun in the gastrohepatic ligament to identify the common bile duct, the portal vein, and the hepatic artery. With traction tapes around each of these, the full length of each of these structures is dissected free so that the right branches can be identified and isolated (Fig. 5-1). These are then held with tapes or ligatures for future identification. Attention is then directed laterally where the right triangular ligament and the peritoneal reflection off the liver are divided. The right lobe of the liver is mobilized medially, exposing the bare area retroperitoneally and the vena cava that runs behind the liver in a groove in the caudate lobe. As the liver is retracted medially and superiorly, a successive number of small hepatic veins come into view which should be individually ligated in continuity and divided. These vary in number from three to eight, but eventually all the smaller outflow tracts are divided and the major veins entering the cava from the right and left lobes are identified (Fig. 5-2). Visualization of this area is extremely important, and the division of the diaphragm down to the vena cava facilitates this particular phase of the operation. If one can, with certainty, identify separate entrances for the major right and left hepatic veins, then a holding ligature is placed around the right hepatic vein. (If, however, there appears to be only a single channel, then identification must be made within the liver dur-

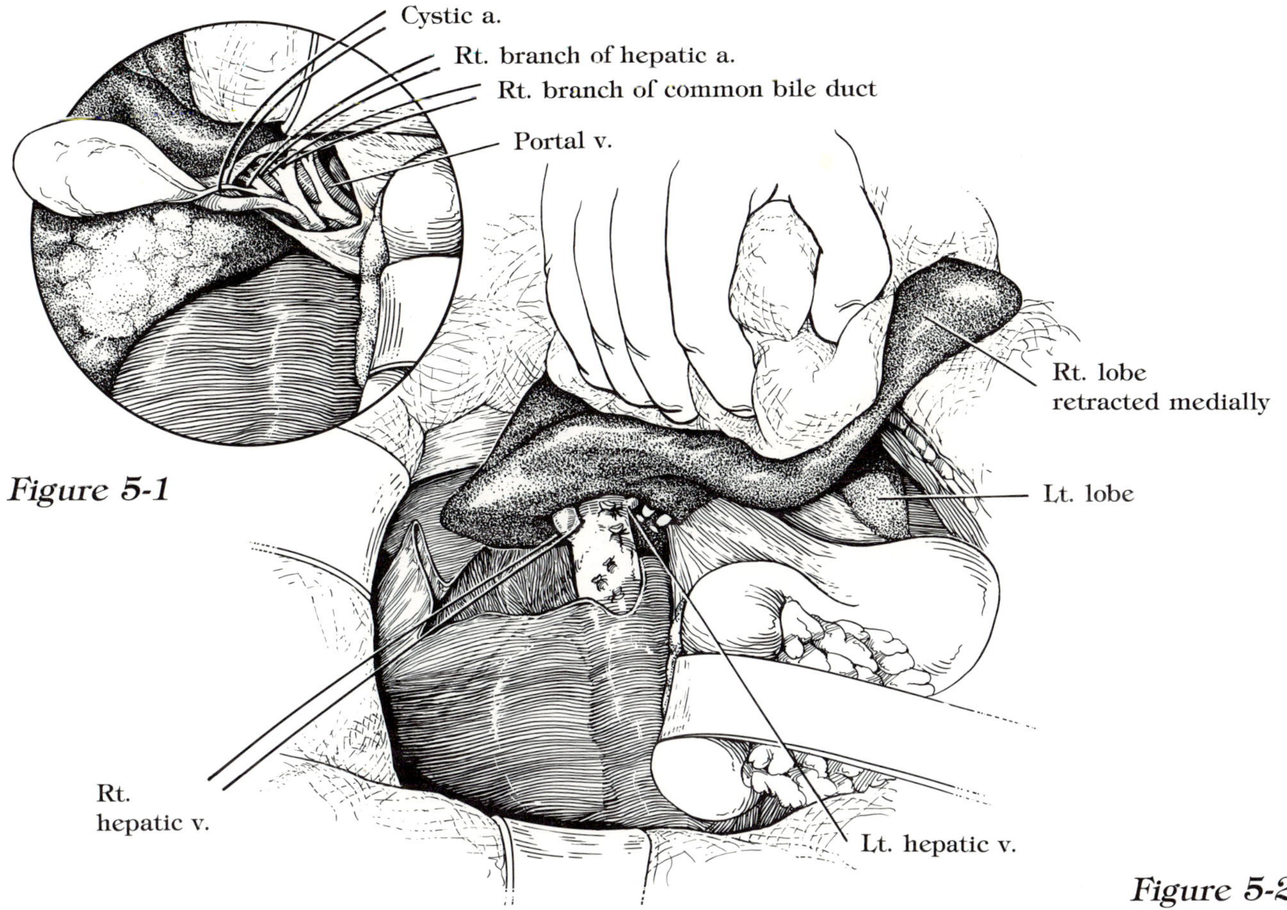

Figure 5-1

Figure 5-2

ing transection to avoid ligating the only outflow tract to the remaining left lobe.) Following this maneuver, attention is redirected to the gastrohepatic ligament, the cystic duct is divided and ligated, and the right branches of the hepatic artery, portal vein, and common hepatic duct are transected and ligated. Again, the surgeon moves posteriorly and ligates and divides the right hepatic vein. Thus, the major inflow and outflow tracts from the right lobe are secured. Demarcation can usually be seen at a point 2 to 4 cm lateral to the attachment of the falciform ligament. Transection of the liver is then begun in the approximate line of the vena cava and along the point indicated by the change in color.

Glisson's capsule is incised with the scalpel. Then, using the handle of the knife for blunt dissection, the surgeon traverses the liver parenchyma, clamping and dividing ducts and vessels as they are encountered during the blunt dissection. Eventually one comes through the substance of the liver to the vena cava, and careful progress is carried on superiorly with attention to preservation of the left hepatic vein (Fig. 5-3). Another technical detail that is sometimes of value involves a choledochotomy and insertion of a metal probe into the left bile duct prior to transection of the liver. This procedure avoids injuring this structure, which sometimes comes quite close to the projected line of transection, particularly if this is extended to include the medial segment of the left lobe. After the right lobe of the liver is removed, all visible ducts and vessels are ligated or cauterized. The round ligament is detached from the anterior peritoneal surface, and the round and falciform ligaments are swung over the liver and sutured posteriorly to reperitonealize the raw surface. A T tube is inserted into the common bile duct as previously described (Fig. 5-4). A suction catheter is placed in the lateral subphrenic area, and a cigarette wick is placed in the hepatorenal fossa below the gastrohepatic ligament. The T tube and drains are brought out appropriately through one or more small muscle-splitting incisions, fixed in position, and the incision is closed. The chest thoracotomy portion is closed with catheter drainage.

Figure 5-3

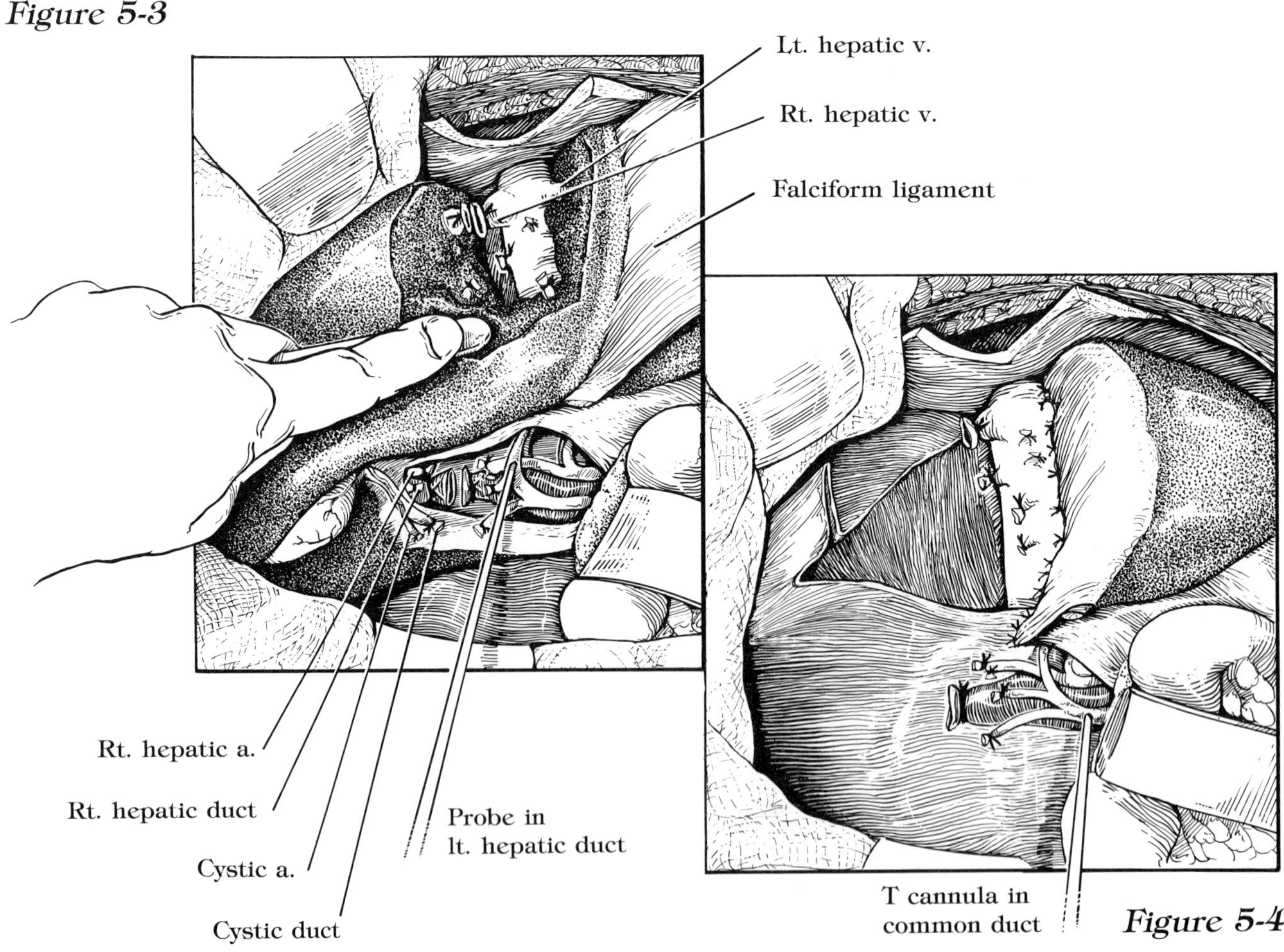

Figure 5-4

Left hepatic lobectomy may be carried out in a formal fashion by identifying and ligating the appropriate left duct and vessels. Ordinarily, however, the anatomic configuration of this lobe lends itself to a wedge resection. The incision is "fishmouthed" in such a way that the transected edge of the liver can be closed with interrupted mattress sutures (Figs. 5-5, 5-6, 5-7). Unless the tumor mass is unusually large, the thoracic component of the incision is not ordinarily necessary.

LEFT HEPATIC LOBECTOMY

The choice of a particular shunting procedure has been the subject of continuing controversy over many years in the literature and does not lend itself easily to oversimplification. Nonetheless, it would be fair to state a few acceptable generalizations: 1) The selective or distal splenorenal shunt is certainly satisfactory for nonalcoholic, presinusoidal block of the type seen in idiopathic hepatic fibrosis or schistosomiasis where a total shunt carries a high incidence of encephalopathy and hepatocellular failure. 2) The presence of significant and intractable ascites mandates a combined decompression with a shunt that provides retrograde flow from the intrahepatic sinusoidal bed as well as the extrahepatic splenic and splanchnic beds. 3) An end-to-side portacaval shunt is probably the simplest and most widely used total shunt and carries with it a high protection against recurrent hemorrhage, but it is as ineffective as the selective shunt in the control of intractable ascites. 4) The

Portal-Systemic Shunts

Split rectus m.
Falciform ligament
Rt. lobe
of liver
Round ligament
Stomach

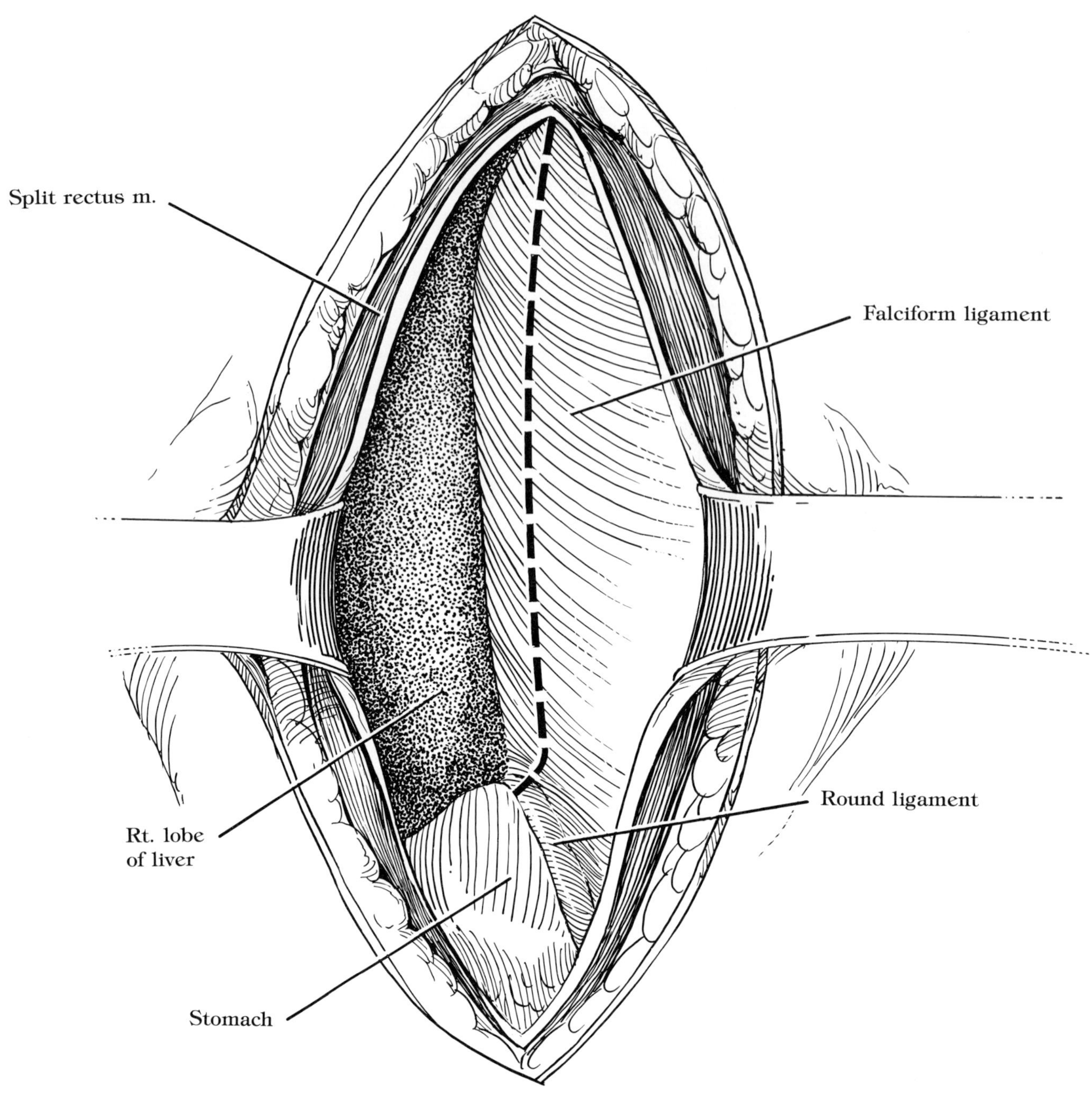

Figure 5-5

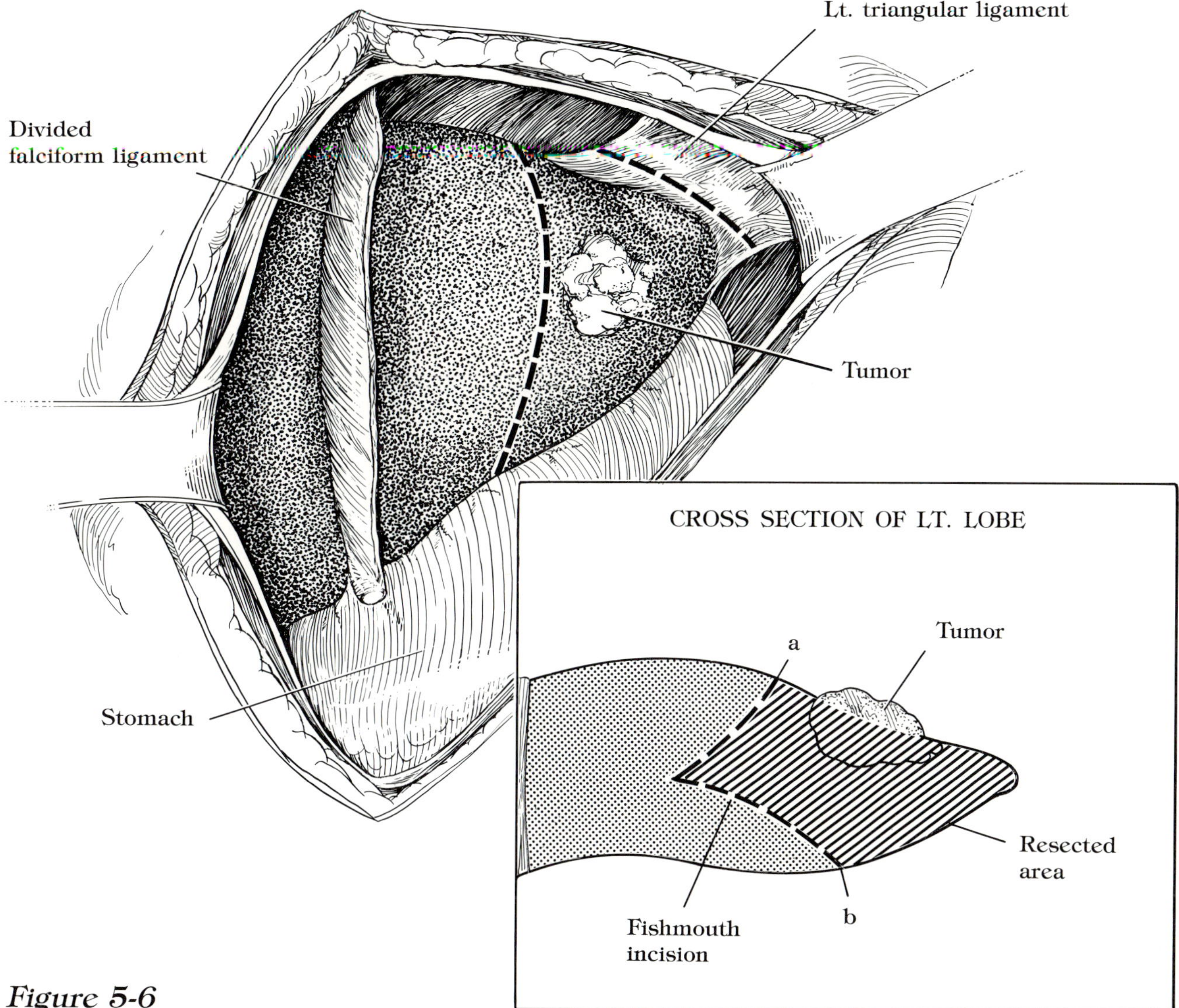

Figure 5-6

mesocaval shunt with an interposition graft has not lived up to the early expectations suggested by Drapanas and carries a relatively high incidence of early and late thrombotic occlusion of the graft; nevertheless, in patients with extrahepatic portal bed block with occlusion of the portal and splenic veins, this may be the only shunt that is technically feasible.

All the portal systemic shunts carry with them the potential hazard of postshunt encephalopathy, a complication that is related both to the shunting of blood from the colon and to the varying degree of decrease in hepatic blood flow occasioned by the shunt. Although this may be a distressing and difficult complication, often it is easily controllable by dietary restriction of protein, increased attention to catharsis in enemas, the use of lactulose or oral antibiotics and, in serious problems, the operative procedures that bypass or remove the greater portion of the large bowel.

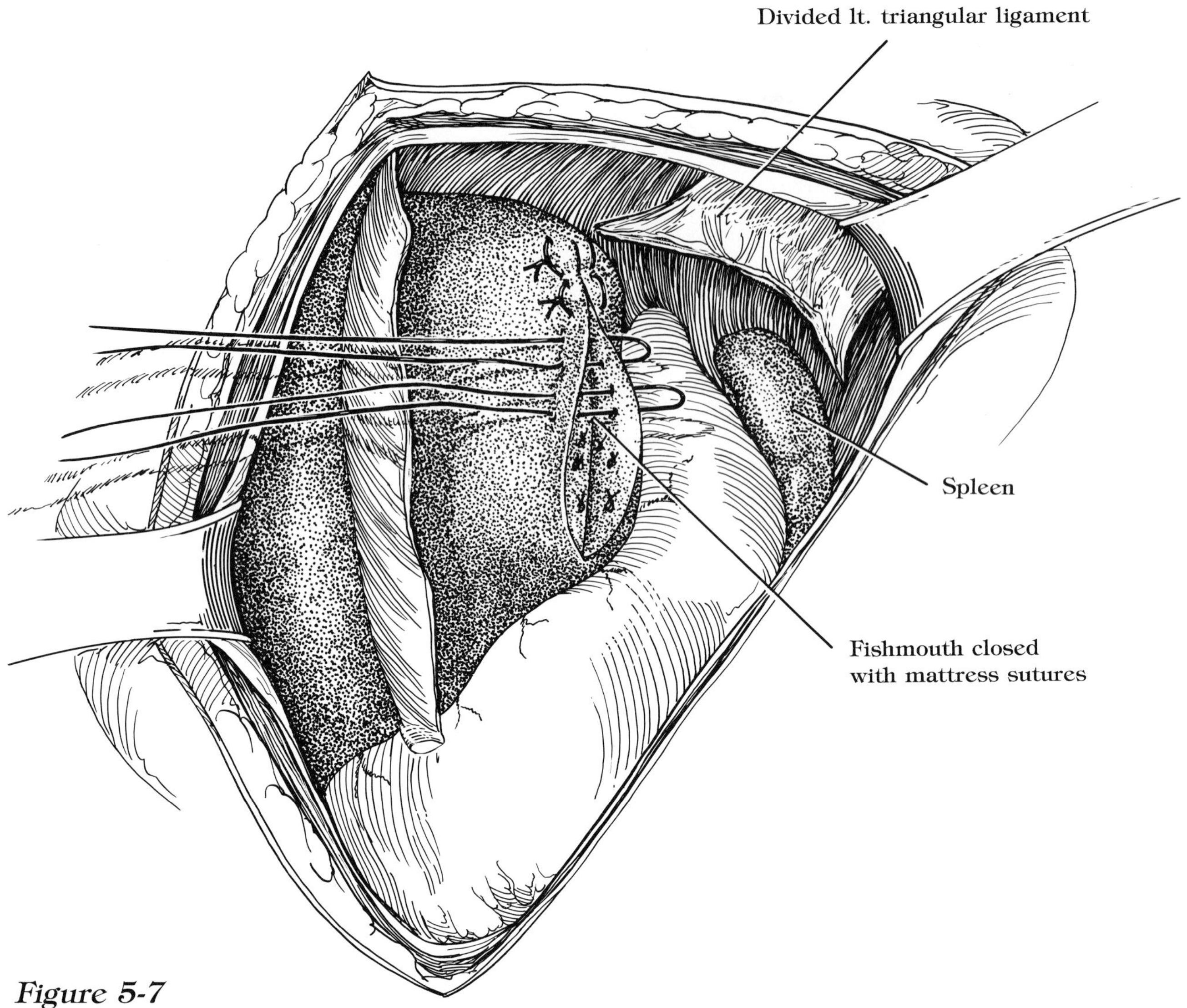

Figure 5-7

Although there are innumerable approaches and variations in the technique of constructing portal-systemic shunts, only one technique will be described in detail for each of the established shunting procedures since it would be nearly impossible and confusing to interject segments of several different methods of achieving the same objective. Utilization by any surgeon of one particular technique, which he may well modify with growing experience, has the advantage of standardization and familiarity, both of which are important to a surgical team intent on performing a quick, effective, and safe operative procedure.

The various types of shunts now in clinical use are shown diagrammatically in Figures 5-8 through 5-17. Only the five shunts most likely to be used by the general surgeon are described in detail.

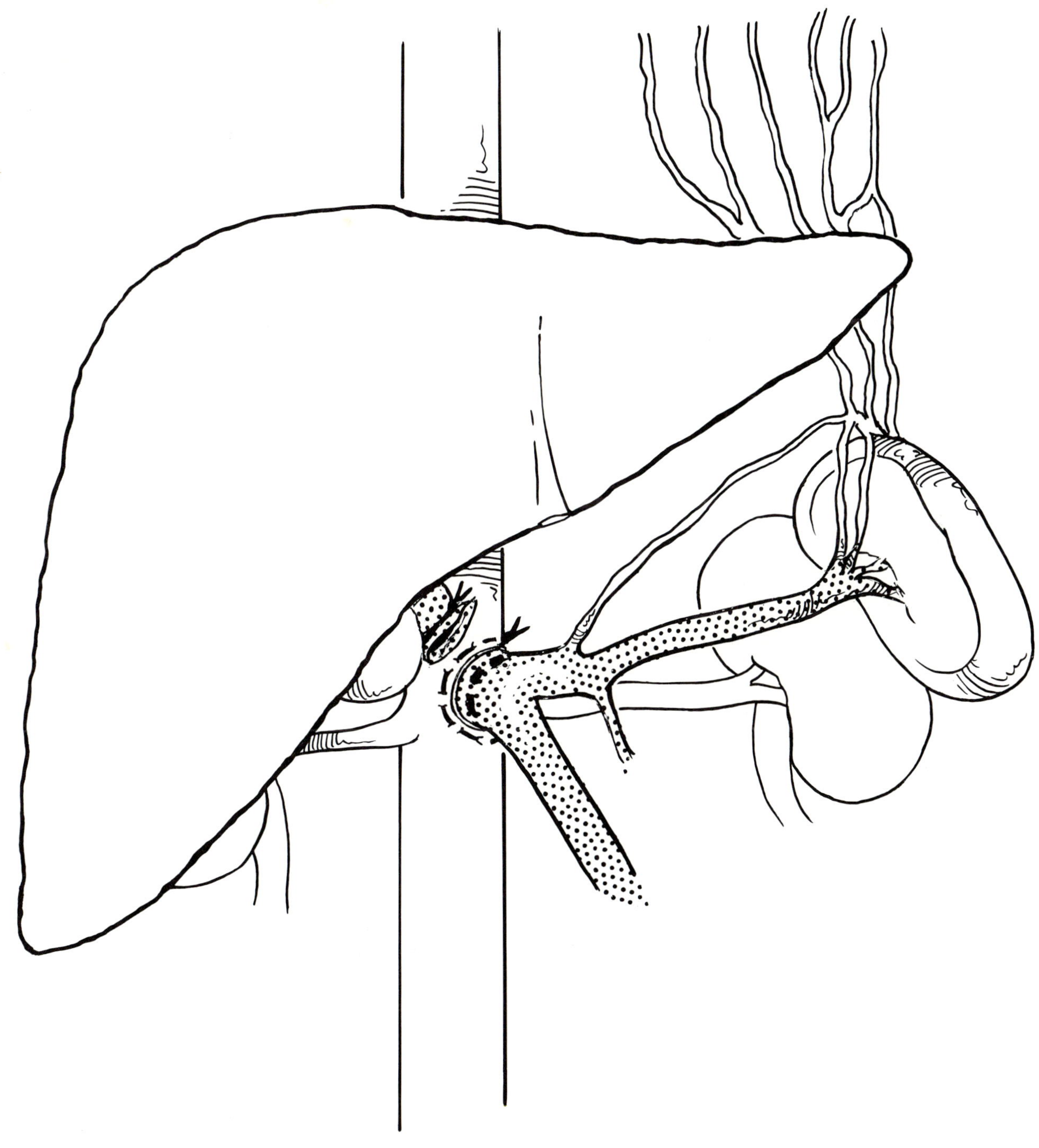

SIDE-TO-SIDE PORTACAVAL SHUNT

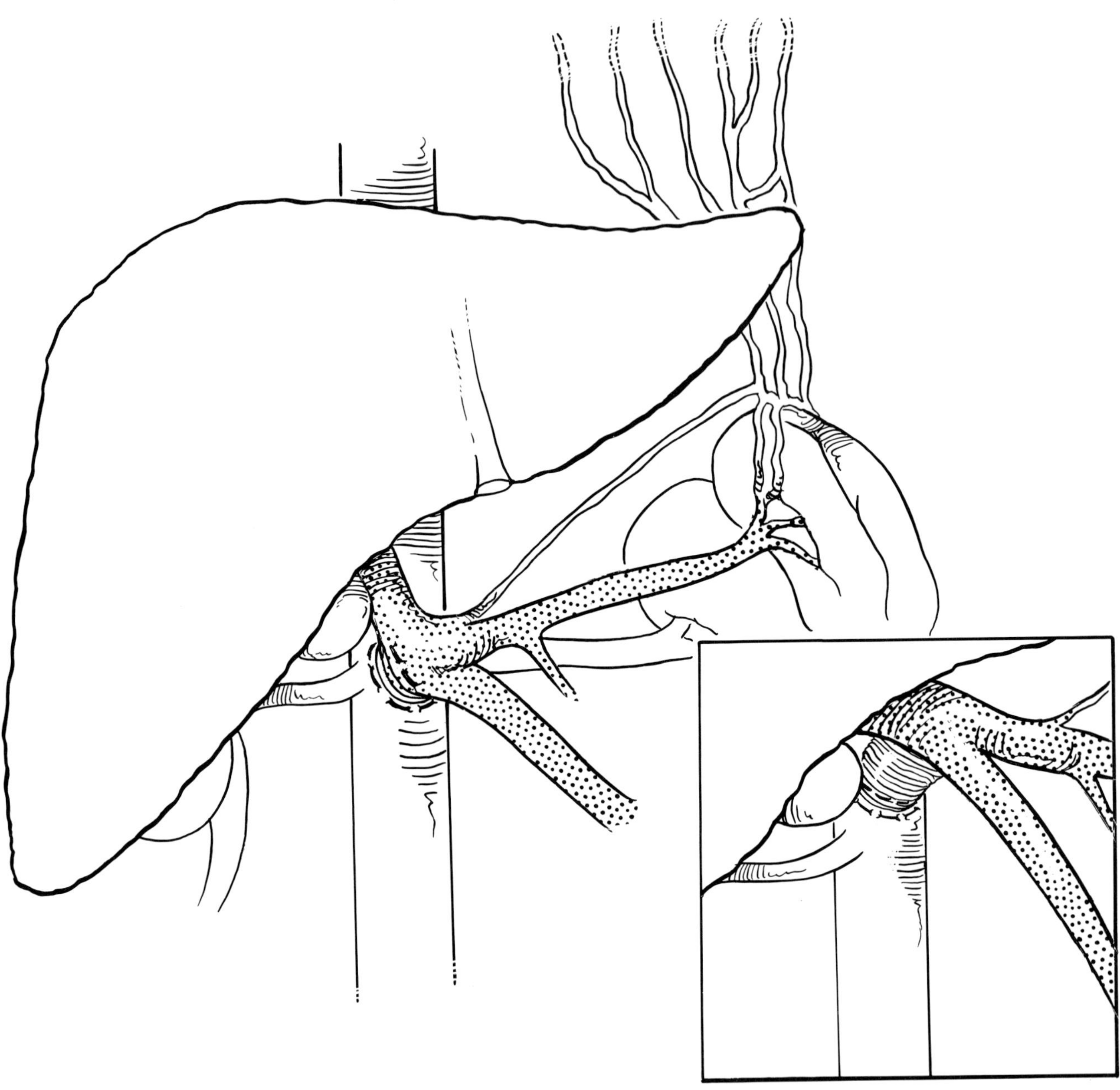

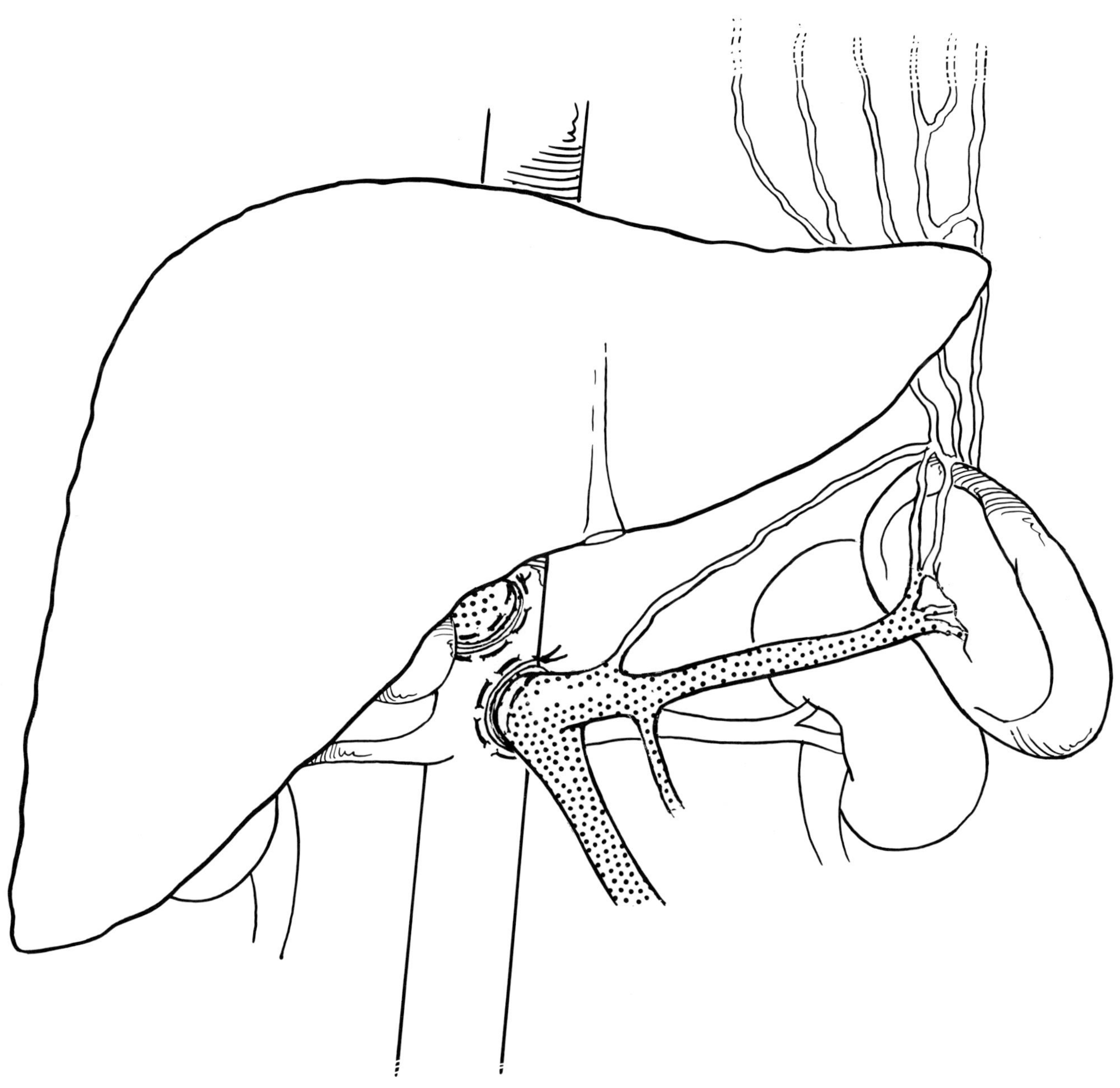

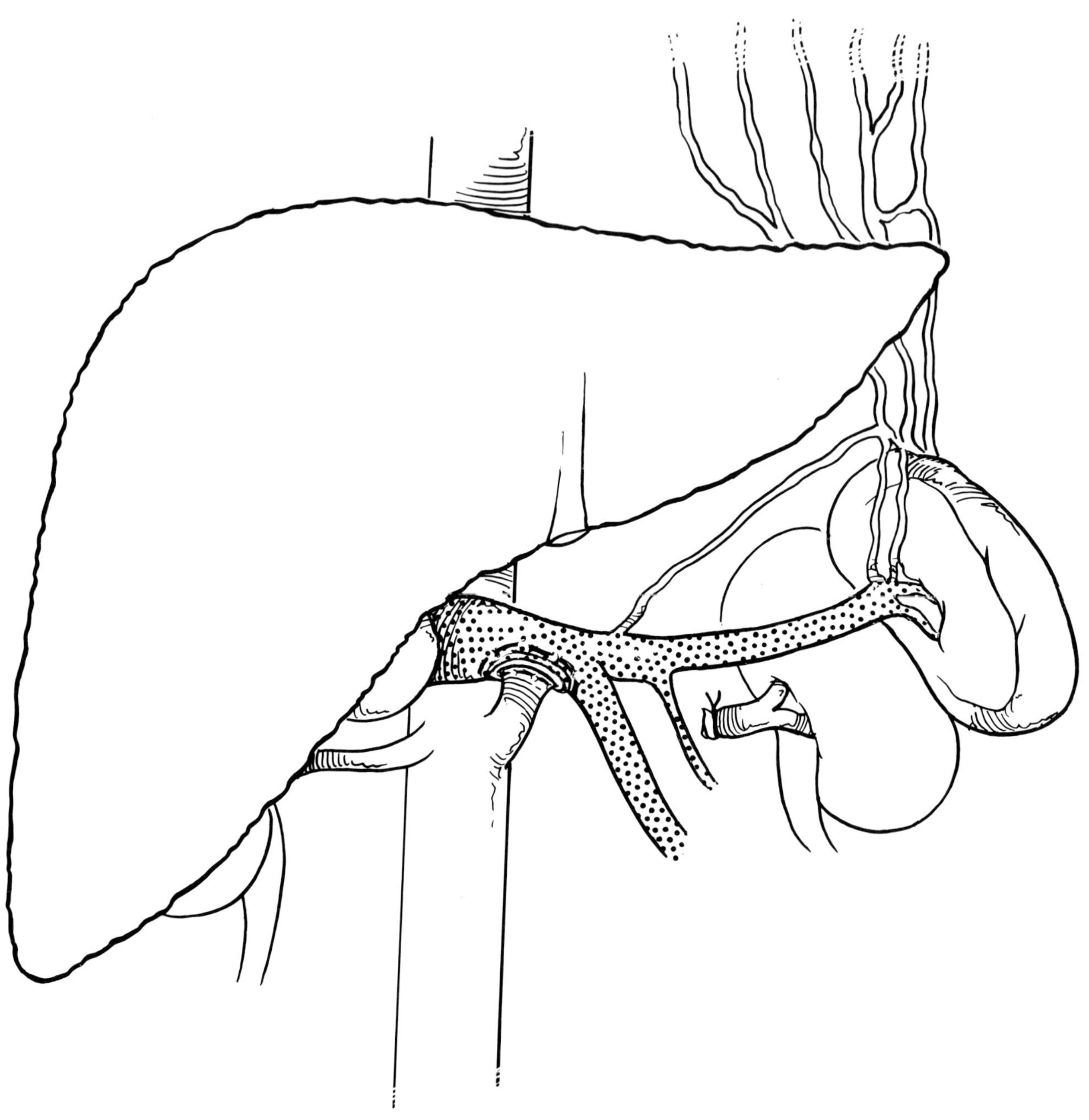

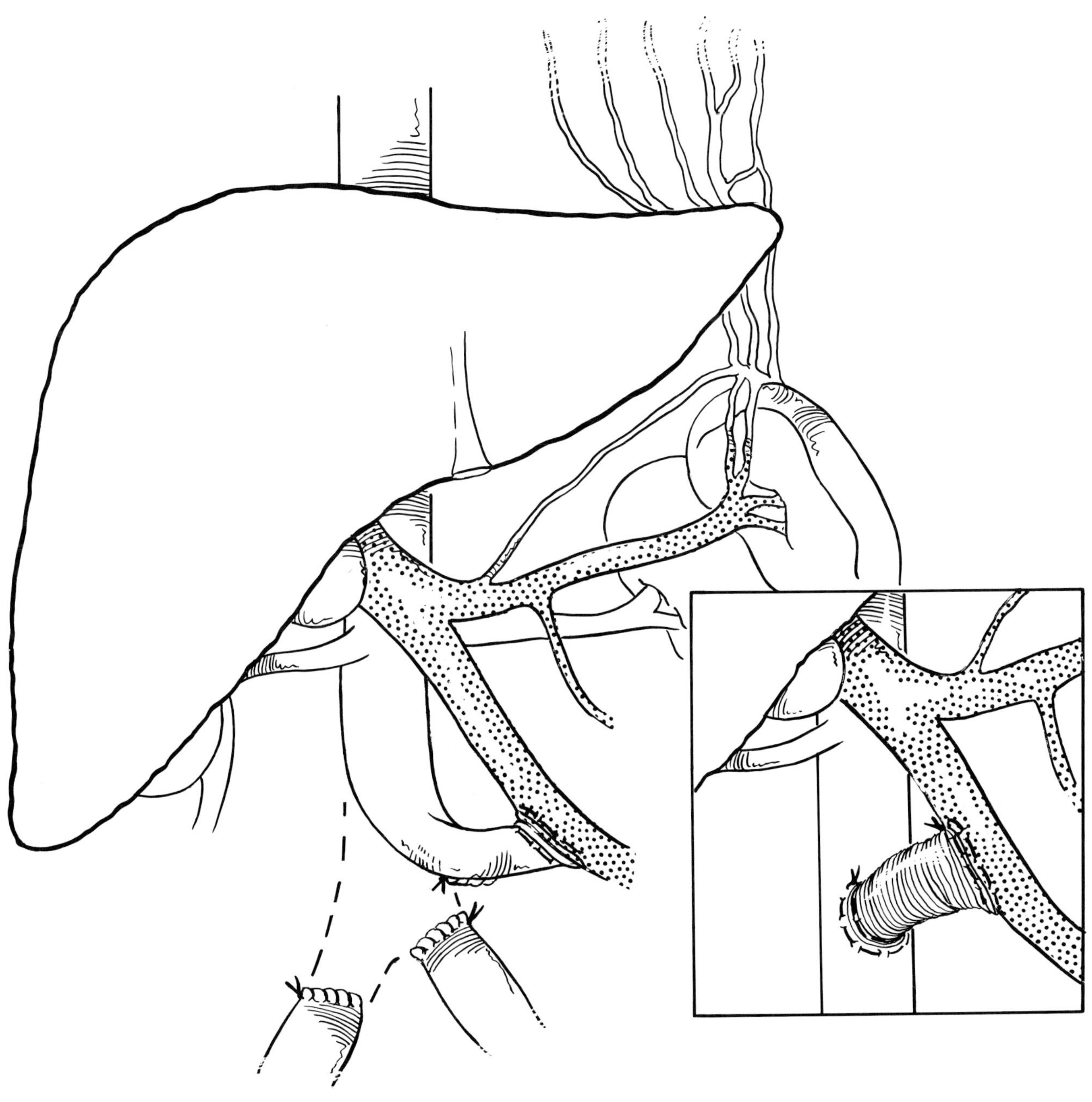

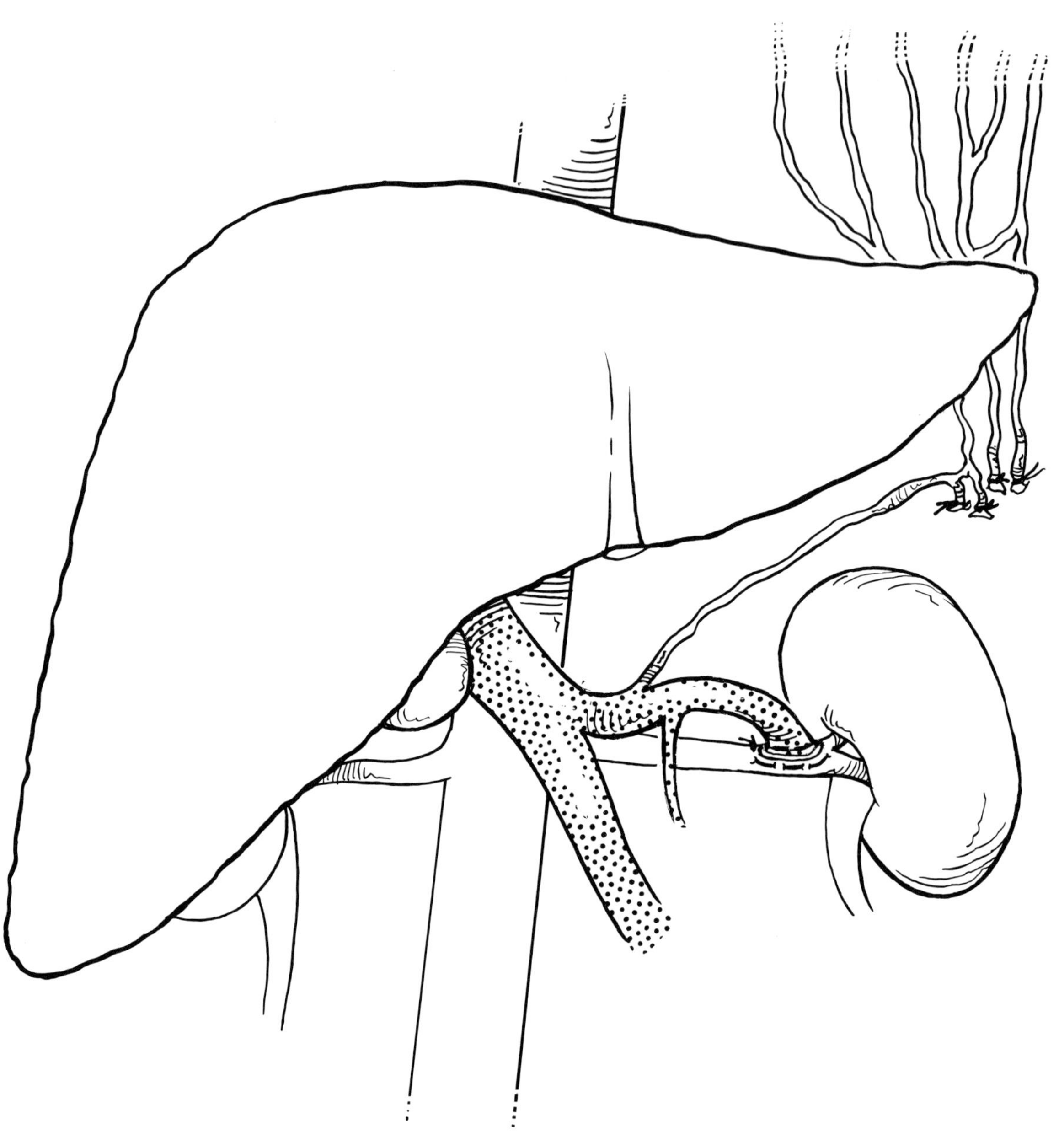

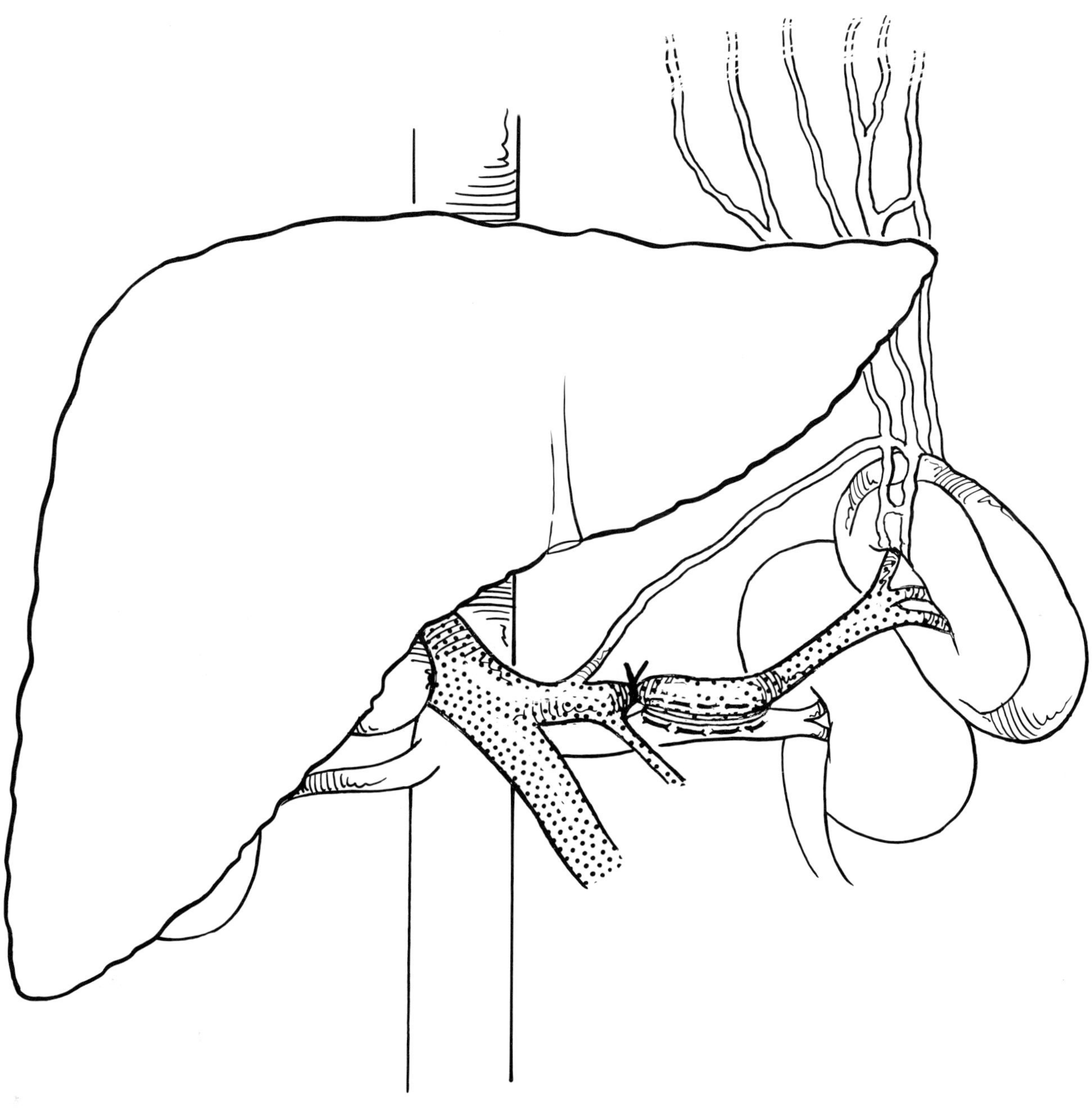

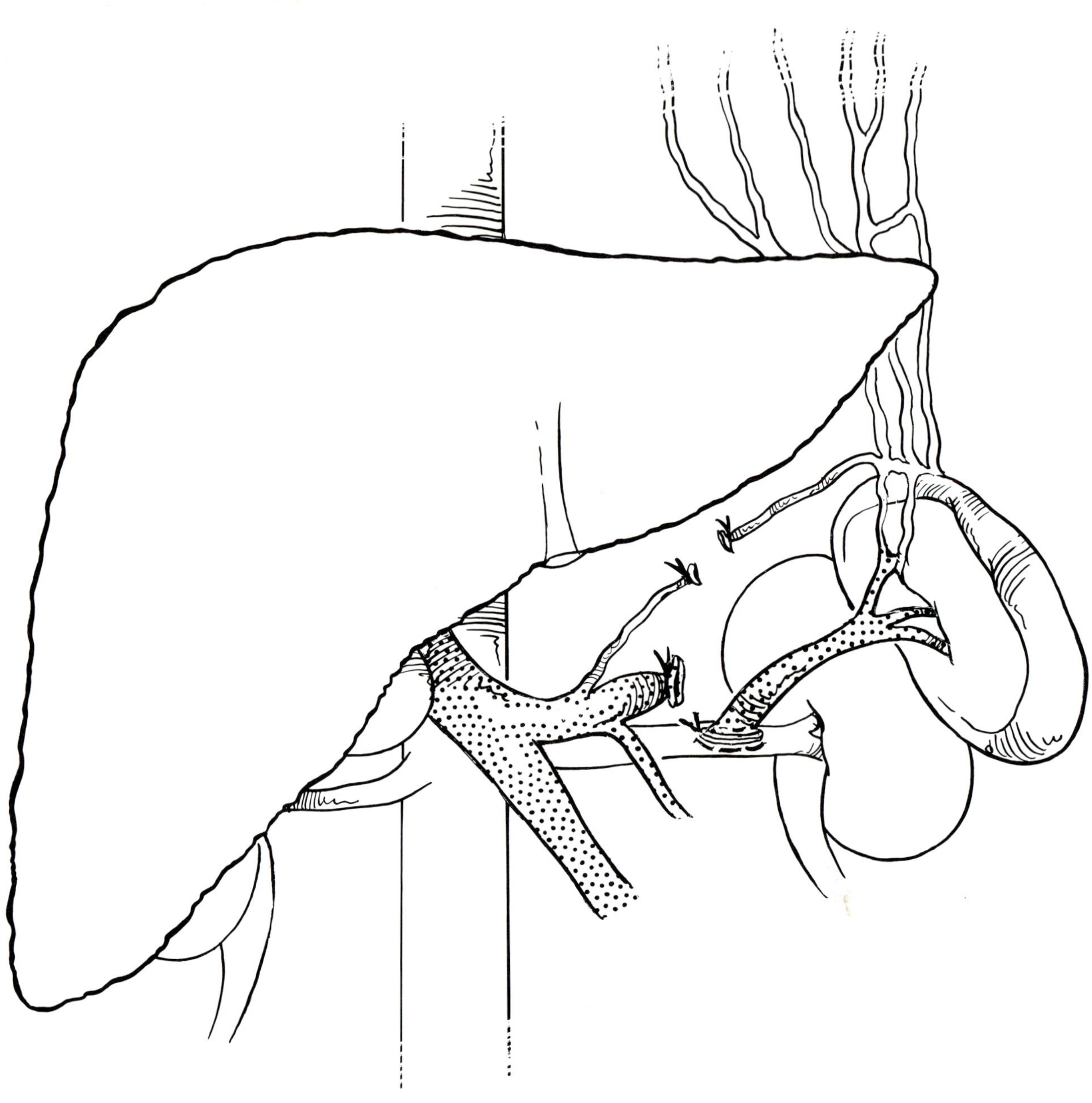

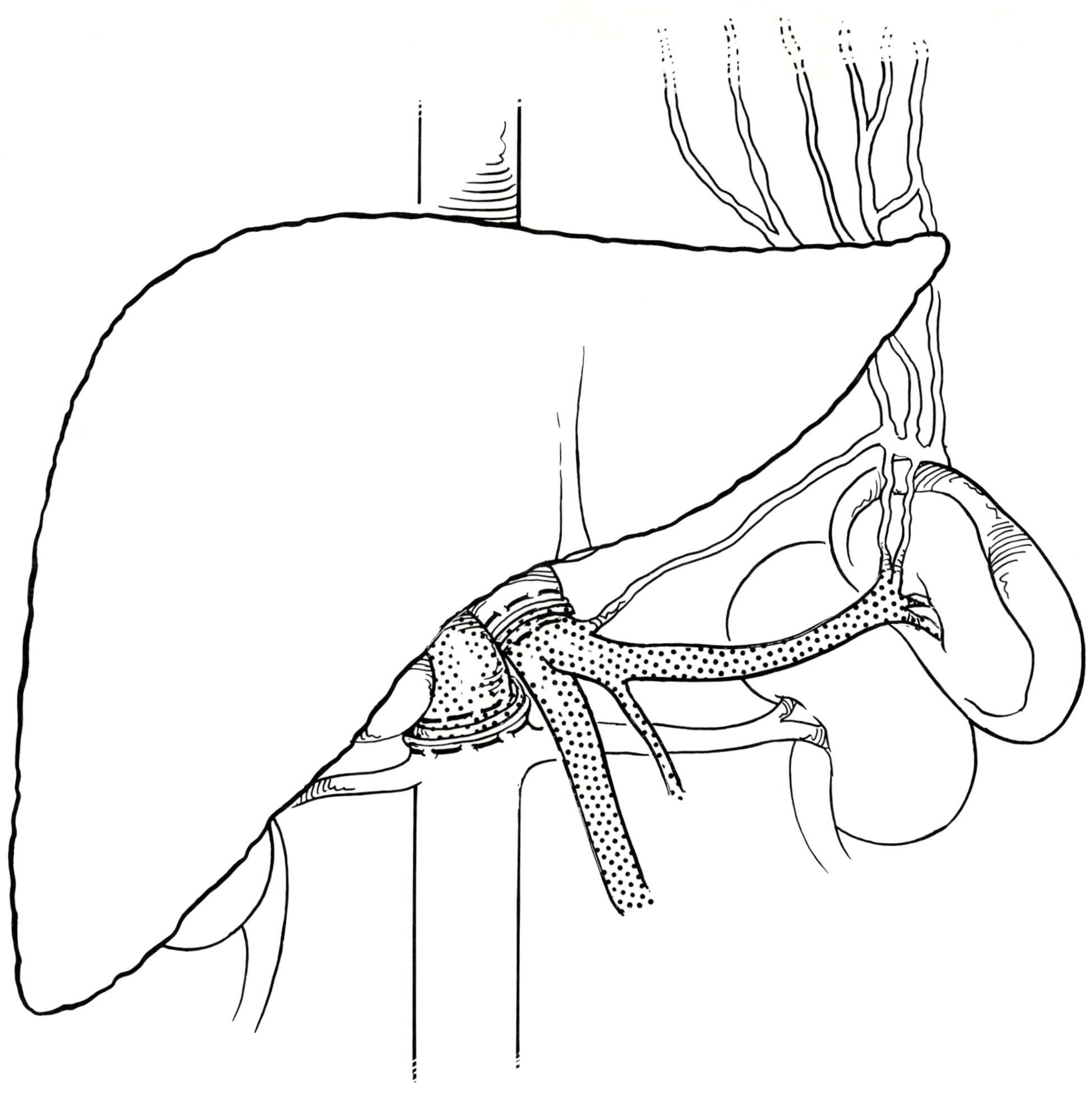

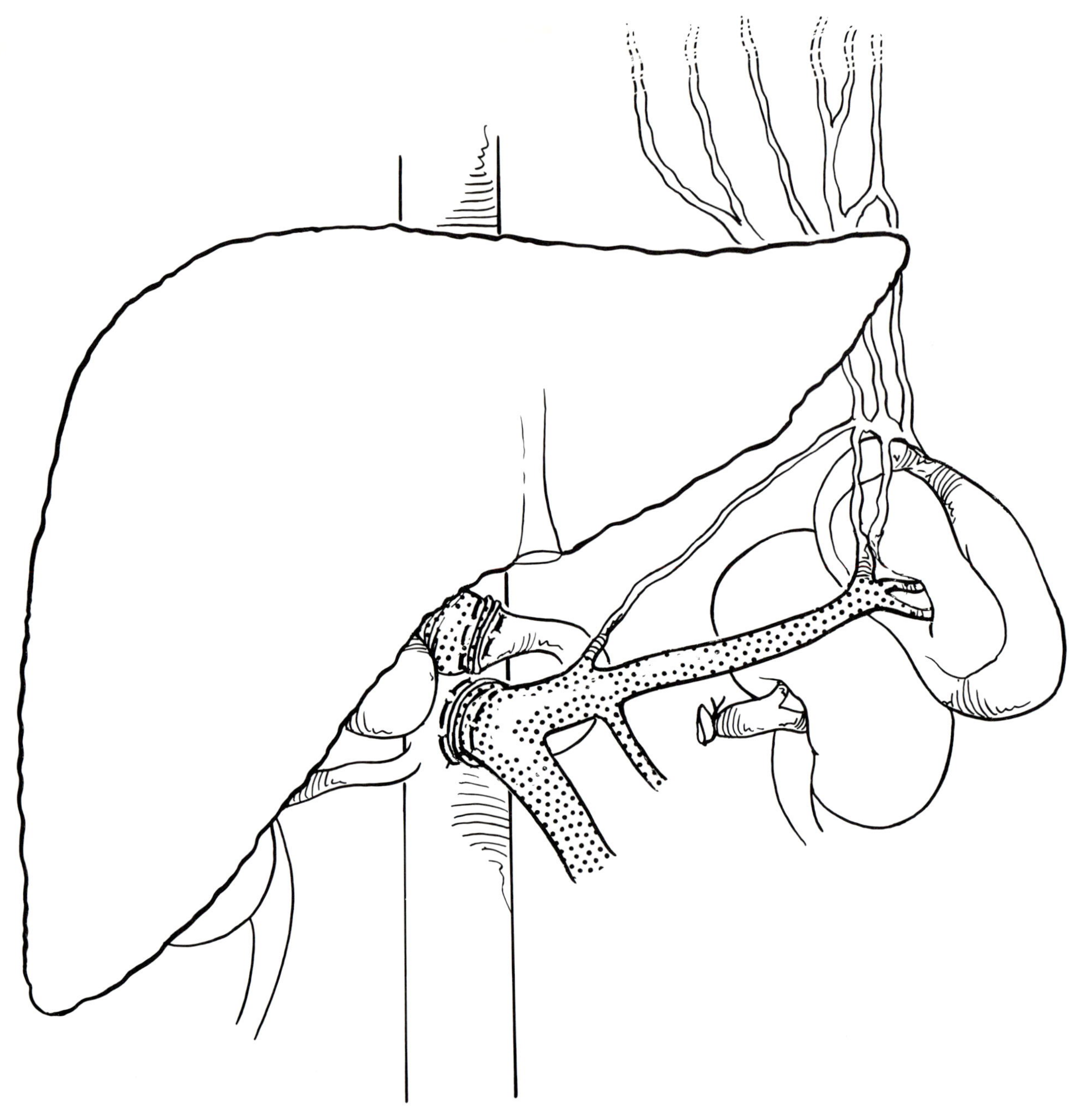

The most commonly employed is the direct end-to-side porta-caval shunt. Because of its relative simplicity and the effectiveness with which it controls bleeding from esophageal varices, it continues to be the operation of general use.

The patient is placed in a 30° oblique angle from the supine position with a break just below the right costal margin posteriorly. A long, lateral, subcostal incision is made, extending from the midline well out into the flank. This permits easy access to and exposure of the underside of the gastrohepatic ligament and to the infrahepatic vena cava. After the duodenum and hepatic flexure are mobilized, the vena cava is identified by retroperitoneal dissection. In obese patients with ascites a thick, edematous, fat layer is often present retroperitoneally; therefore, this maneuver is not always as simple as it appears. By palpation of the right kidney, the aorta, and vertebral column, one can determine the approximate location of the vena cava, and the retroperitoneal opening can be placed accordingly. Because of the extensive spontaneous collateral circulation that develops in portal hypertension, serious bleeding can occur at this point in the operative procedure. Rather than attempt to establish meticulous hemostasis with cautery or ligatures, the surgeon is urged to proceed rapidly to the vena cava, packing the edges of the retroperitoneum with dry gauze used for both retraction and temporary hemostasis. Once the vena cava is identified and the retroperitoneum opened longitudinally, a whipping stitch of chromic catgut can be carried down both leaves of the retroperitoneum, and some of the fatty tissue can be included behind it. This provides rapid, adequate, and satisfactory hemostasis, which might literally take hours if attempts were made to identify individually and to ligate or cauterize the multiple bleeding points (Fig. 5-18).

CAUTION

In dissection and mobilization of the inferior vena cava, the surgeon would be advised to avoid the lateral side of the vena cava above the entrance of the right renal vein because of the risk of damaging the right adrenal vein or the adrenal gland itself. It is also important to identify the first hepatic vein draining the caudate lobe of the liver. During mobilization of the inferior vena cava, the process is expedited by dividing this vein to prevent the possibility of damage and significant bleeding while placing appropriate partially occluding clamps on the vena cava.

Once this maneuver is completed, attention is directed to

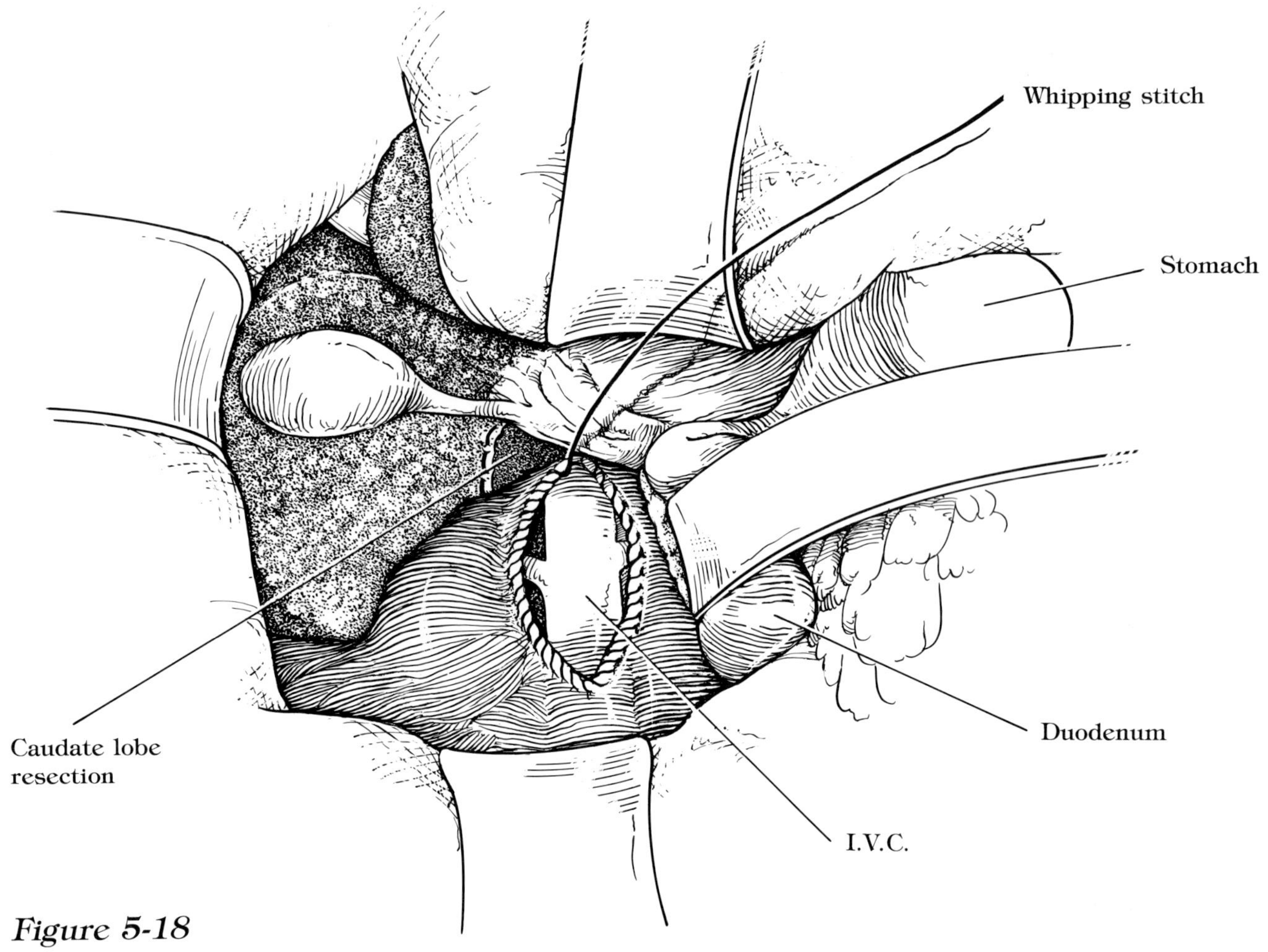

Figure 5-18

the underside of the gastrohepatic ligament where the peritoneal covering is incised posteriorly. Once the portal vein is initially identified and appears patent by palpation, it is carefully dissected out from its bed behind the common bile duct and the hepatic artery. If preoperative arteriography has not been carried out, the surgeon should ascertain that the hepatic artery lies in its normal position rather than assuming a relatively common anomalous course in which the right hepatic artery enters the liver behind the portal vein. Dissection of the portal vein is continued proximally and distally; this dissection is greatly facilitated by the maneuver shown in Figure 5-19 in which two pledgets held in Moynihan clamps are used to keep the gastrohepatic ligament on stretch and to retract the common bile duct from its position overlying the portal vein. Caution should be exercised relative to the location of the pyloric vein: It should be ligated carefully and divided if it appears in the course of the anatomic dissections; otherwise, extremely troublesome bleeding may occur since this vein retracts to an inaccessible position. Once the portal vein has been mobilized satisfactorily from the bifurcation at the hilus of the liver to the point where the portal vein passes behind the pancreas, the surgeon can then determine how much further mobilization of the vena cava is required.

The anatomic relationship of the portal vein to the vena cava is variable and depends on the distortion that has occurred from the process of regeneration in the cirrhotic liver. Frequently, the caudate lobe hypertrophies and presents a barrier between the vena cava and the portal vein; also, the angle at which the portal vein enters the liver relative to the course of the vena cava behind the liver varies considerably. Sometimes they may run nearly parallel courses, but on other occasions they may be almost at right angles to one another.

Further mobilization of the vena cava is then carried out, if necessary, to construct a portacaval shunt without tension; this may necessitate ligation of the lower one or two small hepatic veins and occasionally a wedge resection of a portion of intervening caudate lobe. Although it is important to clean the vena cava by sharp dissection, too vigorous and meticulous an approach to this leaves the cava without a tough adventitial covering, which of course makes it more likely to tear during the construction of the anastomosis.

At this point, splanchnic and hepatic pressure measurements can be taken, not only for general informational purposes, but to use as partial determinants of the type of shunt to be constructed. A medium Blalock clamp is then placed across the portal vein, as it disappears behind the pancreas, in such a way that it does not angulate the portal vein. Next a heavy ligature is placed as high as possible around the hepatic end of the portal vein, and a right-angle clamp is applied proximal to this. The portal vein is then divided with sharp scissors and a suture ligature is fixed around the right-angle clamp before it is removed (Fig. 5-20A).

At this point a Satinsky clamp is placed at an appropriate position on the anterior medial aspect of the vena cava. The exact location is determined by the angle at which the portal vein may be swung down to meet it. Since one of the real disasters of the operation may occur if the Satinsky clamp slips, it is advisable to tie heavy tape around the middle of the clamp so that it cannot be sprung inadvertently during construction of the shunt (see Fig. 5-20A).

CAUTION

If there is any question of the security of the Satinsky clamp on the vena cava, it may be advisable to place two adapted clamps in succession on the cava for greater security.

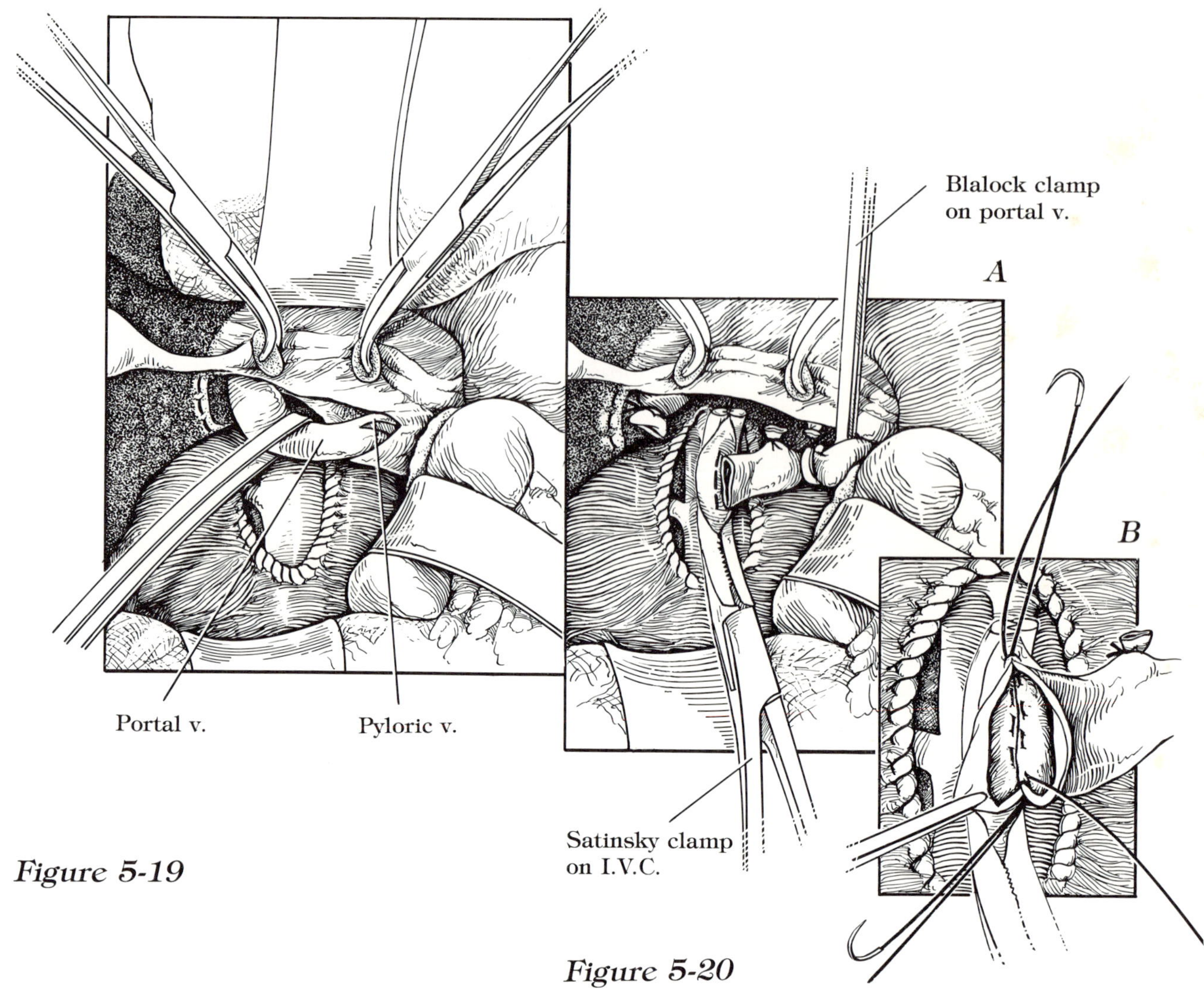

Figure 5-19

Figure 5-20

The size of the ellipse of the wall of the vena cava which is then to be removed for construction of the shunt remains a controversial subject. The high incidence of encephalopathy would indicate that as large a shunt as possible should not be constructed; on the other hand, one must be sure to achieve adequate decompression since the primary objective of the operation is to prevent further bleeding from esophageal varices. We believe the shunt should measure approximately 1.5 cm in diameter; an appropriate ellipse of cava is then removed with a Potts scissors and 5-0 Mersilene is used to construct the anastomosis. A holding suture is placed through the superior end of the two vessels, and an everting continuous mattress suture is carried out from above down. When the lower end of the projected anastomosis has been reached, another holding stitch is applied at the lower junction, and both these holding stitches are tied down securely. By gentle traction on the posterior suture line, the continuous suture can be snugged up and an everting approximation of the intima of the portal vein and vena cava accomplished. The two ends of the posterior row are then tied to the end sutures already placed as indicated (Fig. 5-20*B*).

An anterior row is then begun from above down, using the same technique of everting mattress stitch, which is, of course, easier in the anterior than the posterior row. Rather than continuing the anterior stitch throughout the entire length of the anterior portion of the anastomosis, one should interrupt it at a midpoint and start another continuous everting suture from below. When these are in proximity, the Blalock clamps should be released temporarily to flush out any potential clot that has formed.

A side-to-side portacaval shunt is constructed in a similar fashion, although it is more difficult because of the problem of approximating vessels which are still in continuity. Usually a right-angle Potts clamp is most satisfactory for occlusion of the upper end of the portal vein. A double-bladed Kimoto clamp can be used for this anastomosis if desired, although this has not proved as satisfactory as had been hoped. After appropriate clamps have been positioned, an open anastomosis is then constructed (Fig. 5-21). With a side-to-side shunt, it is usually too difficult to carry out an everting mattress suture on the posterior row, and an over-and-over continuous suture has proved to be satisfactory with no obvious incidence of thrombotic occlusion. If for any reason a side-to-side shunt is desirable and the anatomic configuration precludes the approximation of vessels, a *renoportal shunt* can be constructed by isolating a segment of left renal vein, dividing it, and swinging it up for an end-to-side approximation to the portal vein, thus establishing what functionally amounts to a side-to-side shunt.

CAUTION

A side-to-side anastomosis constructed with too much tension may lead to late stricture. If a renoportal shunt is not feasible or advisable, it is possible to put a short 16-mm knitted Dacron graft between the portal vein and the inferior vena cava. In a limited experience, this shorter graft has not been attended by postoperative thrombosis.

A mesocaval shunt is hemodynamically similar to a side-to-side anastomosis, although the experience of some surgeons has suggested that it may carry a lower incidence of encephalopathy. If this procedure is elected or is necessary because of an

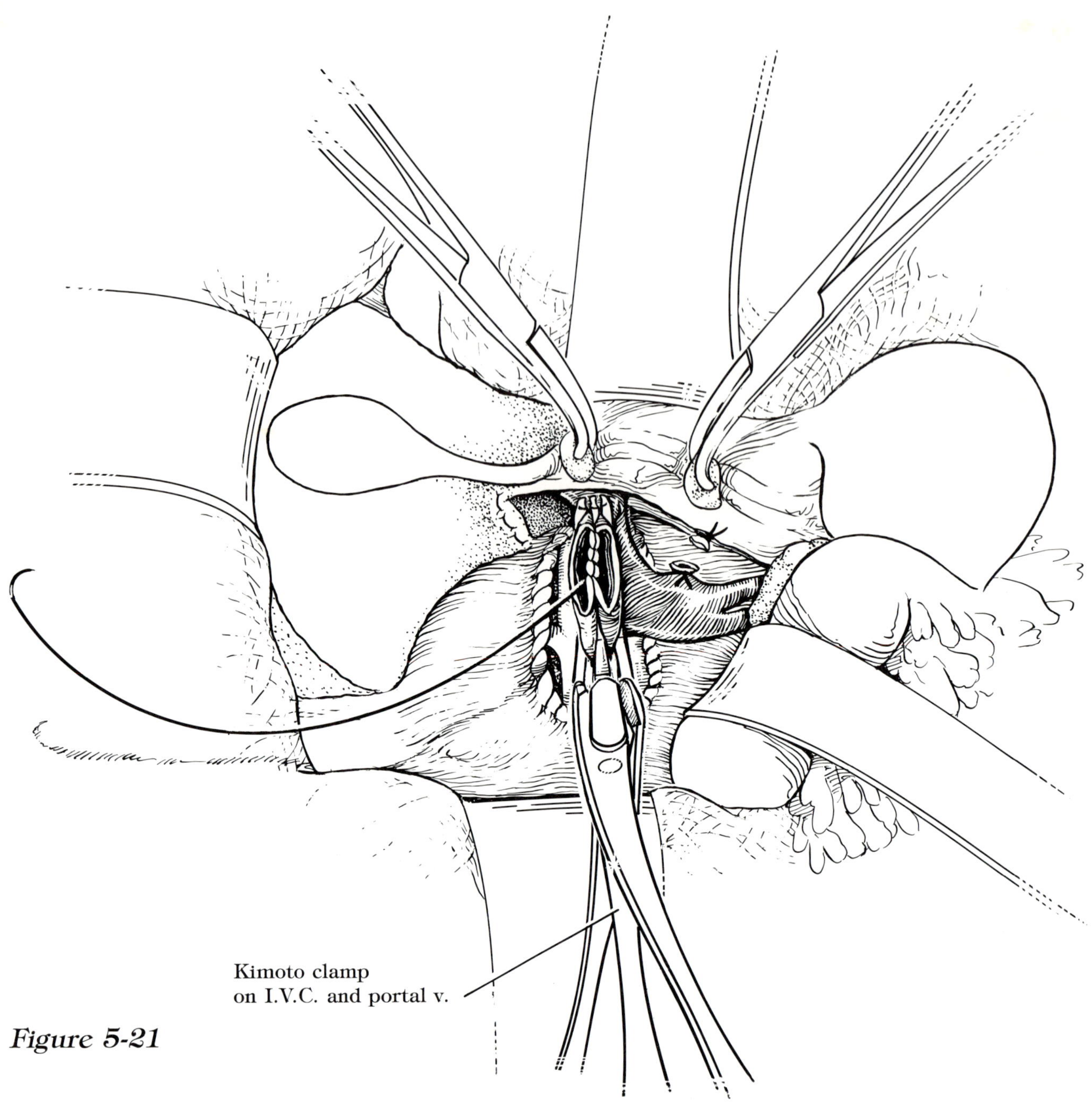

Figure 5-21

occluded portal vein, the operation may be completed by mobilizing the inferior vena cava, dividing the iliac veins, and anasto-
mosing the end of the divided right common iliac vein, which is
drawn through the right mesocolon to the side of the superior
mesenteric vein (Figs. 5-22, 5-23, *A, B*).

An interposed knitted Dacron graft, introduced by Drapanas,
will probably replace the type of mesocaval shunt shown in Figures 5-22, and 5-23, and described separately by Marion and by
Clatworthy. Many technical details are similar, but less dissection of the superior vena cava is required.

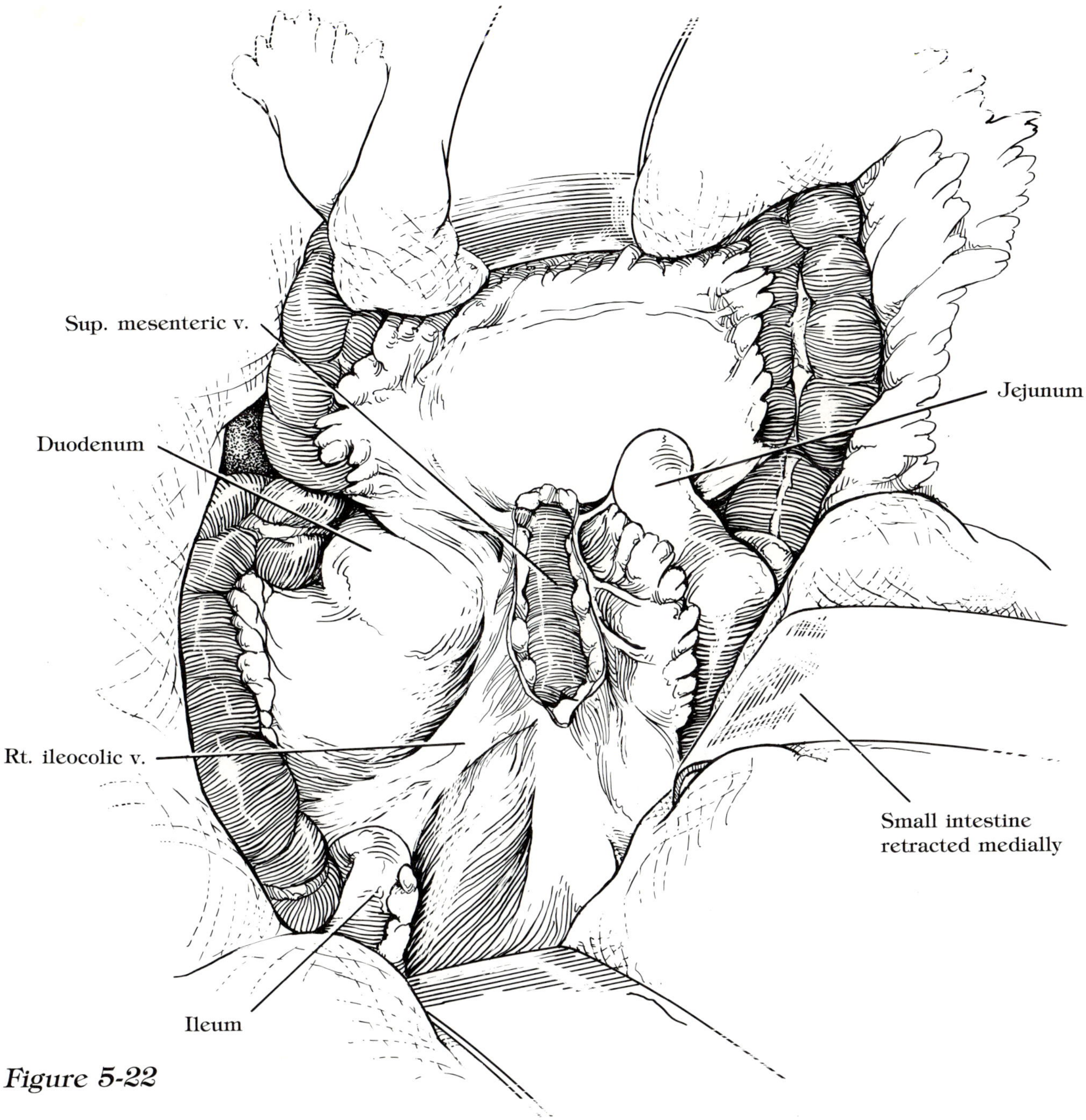

Figure 5-22

The mobilized superior mesenteric vein, with a sufficient number of tributaries ligated, is then occluded, usually with a small Satinsky or Kimoto clamp with one blade removed. A slit corresponding to the size of the graft (usually 16 mm) is made along the anterolateral aspect of the vein, and an anastomosis is constructed with 5-0 Mersilene. The graft is then drawn through the opening in the mesocolon and tailored to fall into a gentle curve below the duodenum and to approximate with slight tension to the anteromedial side of the vena cava. With a partially

occluding Satinsky clamp on the vena cava, an appropriate ellipse is removed, the graft is fixed in position by holding sutures
at each end, and the posterior row is completed with an over-
and-over stitch (Fig. 5-24A). The graft is preclotted (unless
this has been done prior to either anastomosis) and flushed
thoroughly before the anterior row is completed (Fig. 5-24B). It
is imperative that the graft be flushed and irrigated thoroughly
prior to placement of the final sutures of the anastomosis.

PROXIMAL
SPLENORENAL SHUNT

The proximal splenorenal shunt is best approached with the
patient in a semithoracotomy position. One uses an incision that
extends transversely across the abdomen to the ninth or tenth
rib; the rib is removed and the diaphragm is divided in the line
of the incision. The spleen is then mobilized by dividing successively the lienocolic ligaments, the retroperitoneal attachments, and the lienophrenic and lienogastric ligaments and vessels. This dissection is considerably more difficult because of

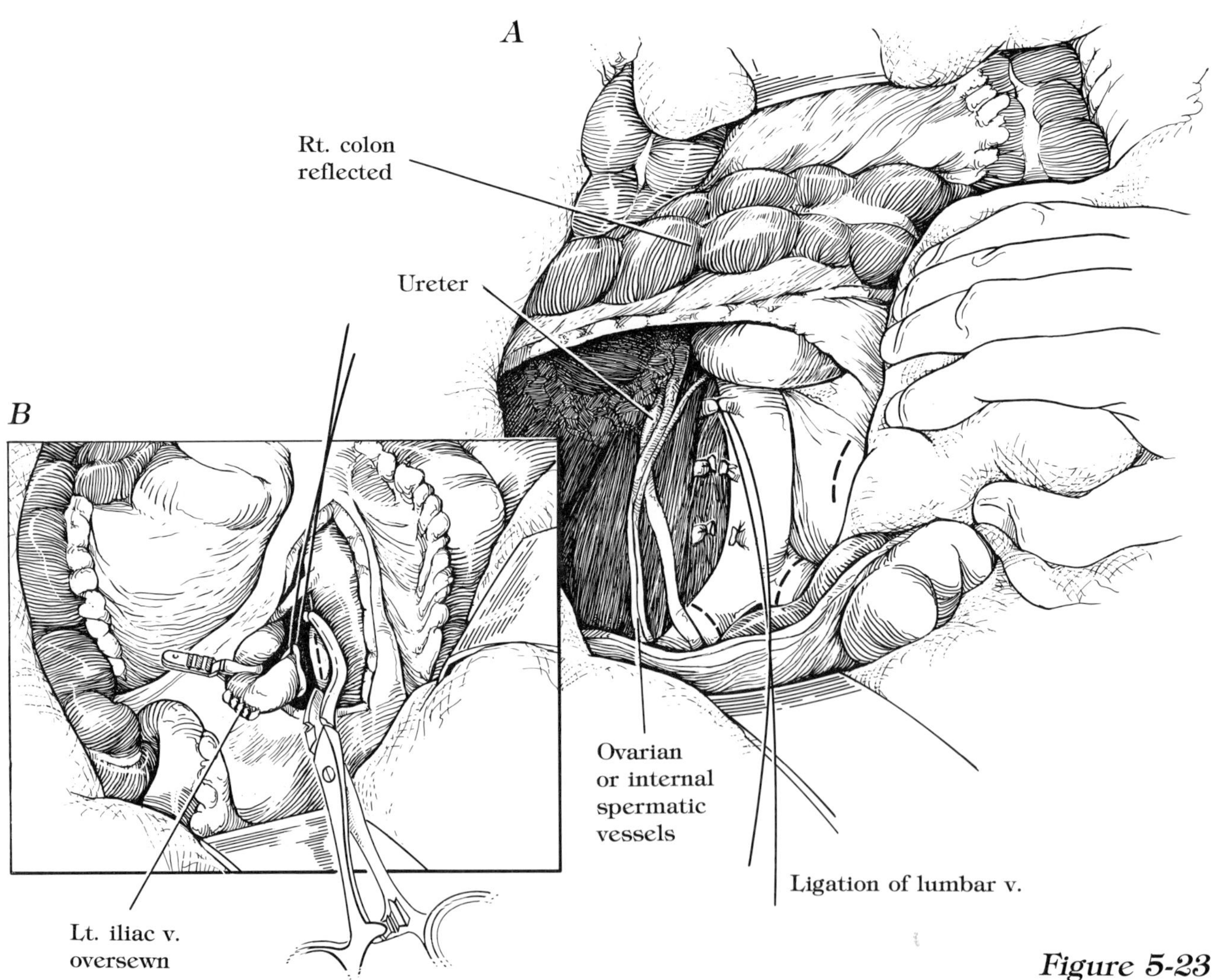

Figure 5-23

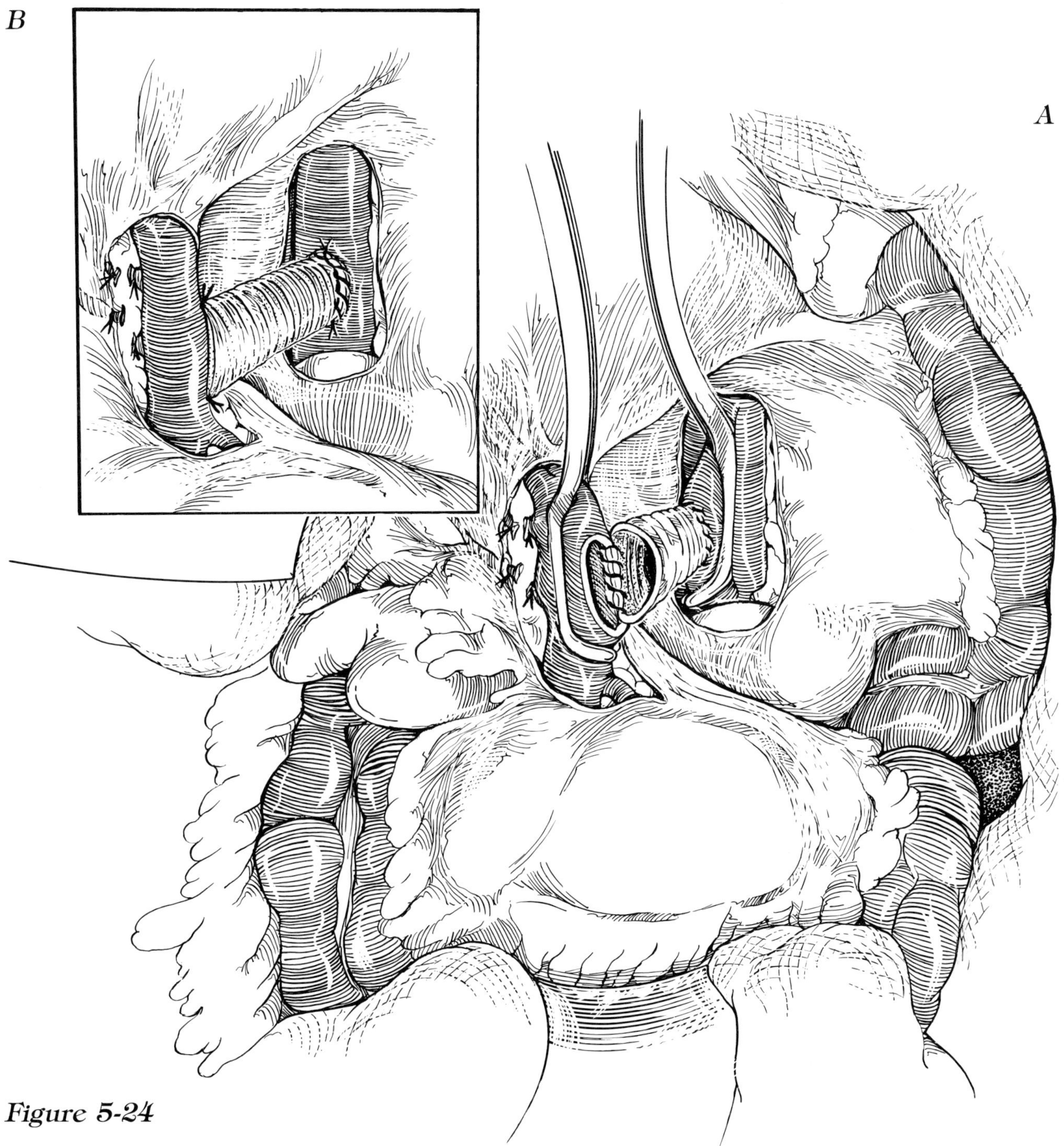

Figure 5-24

the extreme vascularity in portal hypertension, so frequently a
whipping stitch is needed to achieve retroperitoneal hemostasis
as the spleen is mobilized anteriorly. After splenic pulp pressure has been measured, the splenic artery is identified,
clamped, cut, and ligated. Dissection is then begun on the hilum
of the spleen to identify the major right and left bifurcations of

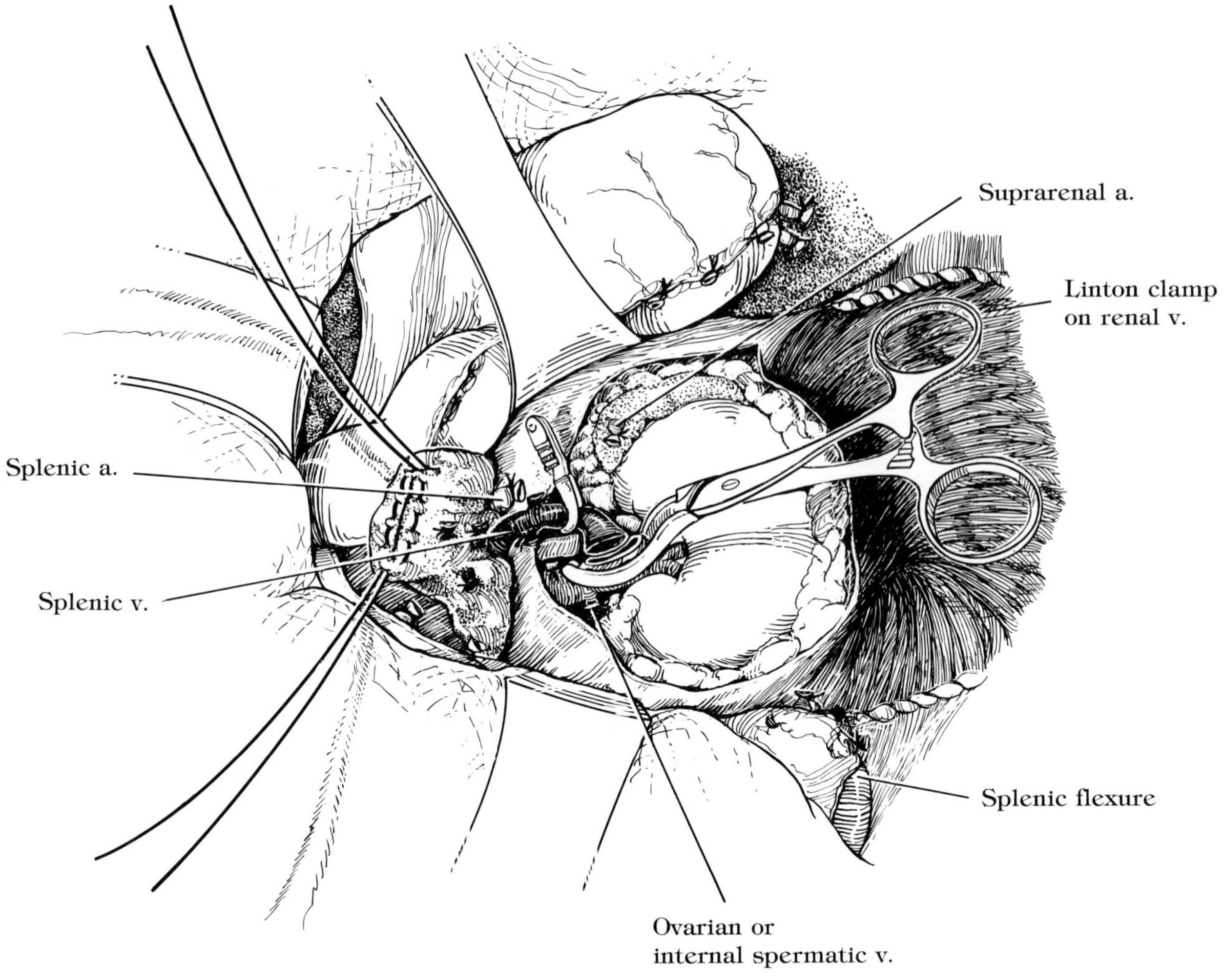

Figure 5-25

the splenic vein. These are both ligated, divided, and held and
the spleen is removed. Attention is then directed to the retroperitoneal area in the hilum of the left kidney where the major
left renal vein and artery can be identified (Fig. 5-25). Anomalies of the renal circulation are relatively common; except for
bifid vessels, the only one that is pertinent to this operation is
the passage of an inferior renal artery branch to the lower pole
of the kidney, thus crossing the renal vein and interfering with
the positioning of the anastomosis. This inferior pole branch
may be ligated and divided to achieve adequate access to the
splenic vein; the occasional renal infarct that results seems to
cause no serious damage. In order to obtain satisfactory mobilization of the renal vein, it is usually necessary to divide the spermatic (or ovarian) vein as it enters from below. A smaller adrenal vein entering superiorly should also be ligated to achieve a
free and mobile renal vein for construction of the shunt.

Once the renal vein is mobilized, one can ascertain whether a sufficient length of splenic vein has been dissected free to swing down to the renal vein in a gently curving arc without tension. Because of anatomic variations, it is sometimes necessary to resect a portion of the tail of the pancreas in such a way that a fishmouth incision permits easy closure of the transected tail of the pancreas. A bulldog clamp is placed across the splenic vein and the ligated end is cut with a Potts scissors at an angle that permits it to lie easily against the anterosuperior surface of the renal vein. A segment of the anterior wall of the renal vein is then drawn up into a partially occluding Linton clamp or a small Kimoto clamp, and an ellipse excised sufficient to match the transected end of the splenic vein. Anastomosis is carried out with an everting, continuous, mattress suture in a fashion similar to that described for the anastomosis of the end of the portal vein to the vena cava (see Fig. 5-25). After liver biopsy and postoperative measurements of splenic vein pressure, the abdomen and chest are closed by the usual method, as described previously. The chest cavity is drained through the tenth or eleventh interspace; the left subphrenic area is not drained unless the tail of the pancreas has been resected.

This particular procedure for control of bleeding from esophagogastric varices was introduced in 1967 by Dr. W. Dean Warren with the objective of providing selective decompression of the esophagogastric varices without diminishing portal flow to the liver. It is not in the province of an atlas to discuss the pathophysiology of disease processes nor to outline the conditions under which various procedures might be applicable, but certainly this particular type of shunt is broadly utilized in the control of bleeding secondary to portal hypertension.

Reference has already been made to the appropriateness of this particular shunt under some circumstances, particularly for the nonalcoholic patient with presinusoidal block due to hepatic fibrosis, schistosomiasis, or some types of posthepatic cirrhosis. Beyond this generalization, a review of the existing controversy of the literature is beyond the scope of an atlas for technical procedures. Certainly in the absence of intractable ascites or a severe degree of postsinusoidal block with retrograde portal flow, this type of shunt provides an acceptable alternative to a total shunt.

Several approaches have been suggested for constructing a distal splenorenal shunt. In order to construct this particular type of shunt, one must 1) expose the splenic vein lying in a groove in the posterior-superior aspect of the pancreas, 2) expose the left renal vein to an extent satisfactory for an anastomosis and, in addition, 3) provide access to the coronary vein and other tributaries leading from the portal circulation along the lesser curvature of the stomach. In the presence of portal hypertension, these tributaries provide a reverse flow that congests the esophagogastric area. One approach has been to enter the retrogastric area through the lesser omental sac above the transverse mesocolon, and another has been to approach this area beneath the transverse mesocolon. We have explored various approaches to this particular surgical problem and believe that a third approach provides maximum access and exposure: a long, lateral, left subcostal incision extending well into the flank with a chevron extension superiorly dividing the right rectus muscle. The splenic flexure is then mobilized by dividing the retroperitoneal attachments and the lienocolic ligaments which, in the presence of portal hypertension, carry a significant number of large collateral channels.

After mobilization of the splenic flexure, the entire left colon and transverse colon are drawn toward the right side of the abdomen. This exposes the whole anatomic area, which includes the retroperitoneal surface of the pancreas, the adrenal gland, left kidney and, at the medial border of the dissection, the inferior mesenteric vein. Once this has been accomplished, the pancreas and spleen can be rotated in such a fashion that the splenic artery and veins are exposed, lying in the posterior and superior aspects of the pancreas. In the absence of preexisting chronic pancreatitis, the splenic vein can be dissected from its bed in the pancreas with relative ease provided careful attention is paid to the multiple tributaries to the superior aspect of the vein which enter the bed of the pancreas. These can be controlled by dura clips or by careful ligation with fine silk sutures. The splenic vein should be dissected to its junction with the superior mesenteric vein, at which point it is divided. The segment of splenic vein toward the portal vein is controlled with a double suture ligature to prevent any disastrous hemorrhage from the medial portion of the vessel.

When the splenic vein has been satisfactorily mobilized as far as the tail of the pancreas and the hilum of the spleen, attention is directed toward the renal vein as it emerges from the hilum of the kidney. When an adequate segment of the renal vein is exposed, a partially occluding clamp is applied and the splenic vein, which had been temporarily occluded with a bulldog clamp, is brought down for an end-to-side anastomosis to the renal vein. This is carried out with a continuous 5-0 Mersilene suture, and the splenic vein is flushed just prior to final completion of the anastomosis to be certain that clotting has not occurred during the period of anastomosis. If necessary, the inferior mesenteric vein can be interrupted to provide further length of the splenic vein. With the completion of the anastomosis, attention is then directed to the retrogastric area where the coronary vein can be identified at its junction with the portal vein, dissected free, and doubly ligated. Since there are multiple tributaries along the lesser curvature of the stomach, in ad-

Figure 5-26
Divided suprarenal v.
Divided coronary v.
Divided splenic v.
Sup. mesenteric v. and a.
Transverse colon
Short gastric v.
Splenic v.
Lt. gastroepiploic v.
Divided gastrocolic ligament
Divided lienocolic ligament
Opened ant. renal fascia
Perirenal fat
Divided inf. mesenteric v.
Divided gonadal v.
Splenic flexure
Divided lienocolic ligament
Avascular dissection of peritoneal reflection
Lt. colic a. ascending branch

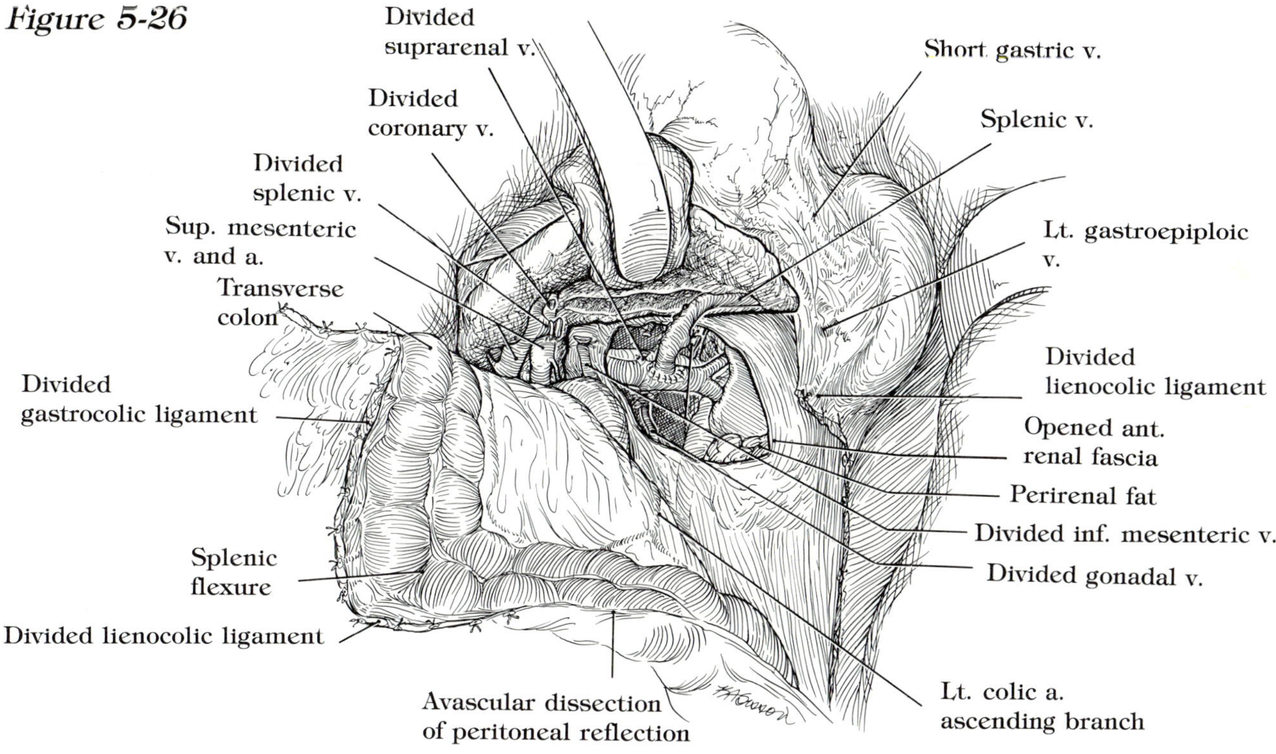

Figure 5-27
Coronary v.
Short gastric v.
Rt. gastric v.
Lt. gastroepiploic v.
Rt. gastroepiploic v.

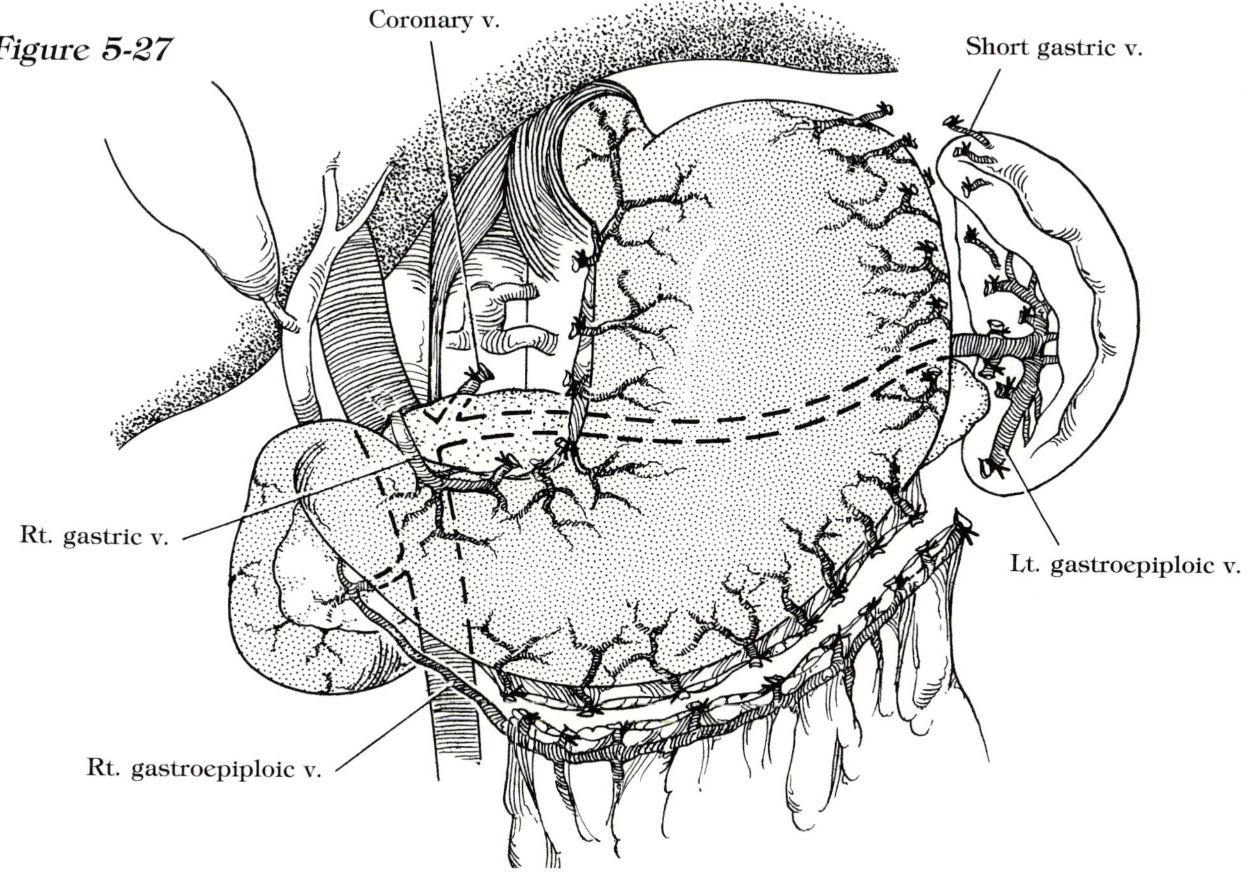

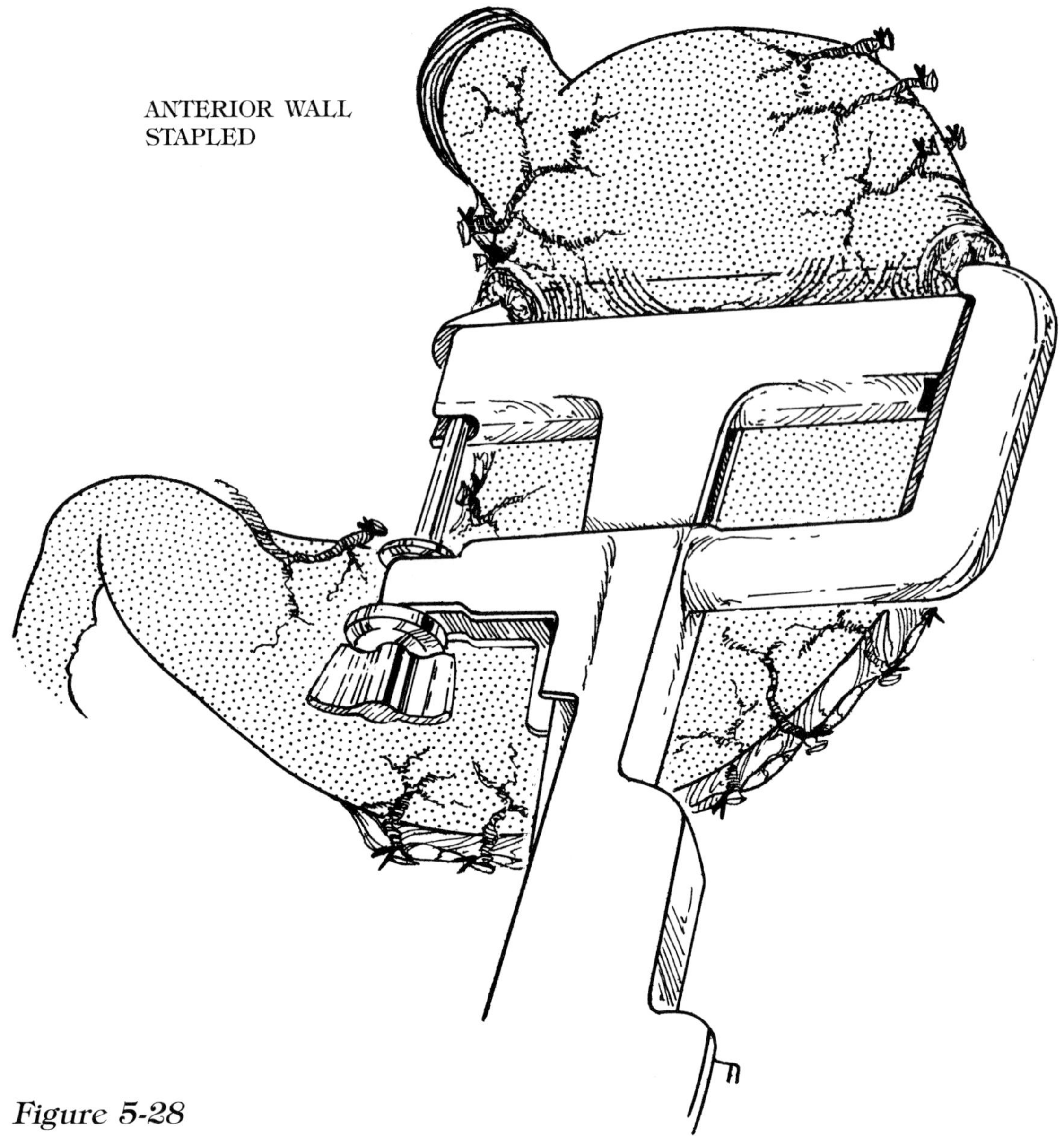

Figure 5-28

dition to the main coronary or left gastric vein, this area should be dissected cleanly to interrupt added collateral channels that may have developed and that feed the esophagogastric area. At the conclusion of the procedure, the transverse colon, the splenic flexure, and the left colon are replaced in their normal positions and the incision is closed (Fig. 5-26).

Portal-Azygous Disconnection Of the various nonshunting procedures that have been suggested for the control of bleeding from esophagogastric varices, we have used the variant to be described 1) in emergency situations, where a portal-systemic shunt was not considered appropriate, and 2) under circumstances of extrahepatic block, where

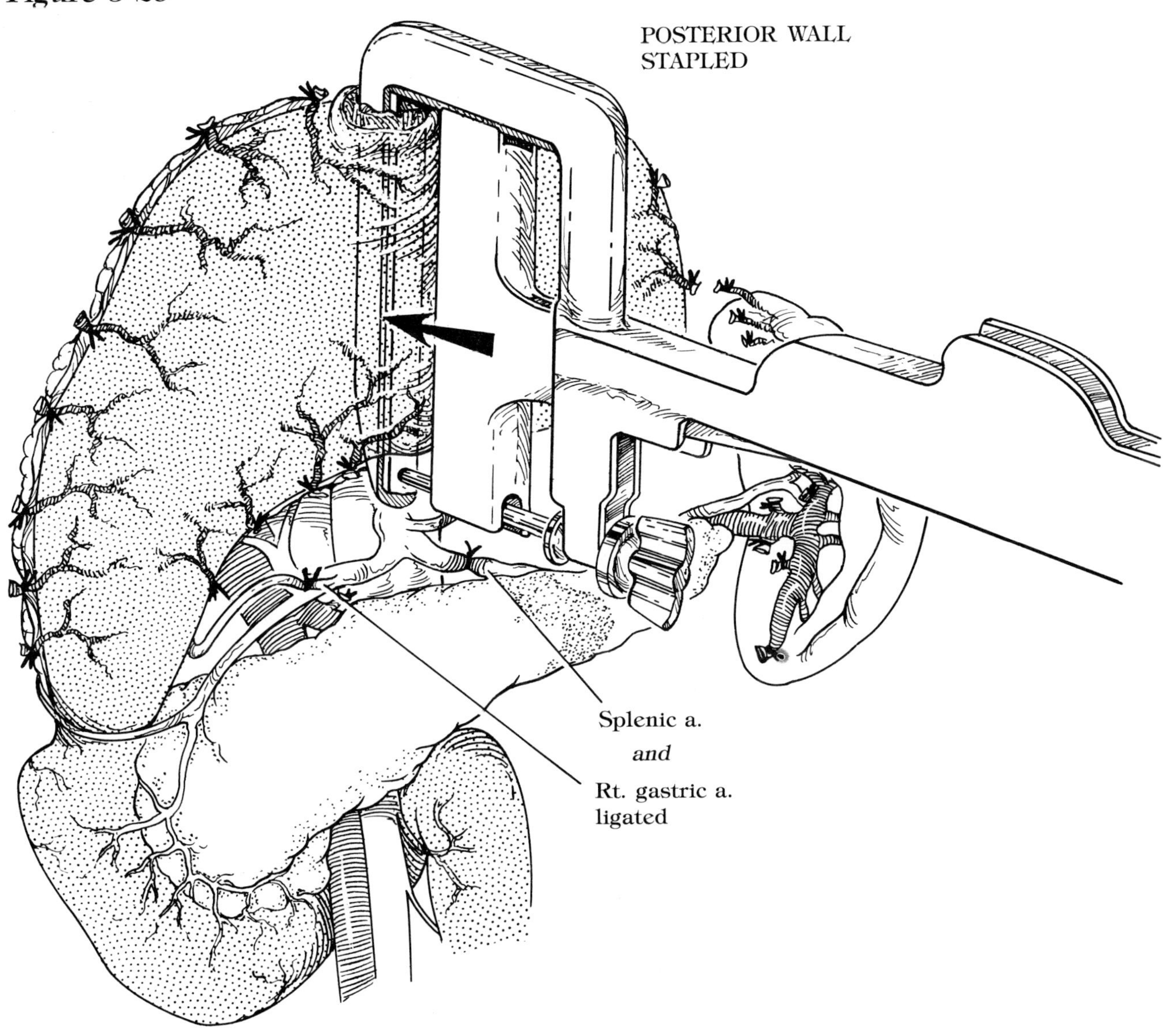

no major vessels in the splanchnic or splenic circulations were patent.

The peritoneal cavity is entered through an upper-abdominal midline incision, and the branches of the gastroepiploic circulation are individually ligated and divided along the greater curvature of the stomach. Dissection is continued to the fundus of the stomach and all the vasa brevia are interrupted. With the stomach thus mobilized and elevated, the left and right gastric and splenic arteries and the coronary and right gastric veins are identified and interrupted. Further dissection along the lesser curvature from the pylorus to the esophagus permits interruption of all other collateral channels leading from the portal circulation to the esophagogastric area (Fig. 5-27).

Small gastrotomies are made on the greater and lesser curvatures, and the TA-90 instrument is introduced to place a double row of staples in the wall in order to interrupt intramural flow (Fig. 5-28). The stapler is withdrawn, the stomach is reflected upward, and the stapler is reintroduced for placement of a similar row in the posterior wall (Fig. 5-29). The small gastrotomy openings and the incision are closed. The completed disconnection and stapling are shown in Figure 5-30.

Figure 5-30

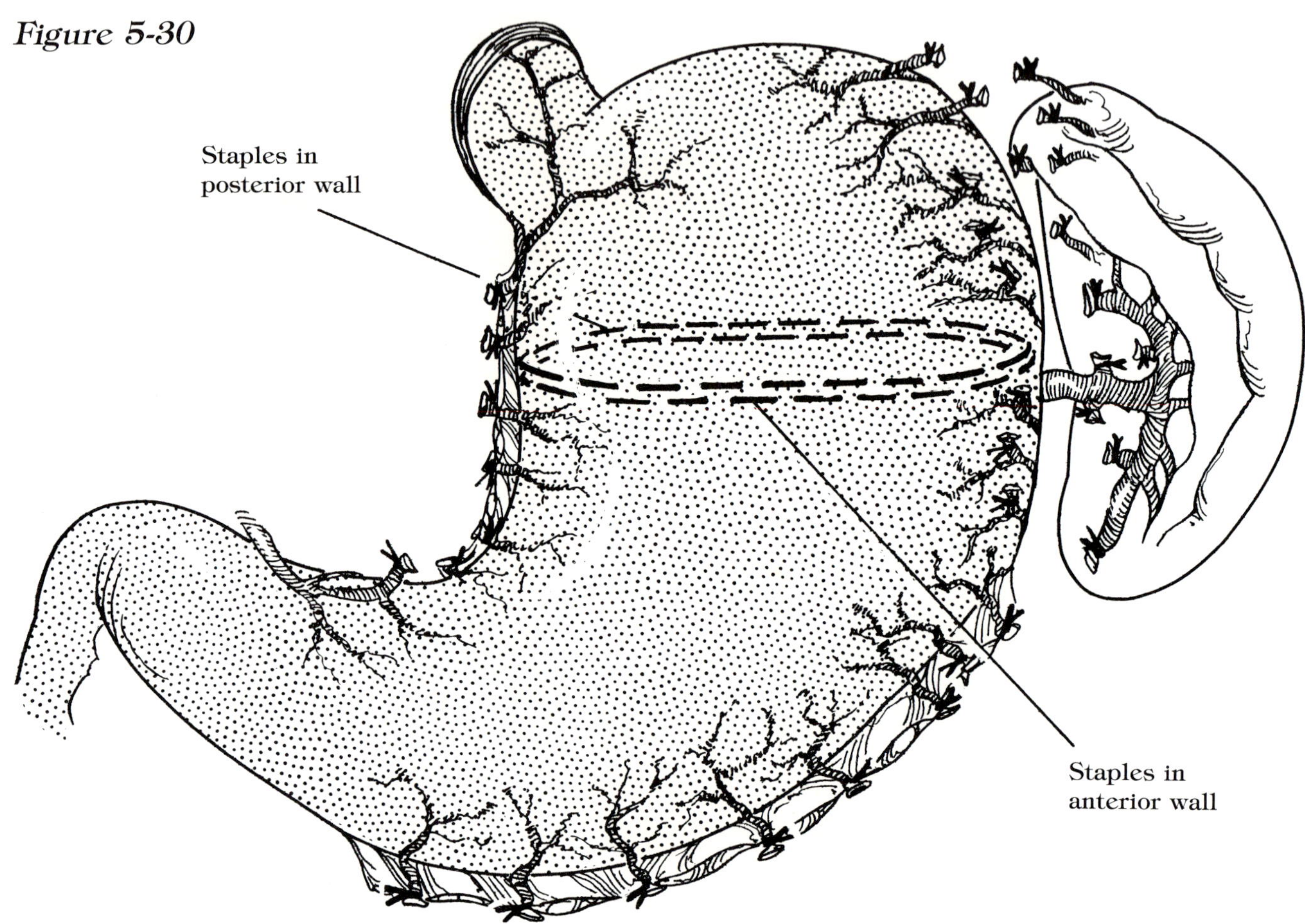

CHAPTER SIX

ENDOCRINE SYSTEM

Surgical removal of one or both adrenal glands is indicated either because of a primary tumor or severe bilateral hyperplasia or, if hormonal ablation is indicated, for the management of widespread carcinoma of the breast. The choice of the anterior or the posterior approach is more related to the experience and the preference of the individual surgeon. Some generalizations can be made as to choice of approach, however. 1) An anterior approach is probably preferable in most types of tumor because of size and the possibility of extension beyond the confines of the adrenal gland, in which case the anterior approach may provide a better opportunity for adequate dissection. 2) If bilateral oophorectomy is indicated at the time of bilateral adrenalectomy, it is simpler to extend the incision downward and remove the ovaries than to turn the patient and perform a separate laparotomy.

With modern radiologic techniques, localization of tumor preoperatively should be quite accurate. Postoperative metabolic support does not present a serious problem if the patient is carefully instructed relative to alteration of maintenance dosage in the event of stress, trauma, or infection.

If the anterior approach is selected, a curved upper abdominal incision is made with an extension downward for exposure of the ovaries (Fig. 6-1). After the peritoneal cavity is entered, the hepatorenal ligament and the peritoneal reflection off the duodenum and right colon are divided in order to mobilize the liver

Adrenalectomy

ANTERIOR APPROACH

Figure 6-1
Transabdominal
Midline extension

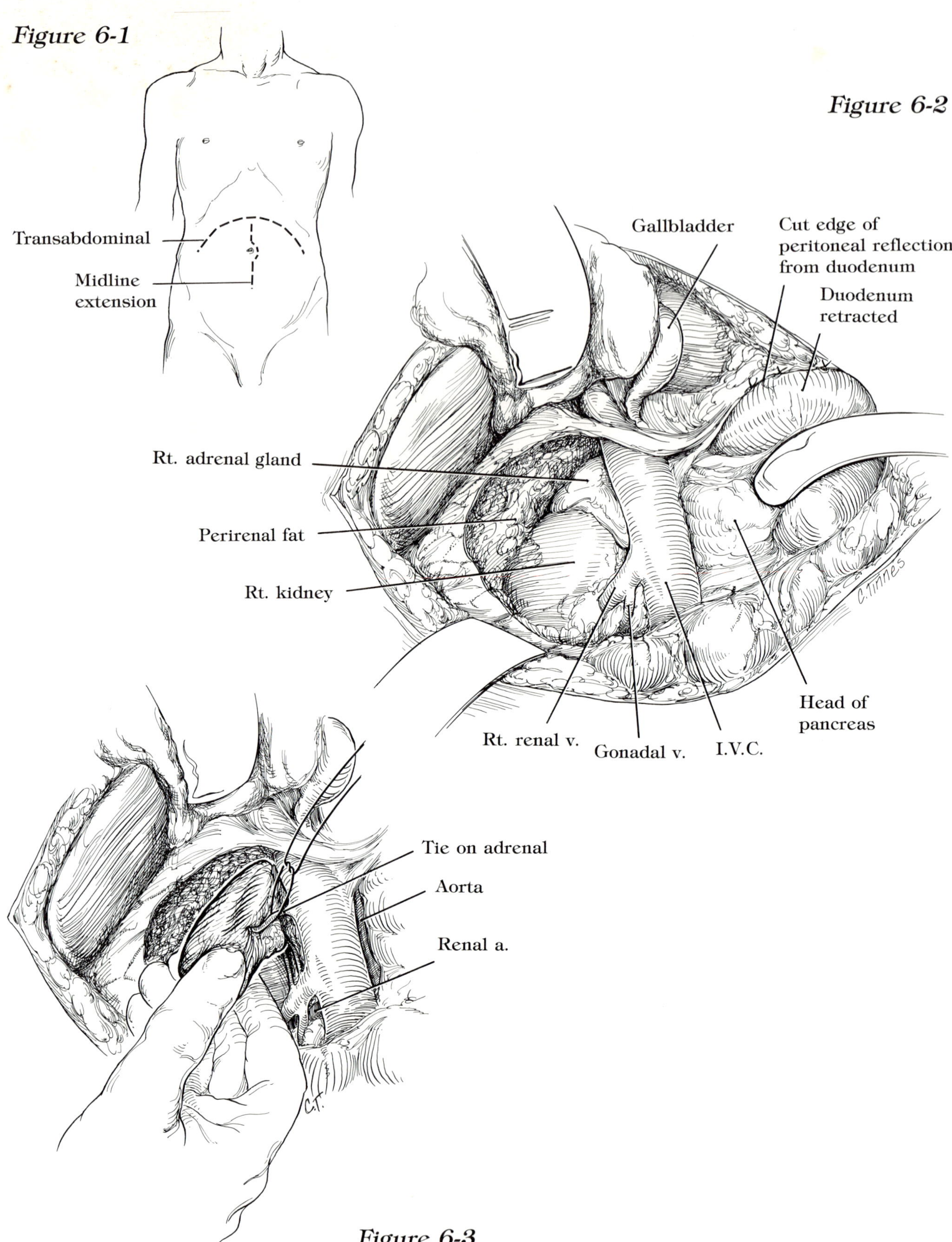
Figure 6-2
Gallbladder
Cut edge of peritoneal reflection from duodenum
Duodenum retracted
Rt. adrenal gland
Perirenal fat
Rt. kidney
Rt. renal v.
Gonadal v.
I.V.C.
Head of pancreas
C. Innes
Tie on adrenal
Aorta
Renal a.
C.I.
Figure 6-3

upward, the duodenum medially, and the hepatic flexure downward. When the inferior vena cava and the right renal vein have been identified, the right adrenal gland should then be seen lying above the renal vein and in close proximity to the vena cava (Fig. 6-2). The major blood supply to the adrenal enters from the medial and inferior sides of the gland and, therefore, dissection is begun by manual retraction of the kidney downward and by sharp and blunt dissection of the gland on its lateral aspect. Once the adrenal gland is dissected free laterally with clips on the few small venous tributaries that may leave the gland at this point, the adrenal may be grasped between thumb and forefinger or drawn down gently with a lightly applied Babcock clamp (the gland is friable, and rough instrumentation may cause fragmentation). This exposes the superior pole where there are many vessels that must be clipped or ligated. Dissection can then proceed between the adrenal gland and the vena cava to identify and ligate the main adrenal vein feeding directly into the vena cava (Fig. 6-3). Often, one or more veins may drain into the right renal vein. In order to avoid annoying hemorrhage, careful and somewhat tedious dissection is necessary since both the gland and its tributaries are fragile and tear easily. When the right adrenalectomy is completed, attention is then directed to the left side where the lesser sac is entered above the transverse colon through the gastrocolic omentum. The splenic flexure of the colon is mobilized downward by dividing the lienocolic ligament and the lateral reflections of the peritoneum. The body and tail of the pancreas should then be visible and the left kidney palpable in the retroperitoneal area, which is now exposed for further dissection (Fig. 6-4). Using these landmarks and with general retraction of the body and tail of the pancreas superiorly, the surgeon should identify the left adrenal vein via sharp and blunt dissection. Again, there are multiple small arterial and venous channels, but the main left adrenal vein courses inferiorly to enter the left renal vein. Because of its longer course, it is more easily dissected and ligated than on the right, and the whole procedure is simpler and less fraught with technical problems (Fig. 6-5).

Bilateral oophorectomy: Since the general surgeon is often involved with general hormonal ablation, the addition of bilateral oophorectomy requires the described extension downward from a curved upper-abdominal incision. With sufficient retraction on this short downward extension and with the patient in Trendelenburg's position, the ovaries can be separately visualized. Using a Babcock clamp with gentle traction, one can place suture ligatures through the infundibulopelvic and tubo-ovarian ligaments, and remove the right and left ovaries (Fig. 6-6).

Since the position of the patient is important in this procedure, it will be described in detail. The patient is placed prone on the

Stomach retracted
Spleen
Divided splenocolic ligament
Divided peritoneal reflection
Gastrocolic ligament retracted, opening lesser omental sac
Cut edge of gastrocolic ligament
Pancreas
Incision of post. parietal peritoneum
Pancreas
Lt. renal v.
Lt. adrenal v.

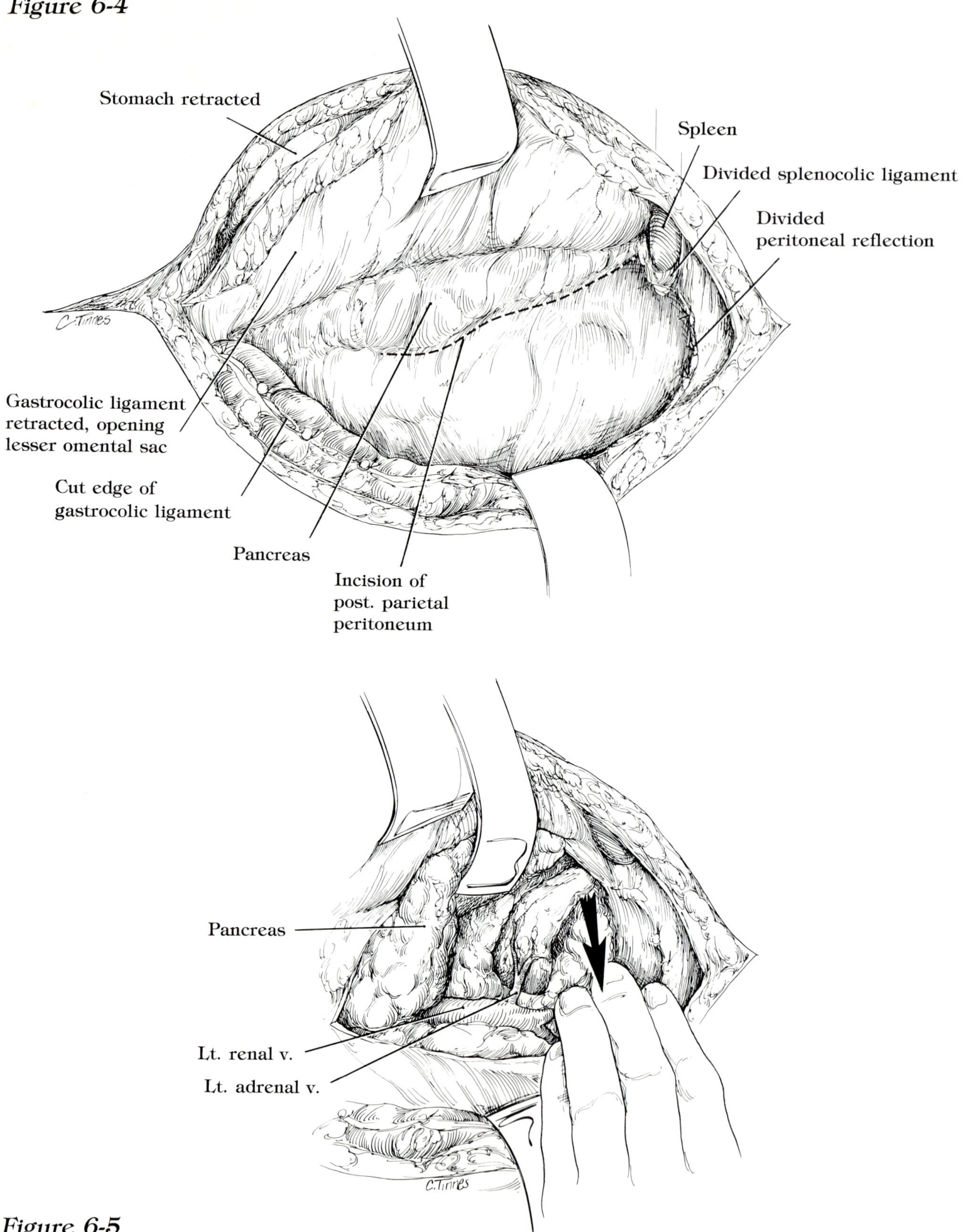

Figure 6-5

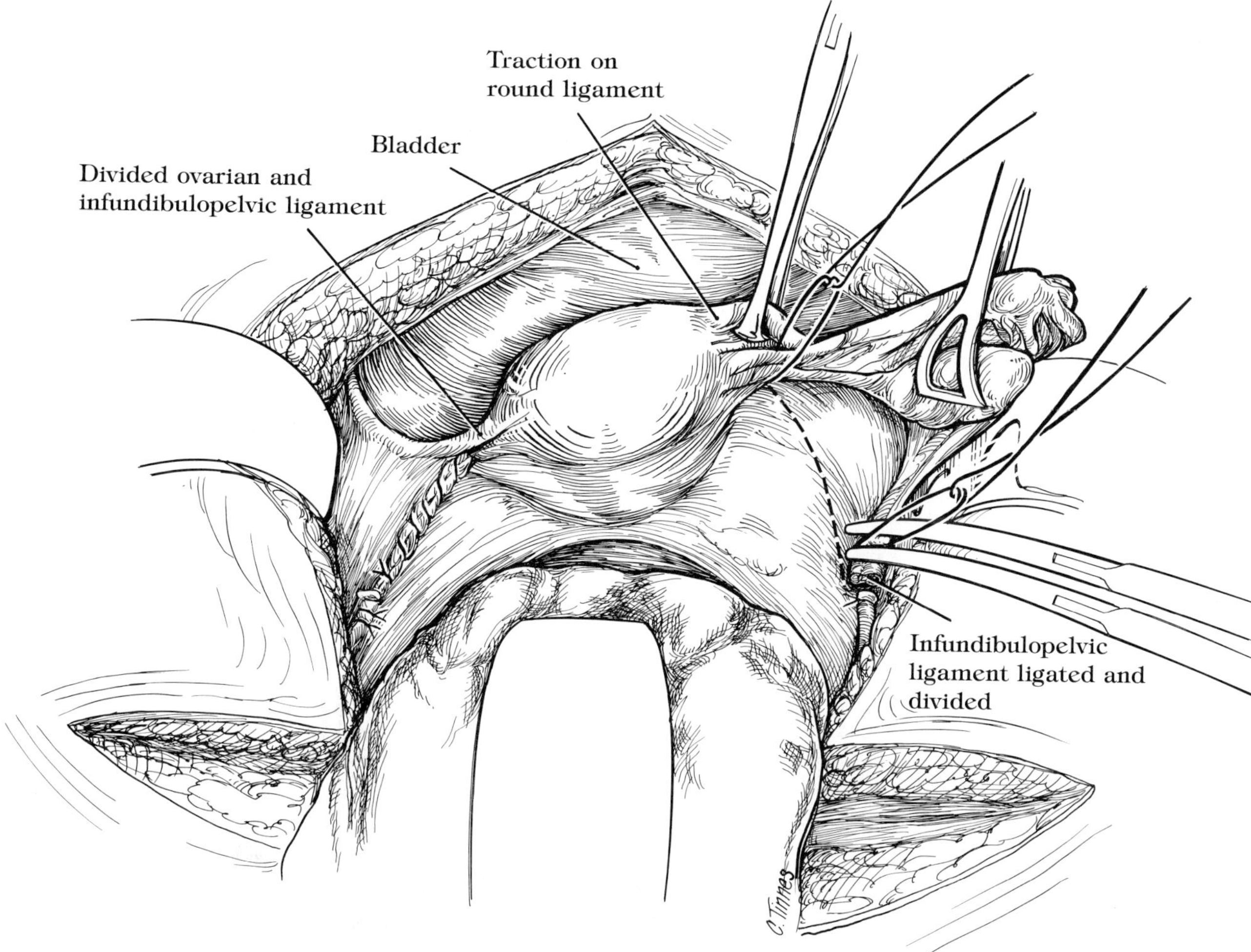

Figure 6-6

operating table, which is then flexed at waist level, thus lowering the feet to about 45°. The level portion of the operating table is then built up to about 4 inches in thickness by hard cushions or blanket rolls placed under the upper chest and pelvis, leaving the abdomen sufficient free space to permit easy respiration (Fig. 6-7). The patient's arms can be placed on arm boards or, in older patients, kept down at the side. The flexion at the hip flattens the lumbar curve and eliminates normal lordosis, which improves the exposure of the adrenal fossa.

Adrenalectomy is normally performed on the right side first since it is more difficult technically than on the left side. The paravertebral portion of the incision is made 4 finger breadths lateral to the spinous processes from a point just below the level of the angle of the scapula (usually about the level of the spinous process of T6). It is carried in a caudal direction until it reaches the soft area of the lumbar fossa where it is turned laterally and obliquely at about a 60° angle with the vertical limb, as far out

Figure 6-7

Trapezius divided
Latissimus dorsi
divided
Erector spinae
Lumbodorsal
fascia
divided
Transversalis
fascia
divided
Gerota's
fascia

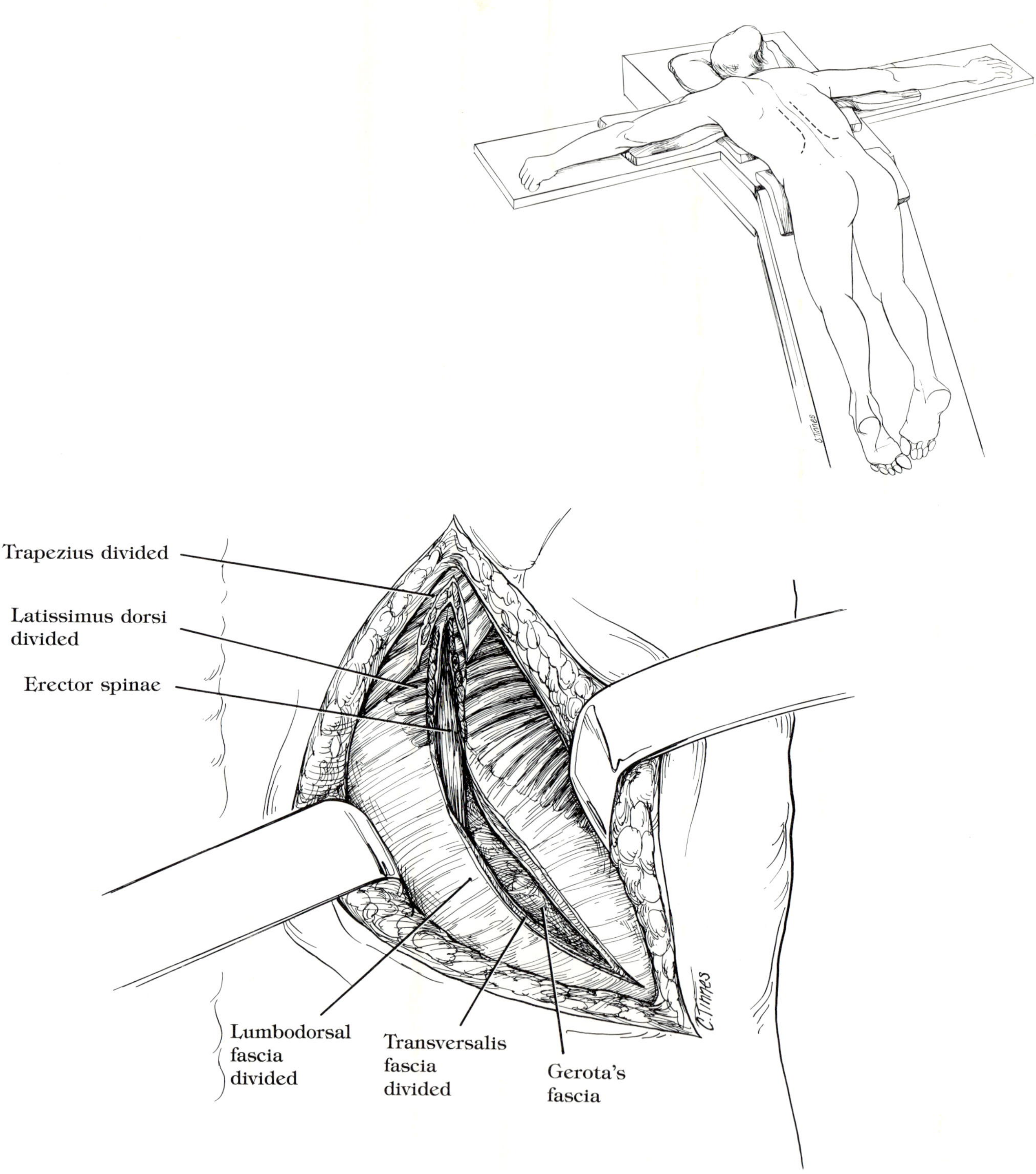

Figure 6-8

as the palpable tip of the eleventh or twelfth rib. The incision is carried through the investing fascia of the *erector spinae group of muscles* and usually divides a few centimeters of the *trapezius muscle* at the upper portion of the incision. The lateral oblique lower extension is carried through the *lumbodorsal fascia,* exposing *Gerota's fascia* as it invests the *perirenal fat* mass (Fig. 6-8). The slips of erector muscles that attach to the ribs in the paravertebral field are then cut or elevated, exposing the eleventh and twelfth ribs. The periosteum of the eleventh rib is then incised and the rib removed subperiosteally, preserving the neurovascular subcostal bundle. Through the pleura and the bed of the eleventh rib, the lung markings can be observed moving with respiration. By gentle blunt dissection, the pleura can then be mobilized from the mediastinal attachment and swept upward from the costophrenic sinus and away from the twelfth rib. This latter serves as a solid structure away from which the pleura can be dissected (Fig. 6-9*A, B*). (If the twelfth rib is excised first, the thin pleura becomes lax and the dissection is more difficult.) Following the dissection of the pleura, the twelfth rib is resected subperiosteally in a fashion similar to that described for the eleventh rib. Diaphragmatic elements can then be divided to whatever degree is necessary to permit wide exposure of the adrenal fossa and the upper half of the perirenal fat mass. The perirenal fat mass is then drawn downward to bring the adrenal gland into view. When the edge of the adrenal

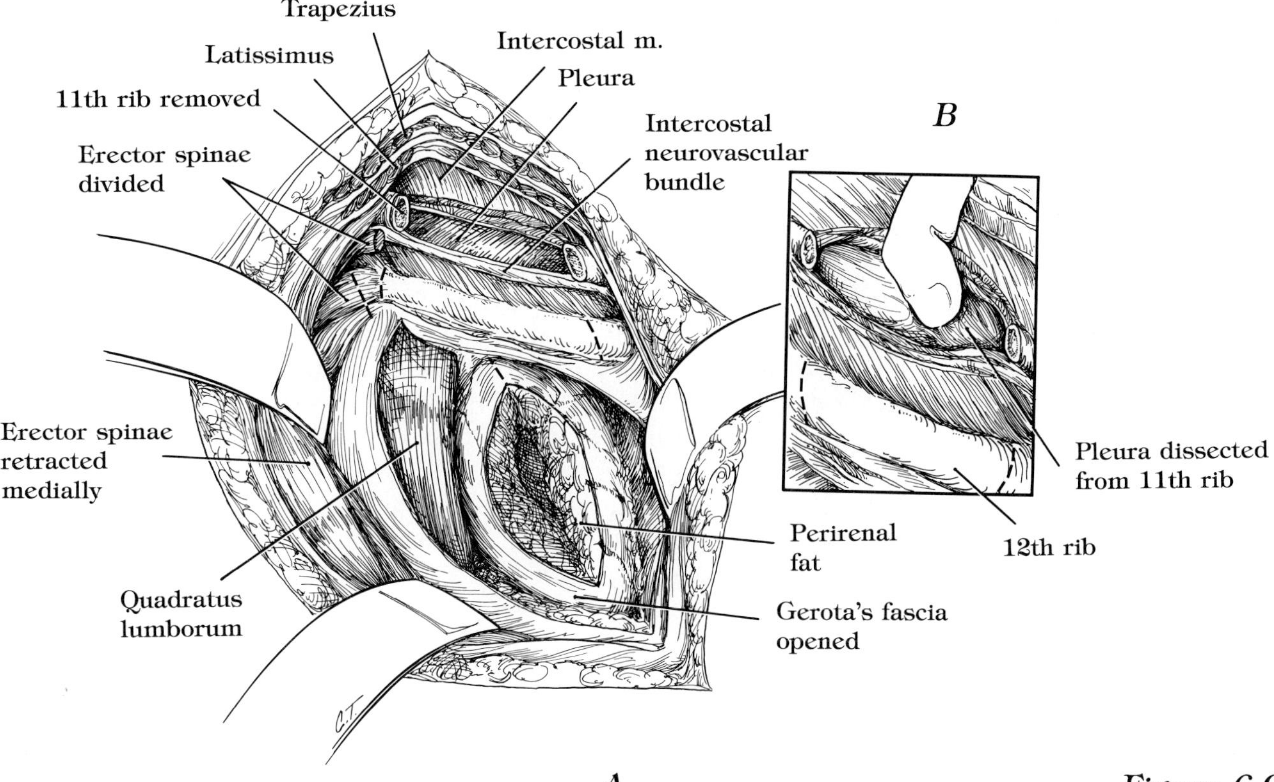

Figure 6-9

gland is identified, the lateral aspect of the gland is sufficiently cleared to permit grasping this friable structure gently with a Babcock clamp or lung forceps. Then, careful sharp and blunt dissection outlines the three sides of the pyramidal gland as it rests like a cap slightly lateral to and beneath the vena cava. The small arterial branches are controlled with small metal clips.

> CAUTION
>
> The critical part of the procedure involves control of the main adrenal vein emptying into the vena cava. Since this vein is often short, it is easy to lose control and be faced with sudden profuse hemorrhage from a tear in the vena cava. A slender right-angle clamp or a small Satinsky clamp can be placed on the cava itself, giving excellent control of any possible tear prior to isolating the adrenal vein. With this precaution, final dissection can then be undertaken to identify the adrenal vein itself and to obtain secure control prior to releasing the clamp on the cava (Fig. 6-10).

Once the gland is removed, the wound is closed with interrupted silk or cotton sutures. If the pleura has been inadvertently opened during the procedure, no special treatment is required other than placing a small catheter through the rent, applying positive pressure, and withdrawing the catheter after all layers except the skin have been closed.

If the right adrenalectomy has been uneventful and the patient's condition is satisfactory, a similar incision can then be made on the left side and identical dissection used to expose the adrenal gland. The operation is easier on the left side because the liver does not intrude in the field and because the venous anatomy does not present the technical problems of the large, short vein that is obscured by the surrounding adrenal tissue in close approximation to the vena cava. The left adrenal vein is more easily identified and controlled than that on the right side (Fig. 6-11). It should be noted that occasionally a superior adrenal vein can be quite large and can represent the main drainage from the adrenal gland. Ordinarily, however, this does not present any great difficulty in identification and ligation. The method of incision is similar to that described for the right side.

Thyroidectomy Because operations on the thyroid gland have been decreasing in frequency during the past two decades, it is even more important for a young surgeon to familiarize himself whenever possible with the technically demanding features of this type of surgical procedure.

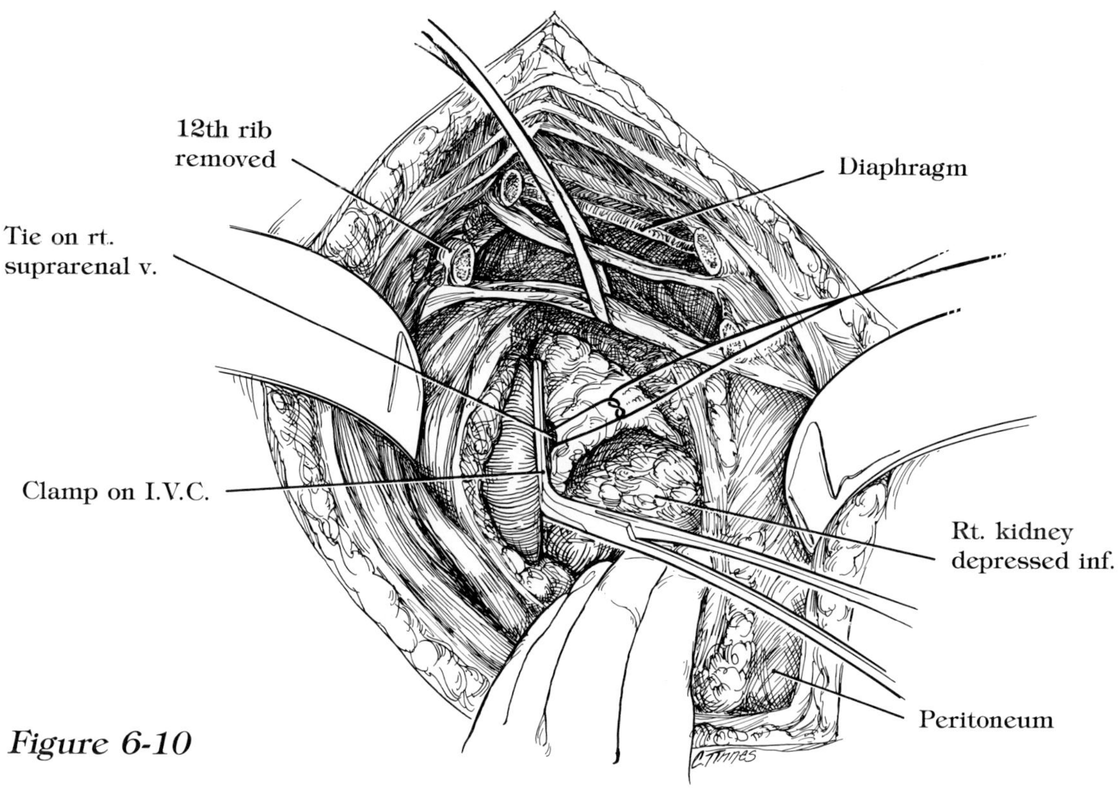

Figure 6-10

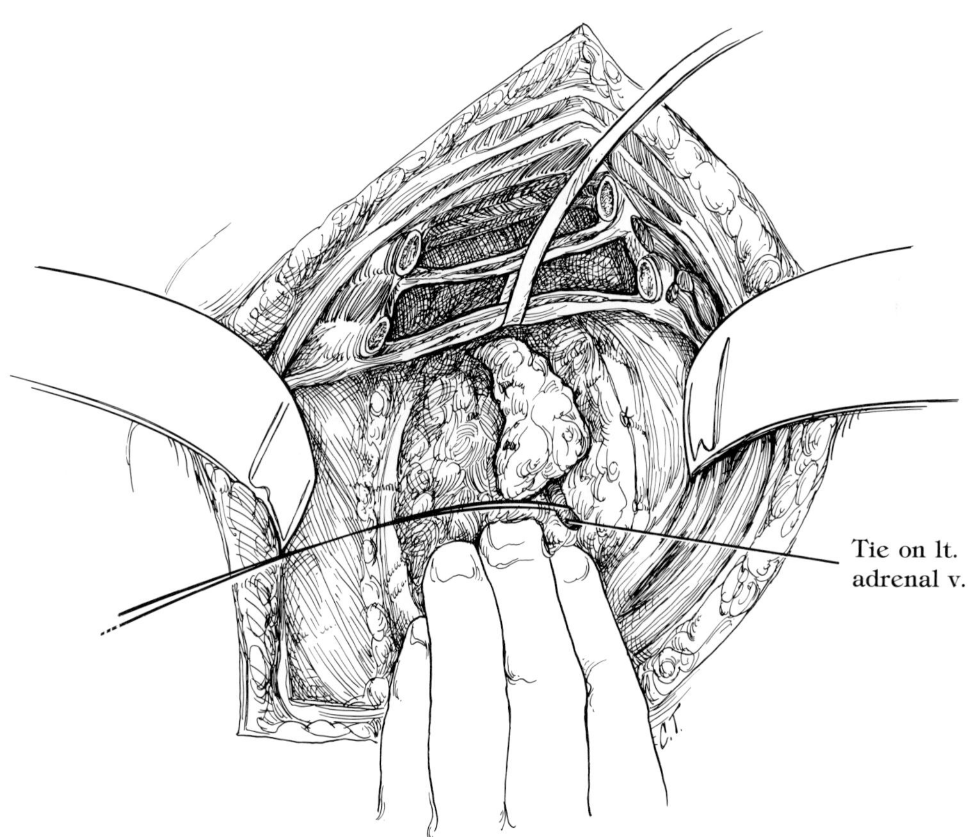

Figure 6-11

Although the use of radioactive iodine has supplanted thyroidectomy in the majority of cases of thyrotoxicosis, there are incidences when the age of the patient, the failure of medical therapy, or the existence of pregnancy may indicate an operative approach to the hyperthyroid patient. Similarly, although iodine-deficient goiter is a rarity and adenomatous goiter may often be controlled by suppressive doses of thyroid, operation is still indicated in certain instances. Certainly, in thyroid nodules where a scan indicates nonfunction, the suspicion of malignancy should be sufficient to warrant exploration. Thus, although the position of thyroidectomy in surgery may be reduced, it nonetheless remains as an important procedure with which to become familiar.

With the head in hyperextension, a transverse collar incision is made about 2 finger breadths above the sternal notch. It curves upward on both sides to just beyond the medial border of the sternocleidomastoid muscles (Fig. 6-12). In order to achieve the proper avascular plane, it is necessary to divide completely the platysma muscle fibers, which are much thicker in the male than in the female. On entering this plane, one can carry dissection upward and laterally on both sides with little bleeding. Elevating the upper flap, the surgeon dissects the midline upward off the pretracheal muscles above the level of the cricoid cartilage, ligating and dividing a few small bleeding vessels. The superficial veins are left on the fascia of the pretracheal muscles. Attention is then directed to the lower flap; with blunt dissection inferiorly to the sternal notch and with elevation of the flaps laterally with sharp dissection, the entire area of the thyroid is exposed. The pretracheal muscles are then divided high in the field between clamps (Figs. 6-13, 6-14). This maneuver is facilitated by blunt finger dissection. If carcinoma is suspected, the cervical nodes in the jugular chain can be inspected and one or more removed for biopsy. The supraisthmic area should also be inspected since a small cluster of lymph nodes in this location is a potential site for metastases. At this point, the thyroid isthmus can be mobilized off the trachea and, if the proper plane is entered, little or no bleeding should be encountered. The pyramidal lobe, arising from the left or right side of the isthmus, must be identified as it extends upward toward the hyoid bone and freed up for removal with the isthmus.

CAUTION

Failure to remove the pyramidal lobe may result in compensatory hyperplasia and the development of an unsightly nodule in front of the trachea and larynx under the upper flap.

Figure 6-12

Figure 6-13

Figure 6-14

Figure 6-15

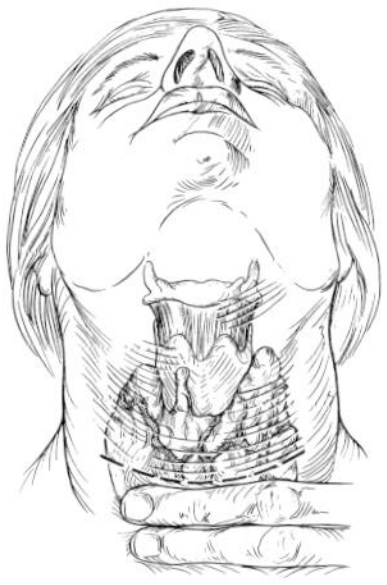

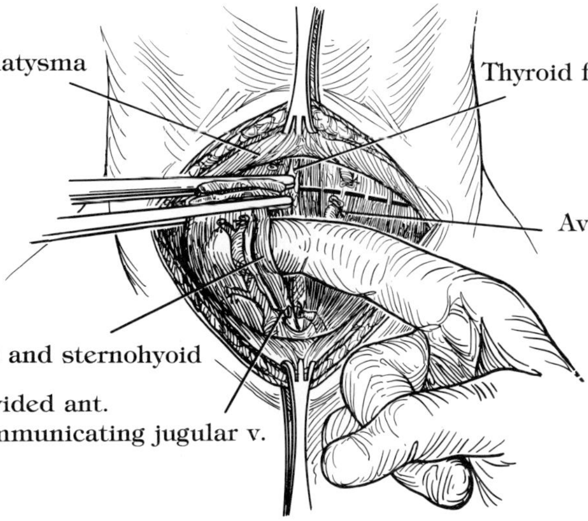

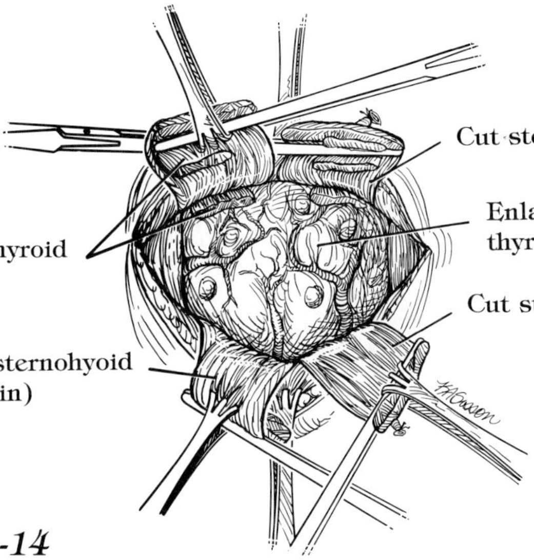

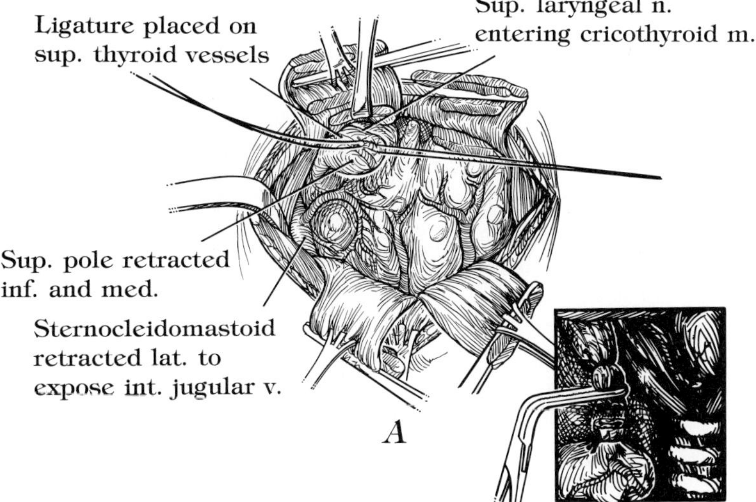

Attention is then directed to the upper pole of the appropriate lobe, depending on the nature and location of the disease. A figure-of-eight heavy stitch of 0 silk is then placed for traction near the upper pole of the gland. With the upper flap elevated and traction maintained on the lobe of the thyroid, the upper pole can be dissected under direct vision. It is often possible during this maneuver to visualize and preserve the superior laryngeal nerve as it diverges from the superior thyroid vessels to enter the larynx (Fig. 6-15*A, B*). Because loss of control of superior thyroid vessels is a serious threat, the division is accomplished by placing heavy ligatures in continuity, positioning a right-angle clamp just below the upper ligature, and dividing the vessels. A second ligature is then placed around the right-angle clamp. After this ligature is cut, the superior pole vessels retract upward. A similar figure-of-eight stitch is placed near the lower pole of the thyroid for traction. The middle and inferior thyroid veins can be clamped, cut, and ligated at this point, which permits full retraction medially of the mobilized thyroid lobe. Dissection of and anterior traction on the inferior thyroid artery are valuable for identification of the recurrent laryngeal nerve since this nerve passes between the bifurcation of the inferior thyroid artery just behind the lower pole of the thyroid on the right. With traction on the inferior thyroid artery, careful dissection should visualize the recurrent laryngeal nerve so that it may be preserved during further steps of the procedure (Fig. 6-16). An inferior parathyroid gland, which often lies in this immediate area, should also be identified when possible and its blood supply carefully preserved (Fig. 6-17).

CAUTION

The parathyroid glands are easily damaged, and postoperative hypoparathyroidism may occur purely from damage to the glands rather than from total removal. Thus, the surgeon must be meticulous in avoiding devascularization or even a subcapsular hematoma in any of the glands.

If total removal of the lobe is contemplated, one must maintain full visualization of the recurrent laryngeal nerve as the lobe is dissected off the trachea. If subtotal thyroidectomy is contemplated, a ring of hemostats can be placed along the thyroid lobe pointed in the projected line of resection toward the anterior border of the trachea. With a sharp knife and the placement of successive hemostats, the major portion of the lobe can be completely mobilized with the already free isthmus and

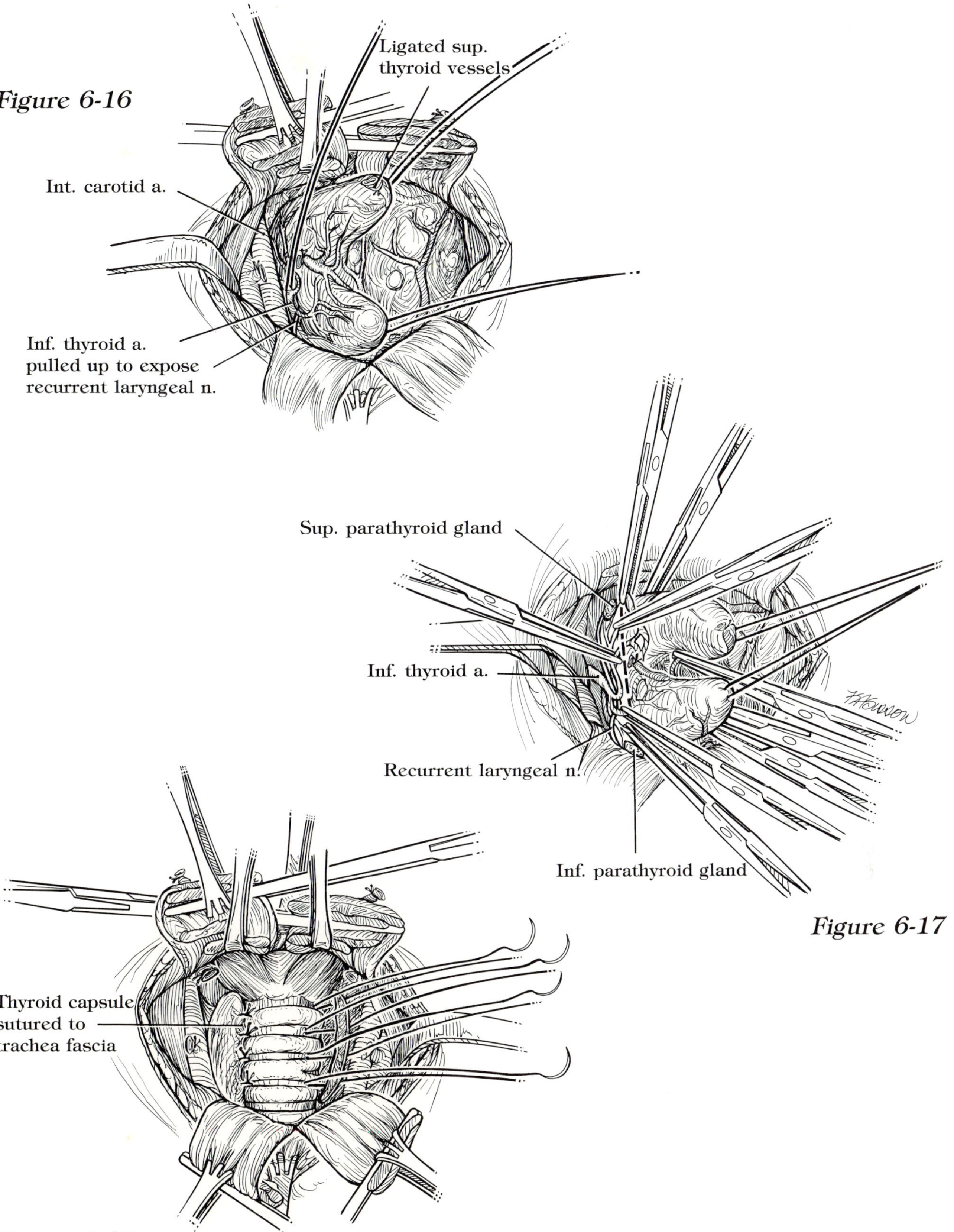

Figure 6-16

Figure 6-17

Figure 6-18

turned backward toward the opposite side (see Fig. 6-17). If hemithyroidectomy is planned, the thyroid isthmus is divided near the opposite lobe and suture ligatures are placed. The hemostats in the partially resected lobe are then removed after ligatures are placed around them. The lobe can be turned medially toward the trachea and sutured in position. The stitches are placed through the thyroid capsule and the layer of tissue overlying the cartilage of the trachea (Fig. 6-18). The pretracheal muscles are reapproximated. Closure is effected by interrupted fine sutures on the platysma and skin. Adequate hemostasis is essential in thyroid surgery; if this is achieved, as it should always be, drainage is not necessary.

Parathyroid Surgery

Exploration of the neck for visualization and possible removal of the parathyroid glands may be indicated because of primary or secondary hyperparathyroidism. In the former instance, excess function may be due to a parathyroid tumor (only rarely are these malignant) or to a generalized hyperplasia of the glands secondary to increased parathyrotropic hormone. In both instances it is important to identify all parathyroid glands because of the possible existence of more than a single parathyroid adenoma and also because of the difficulty in microscopic evaluation of parathyroid tissue removed for frozen section. Thus, under all instances it is imperative to visualize and possibly to take a biopsy of all parathyroid glands while realizing that occasionally there may be a fifth gland in addition to the ordinary pattern of four. If a single parathyroid adenoma exists and three other atrophic glands are visualized, the decision is simple: removal of the tumor-bearing gland. If, however, all four glands are enlarged and apparently hyperplastic, it is probably advisable to perform a radical subtotal parathyroidectomy, carefully preserving a small but well-vascularized segment of one of the parathyroid glands. In the case of secondary hyperparathyroidism usually due to renal disease, it is becoming more acceptable to remove all four parathyroid glands and to implant small segments of parathyroid tissue in the muscle of the forearm with identifying clips or ligatures nearby. The high incidence of recurrence in subtotal parathyroidectomy has led to a general acceptance of the advisability of this particular approach. With this brief summary as a background, a description follows of the technical problems associated with parathyroid exploration.

The incision for a parathyroid exploration is similar to that already described for exploration of or resection of the thyroid gland. Successful parathyroid exploration depends on a precise knowledge of the normal and aberrant locations of the four parathyroid glands, on recognition by gross inspection of the various disease processes with which the parathyroids become involved and, most important, on absolutely meticulous hemostasis dur-

ing the dissection and exploration. The most frequent locations
of these glands are shown in Figure 6-19.

Once the thyroid area has been exposed as described for thyroid surgery, dissection can proceed in terms of successive identification and definition of any disease process in the four parathyroid glands.

As in the technical steps for thyroidectomy, one lobe of the thyroid is mobilized, using traction sutures on the superior and inferior poles and dividing the superior pole vessels if necessary

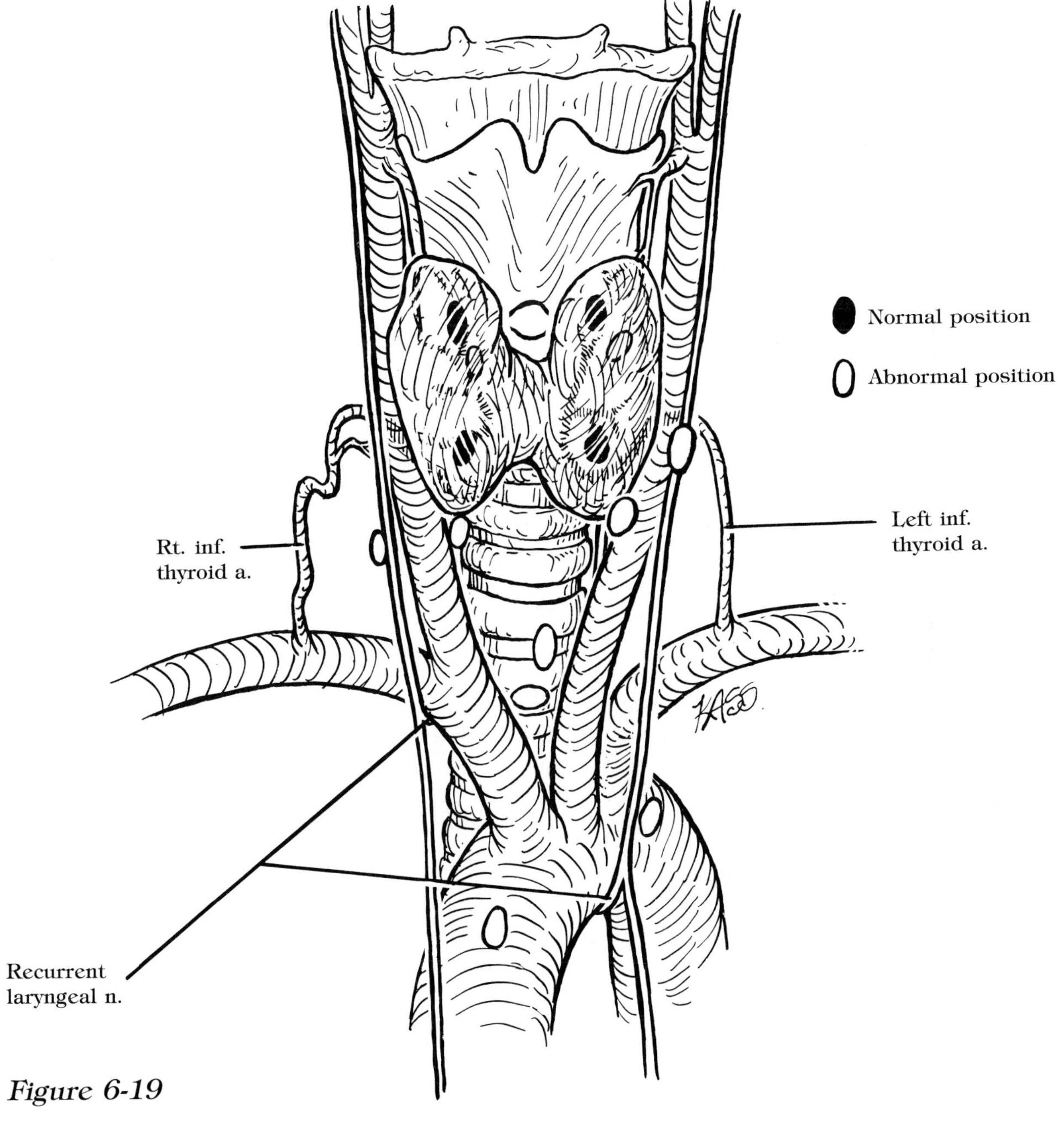

Figure 6-19

for careful inspection of the posterior aspects of the gland. Traction is used on a ligature around the inferior thyroid artery, exactly as previously described for thyroidectomy. With mobilization of the lobe toward the midline, the recurrent laryngeal nerve is identified. By painstaking dissection in a bloodless field, it should be possible to identify the inferior parathyroid gland lying close to the recurrent laryngeal nerve and often supplied by a branch of the inferior thryoid artery. After the inferior gland on the right side is identified, dissection is carried out behind the superior pole of the thyroid. One should carefully inspect the posterior aspect of the gland where it should be possible to identify the superior parathyroid gland on that side. It is probably wise to inspect all four parathyroid glands before removing or taking a biopsy of any. Dissection then proceeds on the left side where the anatomy of the inferior thyroid artery and the recurrent laryngeal nerve are slightly different than on the right and where the inferior parathyroid gland is a little more variable in location but usually is in close approximation to the nerve and artery. The superior gland on the left side lies in a position similar to that shown on the right.

When all four glands have been identified, one is then in a position to define the nature of the pathology by ascertaining the presence of an enlargement of a single gland (indicating an adenoma), or the presence of atrophy in the remaining glands, or enlargement of all four (indicating the likelihood of a generalized hyperplasia). At this point, a suspected adenoma should be removed with the entire gland and submitted for frozen-section diagnosis. Simultaneously, a biopsy should be taken from one of the other glands to determine the presence or absence of atrophy. If all four glands are enlarged and a frozen-section diagnosis of hyperplasia can be made, three of the glands should be totally removed and the fourth gland partially resected carefully to prevent infarction of the remaining parathyroid tissue. If one or more of the glands are not presentable by this approach, the search should be extended laterally in the groove between the trachea and esophagus on both sides and in the tissue immediately below the isthmus and the inferior poles bilaterally. If one or more glands are still missing, the upper mediastinum can be dissected through the neck incision by removing a large portion of the fatty tissue behind the manubrium. If a careful search through this tissue and a meticulous dissection throughout the entire neck as described do not define the extent of the disease and all four parathyroids, the wound should be closed. Plans should be made for a later mediastinotomy with resection of the thymus and the surrounding tissue, which sometimes contains one or more aberrant parathyroid glands.

The general size of parathyroid glands approximates that of a small pea. They are brownish in color in youth, becoming more yellowish with age. They vary in configuration from an attenuated linear structure to a fat shape approximating that of a small lima bean. The disease obviously alters the appearance, since the atrophic glands associated with a hyperfunctioning adenoma may be difficult to identify. The slight variation in color and consistency from surrounding fat should lead the experienced surgeon toward identifying a parathyroid gland. The fine reticular network of vessels lying under the parathyroid capsule provides further confirmation. Delicacy in handling the parathyroid glands is imperative because they are prone to injury from the development of a dissecting hematoma beneath the capsule.

Although the identification and removal of a large parathyroid adenoma may be surprisingly easy, the operation may be tedious and difficult under many circumstances. As a technical procedure, it should be reserved for surgeons with a reasonable degree of experience in this highly specialized area of neck surgery.

CHAPTER SEVEN

LYMPH NODE DISSECTIONS

Until two decades ago lymph node dissections were commonplace and were related to the generally accepted orthodoxy that cancer could only be adequately controlled by extending the operation beyond the primary location to encompass all the accessible lymph nodes draining the area. Although increasing understanding of the biological nature and patterns of malignant disease has brought a more conservative approach, less radical surgery, and fewer indications for radical lymph node dissections, there are, however, still instances when the neck, groin, and axilla should be widely explored and dissected. Even if the occasions for the utilization of these operations are few, a knowledge of the surgical anatomy of these areas is useful to the operating surgeon because of the diverse occasions in which he may be led into these areas either as a defined operation or as an extended portion of some other procedure. Thus, the four operations concerned with approaches to node-bearing areas are described in detail.

The incision applicable to a radical neck dissection is shown in Figure 7-1. It is carried down through the skin and subcutaneous fat to the platysma myoid muscle. Skin flaps are dissected widely in all directions: superiorly to just below the lower border of the mandible, posteriorly to the border of the trapezius muscle, anteriorly to the sternohyoid, and inferiorly to the clavicle. The platysma muscle is thus exposed and incisions are made through the muscle and underlying fascia, as indicated by the dotted line in Figure 7-2. This portion of platysma and the underlying fat are dissected upward. The two heads of the sterno-

Radical Neck Dissection

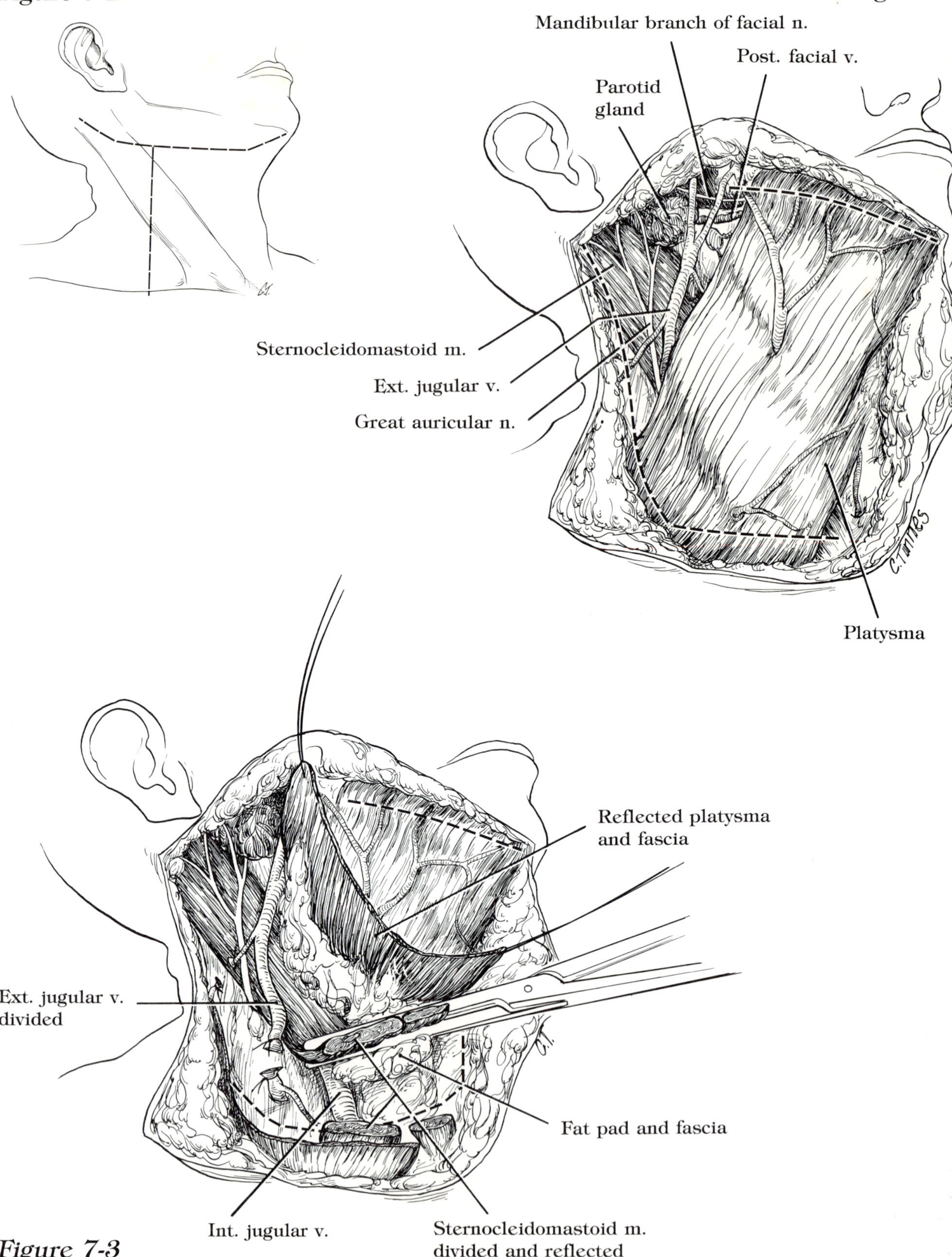

Figure 7-1
Figure 7-2
Mandibular branch of facial n.
Post. facial v.
Parotid gland
Sternocleidomastoid m.
Ext. jugular v.
Great auricular n.
Platysma
Reflected platysma and fascia
Ext. jugular v. divided
Fat pad and fascia
Int. jugular v.
Sternocleidomastoid m. divided and reflected
Figure 7-3

cleidomastoid muscle are evident and are divided close to their
origin (Fig. 7-3). This muscle is then retracted upward with the
platysma. The internal jugular vein is exposed in the depths of
the wound (see Fig. 7-3). After the external jugular vein is then
divided, dissection of the node-bearing fat is carried laterally
toward the anterior border of the trapezius muscle. The internal
jugular vein is divided and ligated preserving the vagus nerve
which lies just behind the vein. As the nodes are dissected at the
lower end of the wound, care is taken not to injure the thoracic
duct on the left or the major lymphatic trunk on the right (Fig.
7-4). Continued dissection exposes the scalene muscles in the
depth of the wound, and the vagus and phrenic nerve trunks are
carefully preserved. The omohyoid muscle is exposed in the posterior part of the dissection and divided near its origin from the
scapula. In the posterior part of the dissection, several cervical
sensory nerves are divided, but the spinal accessory nerve can
be preserved as it crosses the field and enters the trapezius
muscle. The entire area between the trapezius posteriorly and
the lateral border of the sternomastoid anteriorly is dissected
cleanly and, as the mass is swept upward, the bifurcation of the
common carotid artery comes into view. At this point, the hypoglossal nerve is encountered and identified. The omohyoid muscle is then divided near its insertion on the hyoid bone. Anteriorly and posteriorly, the upper end of the sternocleidomastoid
muscle is also divided close to the mastoid bone for removal
with the specimen. Posteriorly, one can then dissect the upper
nodes of the inferior jugular chain dividing the lower pole of the
parotid gland if necessary for adequate exposure.

CAUTION
   Care should be taken to avoid injury to the parotid
gland. An annoying fistula may develop postoperatively if
the gland is transected or damaged.

As the dissection is carried anteriorly and superiorly, the
stylohyoid muscle and the posterior belly of the digastric can be
retracted upward to permit dissection posterior to these muscles. Here the internal jugular vein is divided to be removed
with the mass of node-bearing fat. Dissection is then carried
superiorly over the posterior belly of the digastric and into the
submaxillary triangle (Fig. 7-5). The facial artery is ligated as it
emerges from the deep fascia. Blunt dissection in the submaxillary triangle frees up that particular salivary gland from below.
At this point, it is best to proceed to the superior margin of the
dissection, carefully identifying and preserving the inframandibular branch of the facial nerve.

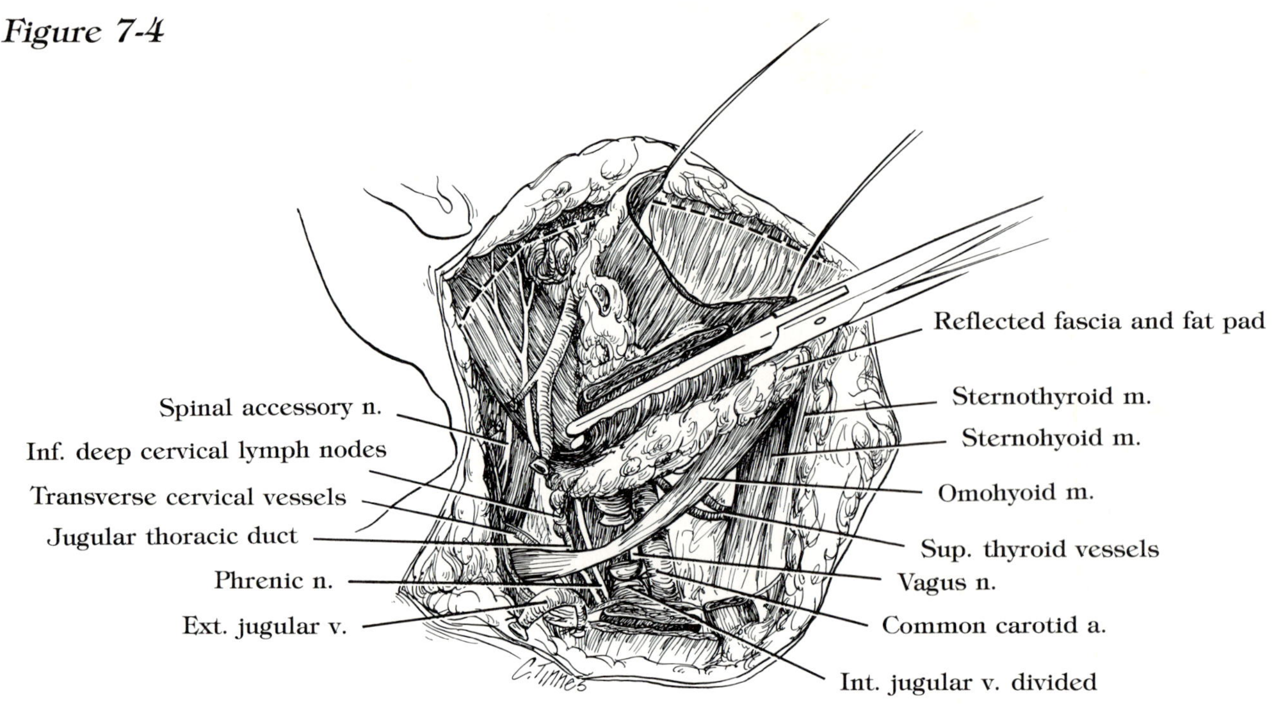

Figure 7-4

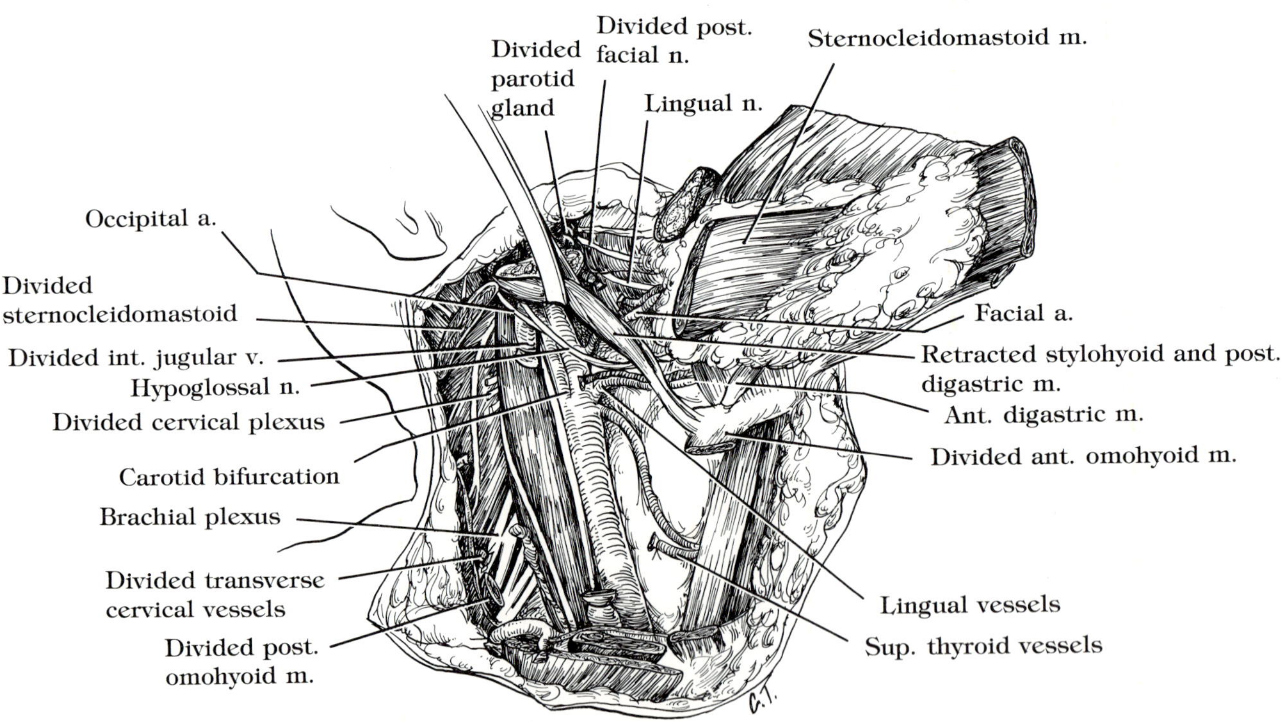

Figure 7-5

The submaxillary triangle is then entered from above; the mylohyoid muscle is visualized; Wharton's duct is clamped, cut, and ligated; and the submaxillary gland is included in the specimen (Fig. 7-6). During the dissection of the submaxillary duct, the lingual nerve lies in close proximity to it, and should be preserved. Dissection proceeds forward to the anterior belly of the digastric muscle and into the submental triangle, which is dissected, cleanly exposing the mylohyoid muscles. The dissected mass is then completely freed and removed en bloc. The anatomy following completion of the radical neck dissection is shown in Figure 7-7. Hemovac catheters are inserted, and the skin is closed with interrupted silk sutures.

Supra Omohyoid Neck Dissection

Incision for the supraomohyoid neck dissection, shown in Figure 7-8, is the transverse portion of the incision for the radical neck dissection. Flaps of skin are dissected upward and downward to expose the field of dissection, which extends from the omohyoid muscle inferiorly to the sternomastoid muscle posteriorly, to the mandible superiorly, and to the submental triangle medially. The platysma muscle is then incised at all these boundaries, and dissection is begun posteriorly and superiorly where the lower pole of the parotid is retracted. The dissection is deepened along the anterior border of the sternomastoid muscle to expose the internal jugular vein. Platysma, fat, and fascia are retracted medially and superiorly to remove all the node-bearing fat from the lateral, anterior, and medial aspects of the vein. An arbitrary division across lymphatic pathways is made behind the omohyoid muscle. The facial or maxillary vein is divided and the tissue mass retracted upward, beginning the exposure of the posterior belly of the digastric muscle (Fig. 7-9). As the inferior border of the dissection is carried medially along the omohyoid muscle, the hyoid bone is encountered. At this point, the digastric and stylohyoid muscles come into view. The hypoglossal nerve lies posterior to them and curves medially and upward in the neck behind the border of the mylohyoid muscle. The superior border of the dissection is defined along the inferior border of the mandible. The surgeon identifies and preserves the inframandibular branch of the facial nerve as it curves downward from the parotid area and then swings upward toward the angle of the mouth. As the submaxillary triangle is entered, the

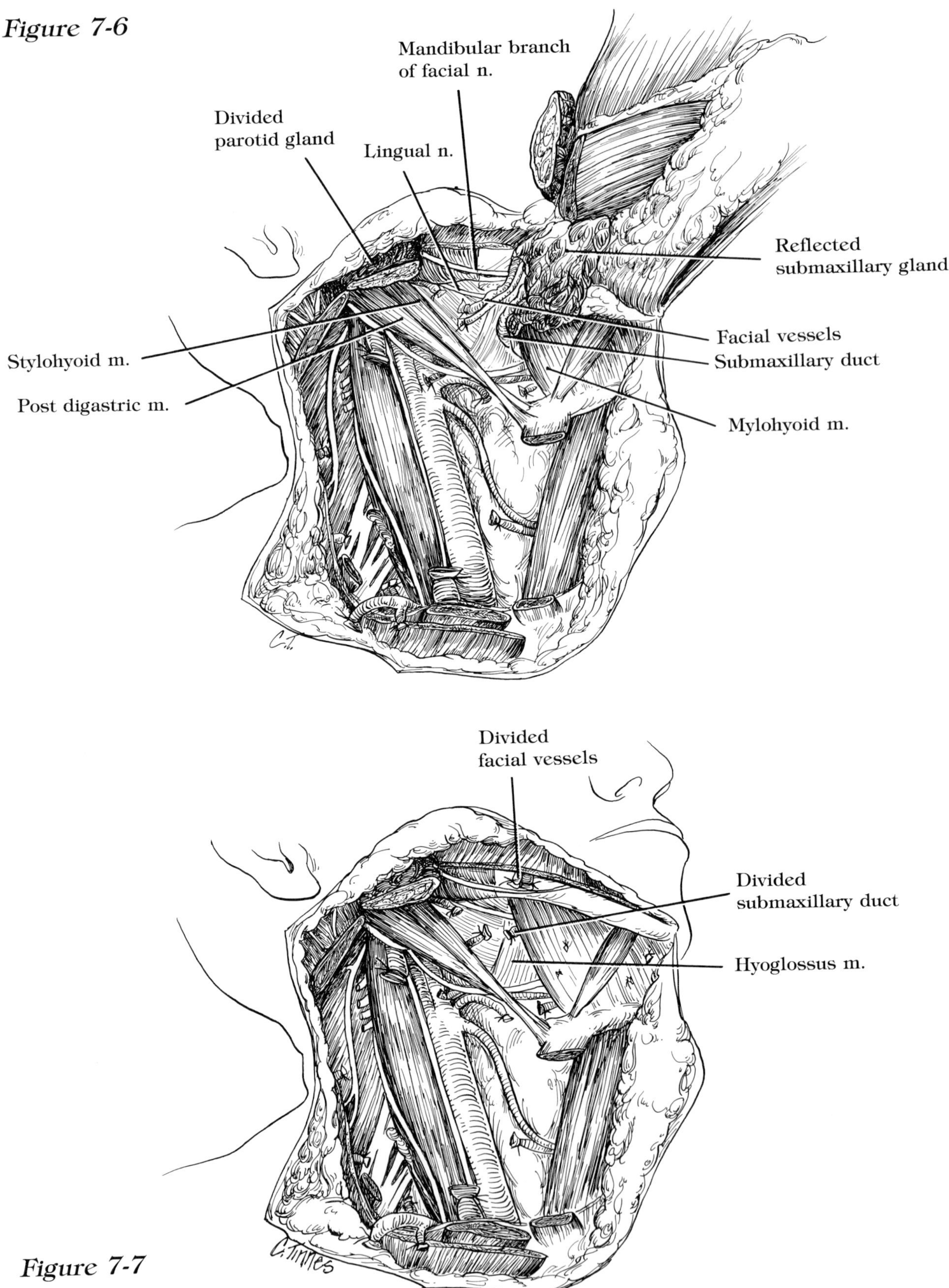

Figure 7-6
Mandibular branch
of facial n.
Divided
parotid gland
Lingual n.
Reflected
submaxillary gland
Stylohyoid m.
Facial vessels
Submaxillary duct
Post digastric m.
Mylohyoid m.
Divided
facial vessels
Divided
submaxillary duct
Hyoglossus m.
Figure 7-7

Divided parotid gland
Reflected platysma
Post. belly of digastric m.
Dissected nodes, veins, and fascia
Stylohyoid m.
Spinal accessory n.
Tie on facial v.
Lingual v.
Int. jugular v.
Sup. thyroid v.
Common carotid a.
Ant. belly of omohyoid m.
Jugular thoracic duct
Sternocleidomastoid m. retracted
Divided ext. jugular v.

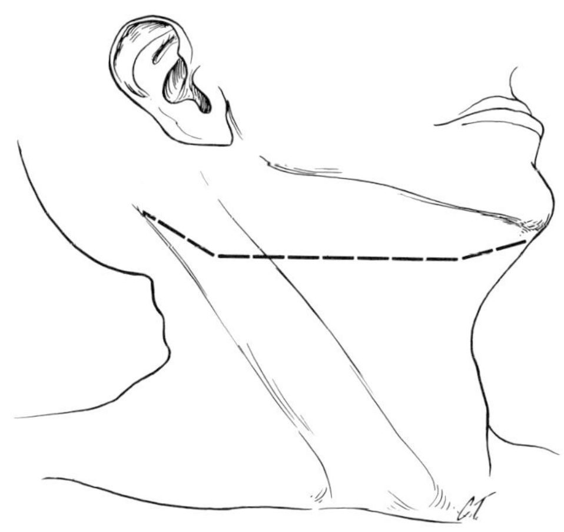

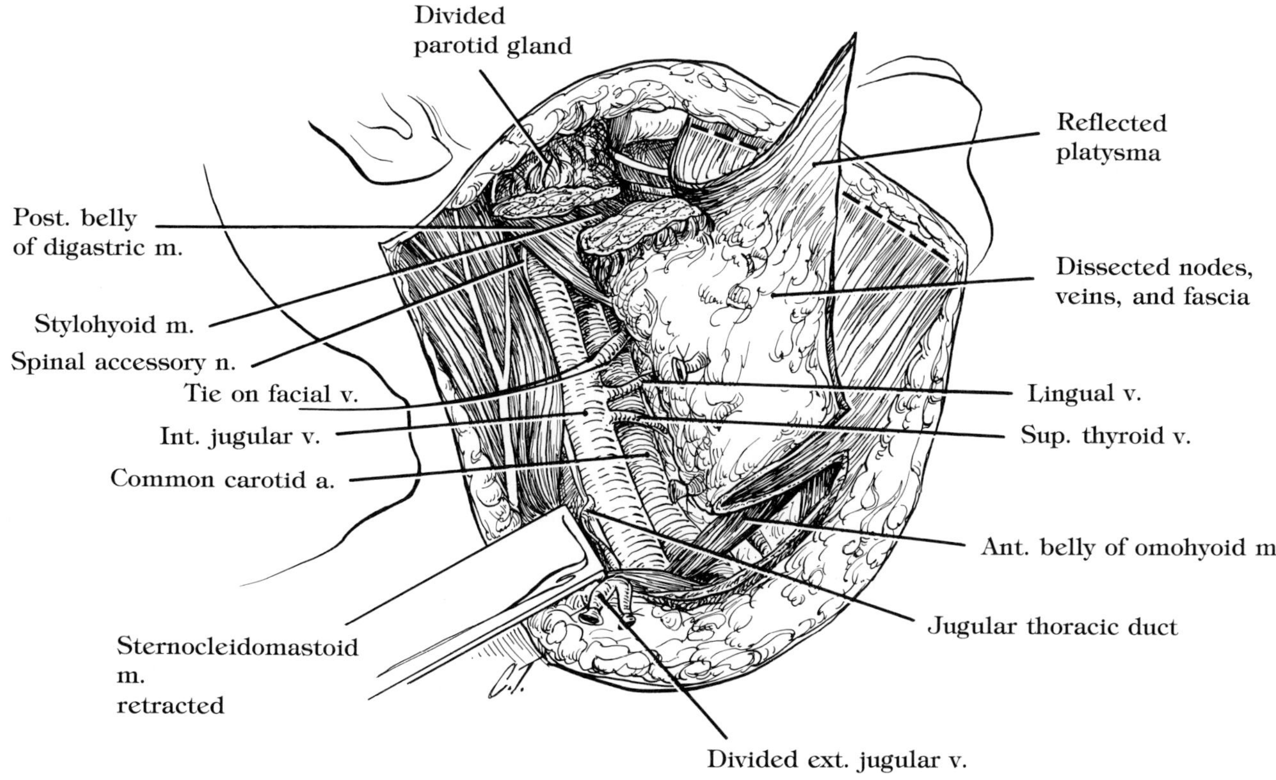

Figure 7-9

submaxillary gland becomes apparent and can be freed up and drawn into the field with blunt dissection. Multiple small veins that may be encountered in this area are ligated (Fig. 7-10). The lingual nerve lying superior to Wharton's duct is identified and preserved, and then the duct itself is clamped, cut, and ligated. The dissection may be carried over the mylohyoid muscles and the submental node-bearing fat included with the dissection, but this is not a necessary part of this limited operation. At the conclusion of the procedure, the dissection appears as shown in Figure 7-11. The skin is closed with interrupted silk sutures, and drainage is achieved through insertion of Hemovac catheters.

Radical Groin Dissection

The operative incision for the radical groin dissection is shown in Figure 7-12. It is made in a straight line on the interior thigh overlying the course of the femoral artery. Then, as the incision crosses the inguinal ligament, it is curved medially toward the umbilicus and extends about half the distance from the inguinal ligament to this point.

Skin flaps are dissected laterally and medially to the limits of the planned dissection, which should be, in the thigh, the sartorius muscle laterally and the long adductor muscle medially. Deep dissection is begun at the lowest angle of the saphenous triangle where the superficial femoral artery and vein are identified. One dissects upward, removing the areolar tissue lying near and anterior to these vessels. Several vessels that are encountered in the dissection through the saphenous triangle are shown in Figure 7-13. The saphenous vein is divided at the beginning of the dissection and again as its entrance into the superficial femoral vein is identified just below the inguinal ligament (Fig. 7-14). The femoral nerve, which is identified lying lateral and deep to the artery, is preserved. As one proceeds across the inguinal ligament, an incision is made in the external oblique fascia over the inguinal canal, just as would be done in a herniorrhaphy (Fig. 7-15). The cord above the ligament is dissected free from the floor of the canal and retracted medially, exposing and dividing the conjoined tendon in the line of its fibers (Fig. 7-16).

The internal inguinal ring is identified. Dissection at its lower limits exposes the deep epigastric vessels, which are clamped, cut, and ligated in order to assist in exposure of the retroperitoneal area over the iliac vessels (see Fig. 7-16). The abdominal wall structures, including the external oblique fascia and the conjoined tendon, are retracted medially. The peritoneum is retracted upward with blunt dissection (Fig. 7-17). This exposes the external iliac vessels up to the bifurcation of the common iliac. Dissection is begun at this level and is carried downward to remove the areolar tissue that lies anterior and medial to the iliac vein and over the iliac artery and iliopsoas

Figure 7-10

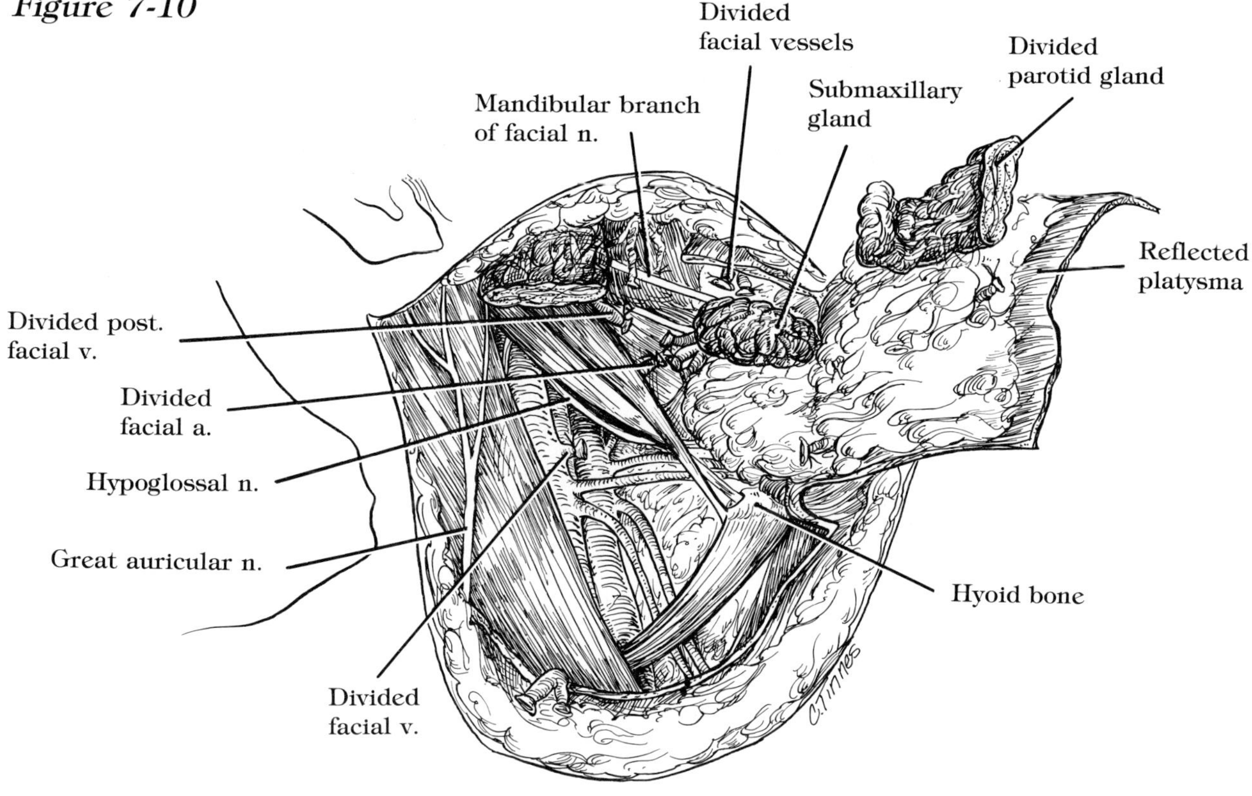
Divided
facial vessels
Mandibular branch
of facial n.
Submaxillary
gland
Divided
parotid gland
Reflected
platysma
Divided post.
facial v.
Divided
facial a.
Hypoglossal n.
Great auricular n.
Hyoid bone
Divided
facial v.

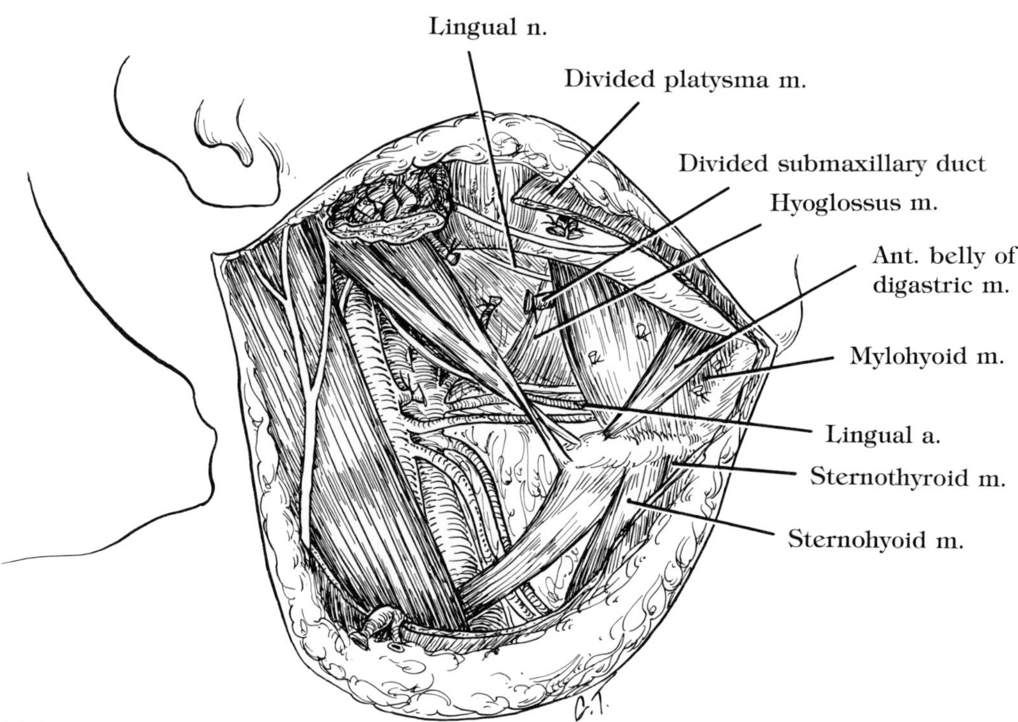
Lingual n.
Divided platysma m.
Divided submaxillary duct
Hyoglossus m.
Ant. belly of
digastric m.
Mylohyoid m.
Lingual a.
Sternothyroid m.
Sternohyoid m.

Figure 7-11

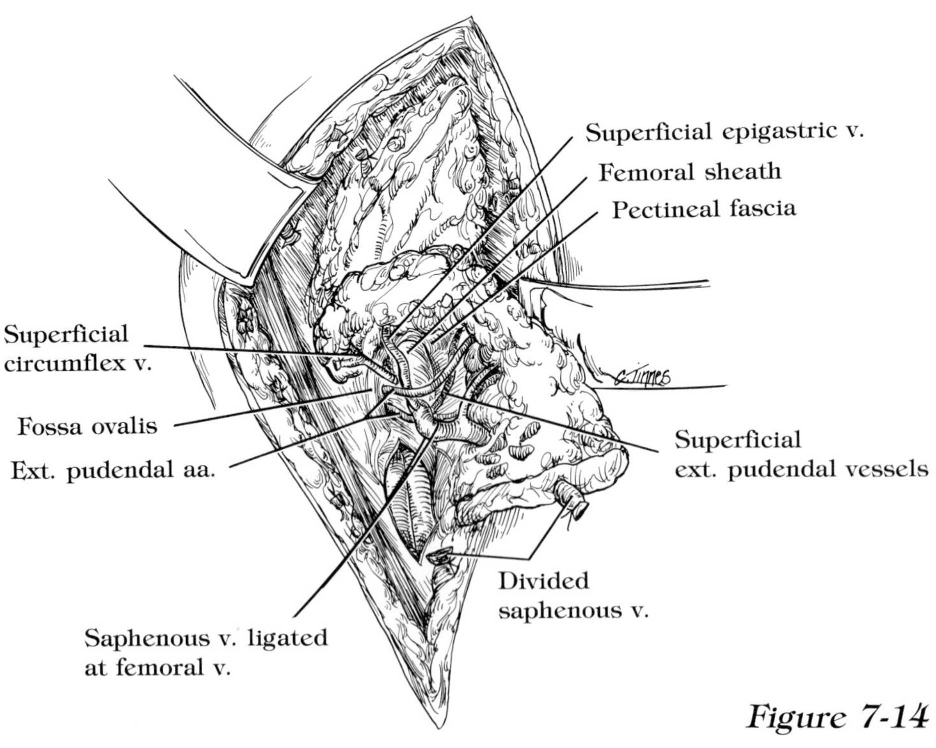

Figure 7-12 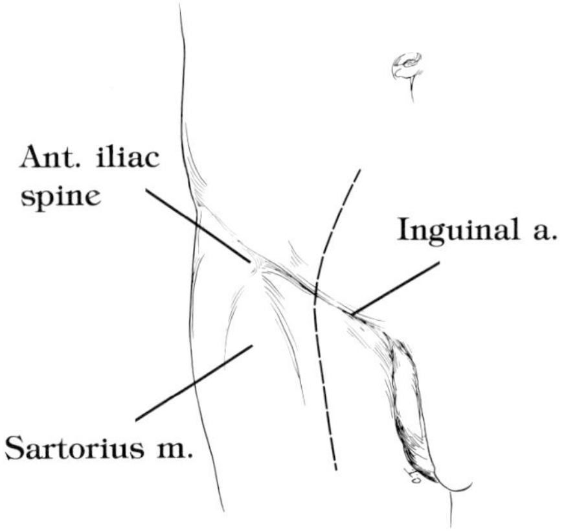
Ant. iliac spine
Inguinal a.
Sartorius m.

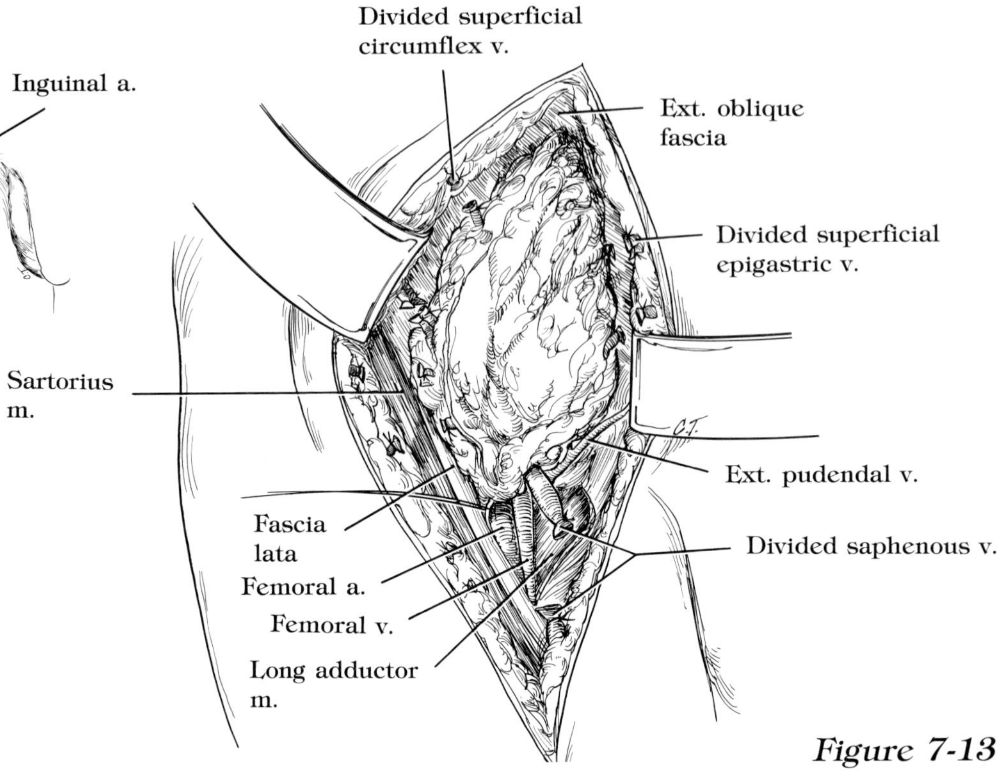

Divided superficial circumflex v.
Ext. oblique fascia
Divided superficial epigastric v.
Sartorius m.
Ext. pudendal v.
Fascia lata
Femoral a.
Femoral v.
Long adductor m.
Divided saphenous v.
Figure 7-13

Superficial epigastric v.
Femoral sheath
Pectineal fascia
Superficial circumflex v.
Fossa ovalis
Ext. pudendal aa.
Superficial ext. pudendal vessels
Divided saphenous v.
Saphenous v. ligated at femoral v.
Figure 7-14

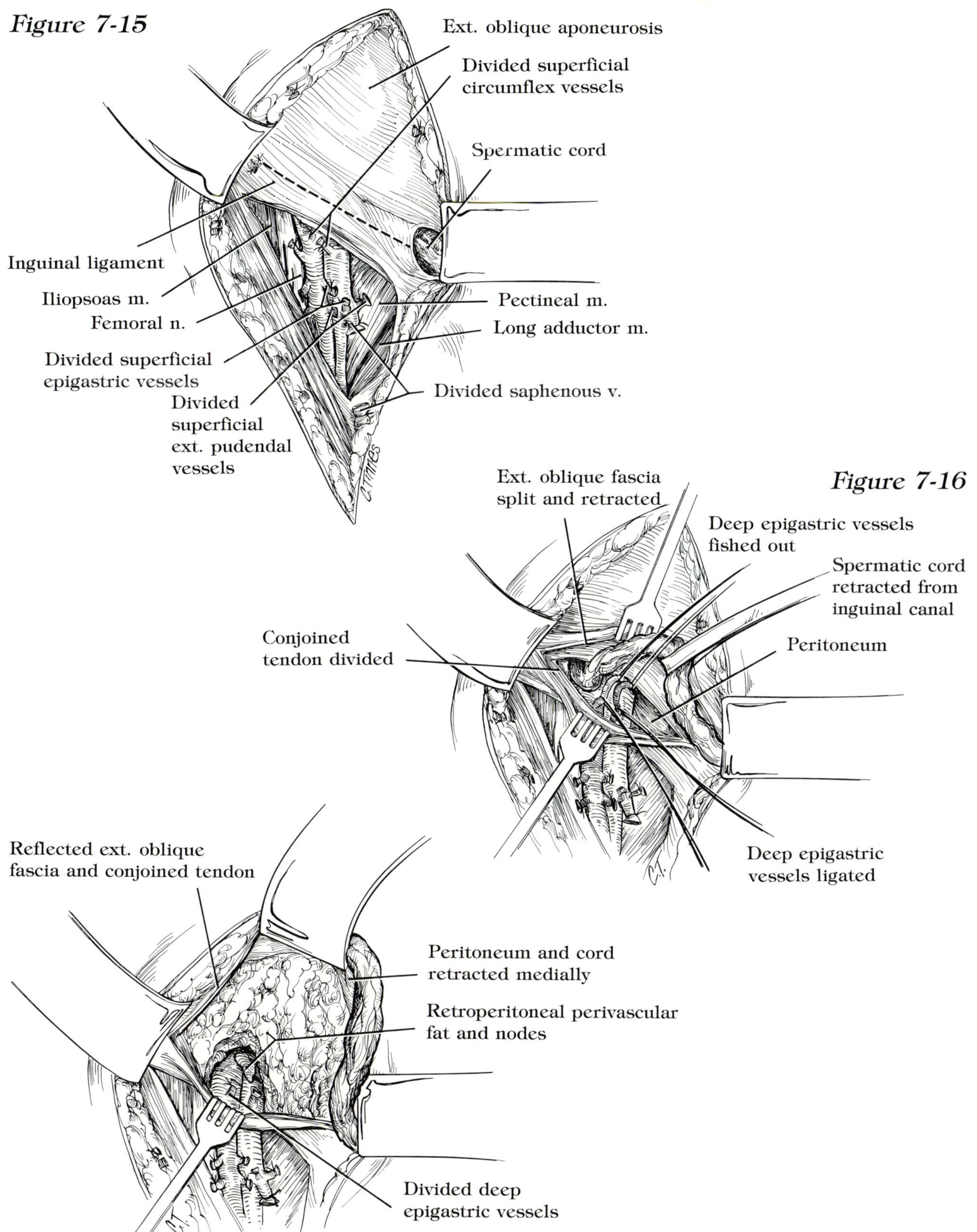

Figure 7-15
Ext. oblique aponeurosis
Divided superficial circumflex vessels
Spermatic cord
Inguinal ligament
Iliopsoas m.
Femoral n.
Divided superficial epigastric vessels
Divided superficial ext. pudendal vessels
Pectineal m.
Long adductor m.
Divided saphenous v.
Ext. oblique fascia split and retracted
Deep epigastric vessels fished out
Spermatic cord retracted from inguinal canal
Peritoneum
Conjoined tendon divided
Figure 7-16
Deep epigastric vessels ligated
Reflected ext. oblique fascia and conjoined tendon
Peritoneum and cord retracted medially
Retroperitoneal perivascular fat and nodes
Divided deep epigastric vessels
Figure 7-17

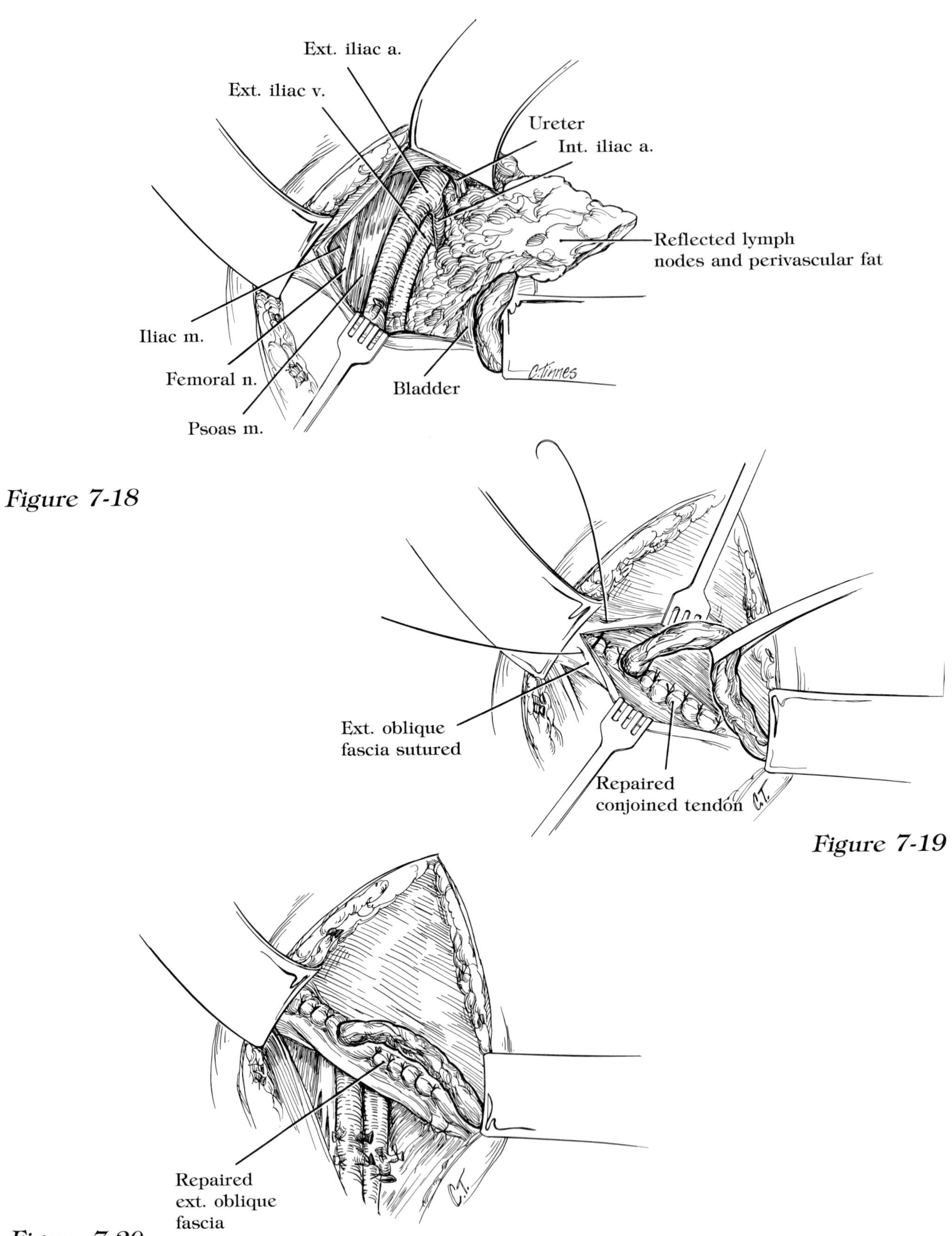

Figure 7-18

Figure 7-19

Figure 7-20

muscle. The femoral nerve should be identified and preserved (Fig. 7-18). In thin individuals, the dissection can sometimes be carried down to the obturator fossa to remove some of the nodes associated with the obturator vessels. The obturator artery and nerve can be palpated and often visualized in the depths of the medial dissection. At the conclusion of the iliac dissection, the conjoined tendon and the external oblique fascia are resutured beneath the cord as in repair of an inguinal herniorrhaphy (Fig. 7-19). It is usually necessary also to close the femoral ring by bringing the inguinal ligament down to the pectinal fascia or to the periosteum of the pubis (Fig. 7-20). One then closes the incision leaving suction catheters beneath the flaps for drainage.

The incision for an axillary dissection crosses the axilla in a location similar to that shown in the lateral portion of the T of the Rodman-Greenough incision. After the flaps have been elevated along the pectoralis and posteriorly to the latissimus dorsi muscle, the entire axillary contents are swept medially, inferiorly, and, later, anteriorly as dissection proceeds. The procedure is similar to the description given in Chapter 8 of the modified radical mastectomy. The pectoral muscles ordinarily do not have to be divided or removed but can be retracted upward, allowing access to all of the axilla except the highest apical point where the vein crosses the first rib. The steps in the anatomy of this procedure can be seen in Chapter 8 (Fig. 8-10). The skin is closed, and suction catheters are used to prevent reaccumulation of fluid under the flaps.

Axillary
Dissection

CHAPTER EIGHT

BREAST

There is still extensive and justifiable controversy relative to the degree of operation designed for adequate control of a proven cancer of the breast. It is not within the province of this text to discuss the merits of a radical or modified procedure for cancer of the breast; therefore, both procedures are described in detail.

Some surgical preceptors may object to the inclusion of the radical mastectomy on the grounds of limited applicability in surgical treatment of cancer of the breast today. On the other hand, occasionally the depth of invasion may indicate more than a simple mastectomy. In addition, many surgeons still utilize a more radical axillary dissection (the Patey procedure) than is done for ordinary axillary sampling. More important, however, for a surgical atlas, is the obvious fact that a pictorial representation of the radical mastectomy presents a view of the entire anatomy of the chest wall and axilla with which the surgeon will be involved, regardless of the extent of the actual operation.

Biopsy of the Breast

A tumor or palpable abnormality of the breast can often be approached through a circumareolar incision (Fig. 8-1), which leaves minimal deformity of the breast and permits adequate removal of tissue. Controversy over excisional versus incisional biopsy is probably inconsequential and depends on the ease and necessity of removal of the total mass. If the tumor or abnormality is not easily accessible through a circumareolar incision, however, it is preferable to make a direct radial incision over the tumor placed to avoid the lines of any projected mastectomy (Fig. 8-2). Once the skin and superficial fascia are incised and the breast tissue exposed, a figure-of-eight traction stitch can be

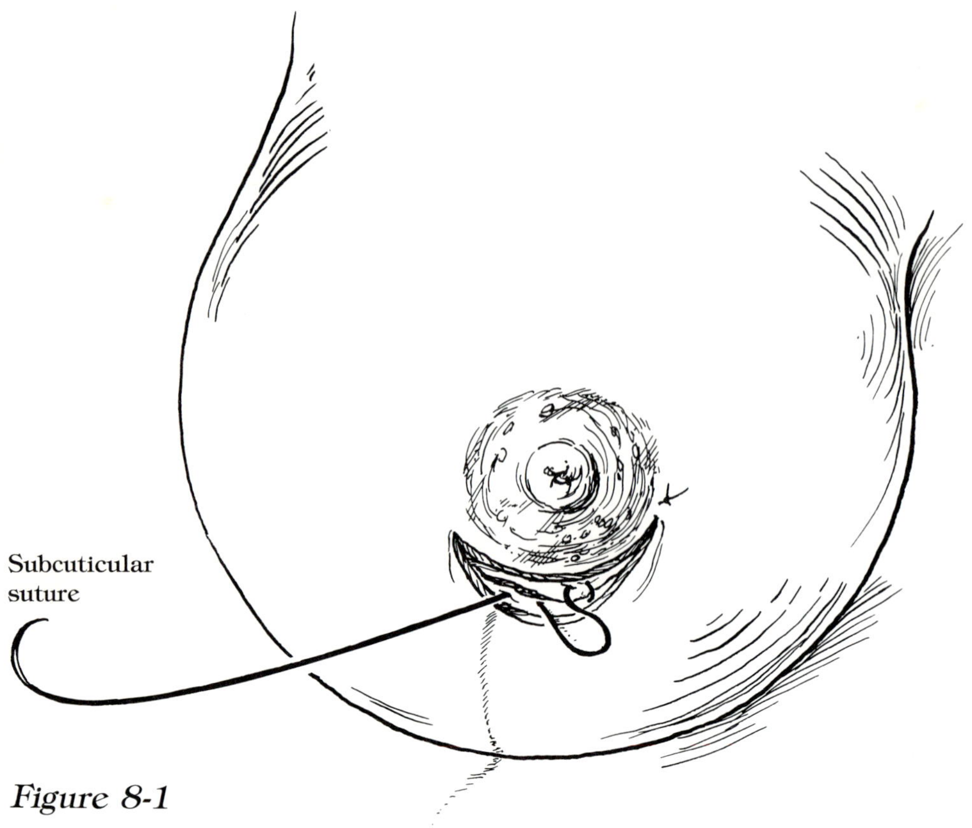

Figure 8-1

placed through the tumor so that it can be drawn easily up into the incision for dissection and removal or for wedge excision of a specimen (Fig. 8-3). Following the procedure within the breast, the breast tissue should be reconstructed with interrupted absorbable suture material (Fig. 8-4), the skin closed with a subcuticular stitch (Figs. 8-1, 8-5), and a pressure dressing applied. Drainage is usually not indicated if adequate hemostasis has been secured.

A special problem in breast surgery warrants mention: the patient whose complaint is discharge or bleeding from the nipple and in whom no tumor is palpable. In these instances, *intraductal exploration* is warranted. Compression or massage of the breast under anesthesia usually produces a drop of the discharge from one of the ductal orifices. A lacrimal duct or fine malleable probe can then be inserted into the specific duct (Fig. 8-6), and a small wedge excision carried out through a circumareolar incision using the inserted probe as a guide (Fig. 8-7). Inspection of the specimen usually reveals the small intraductal tumor that caused the bleeding or discharge, and frozen section can establish the diagnosis and determine definitive treatment. The incision is closed as described previously (see Fig. 8-5).

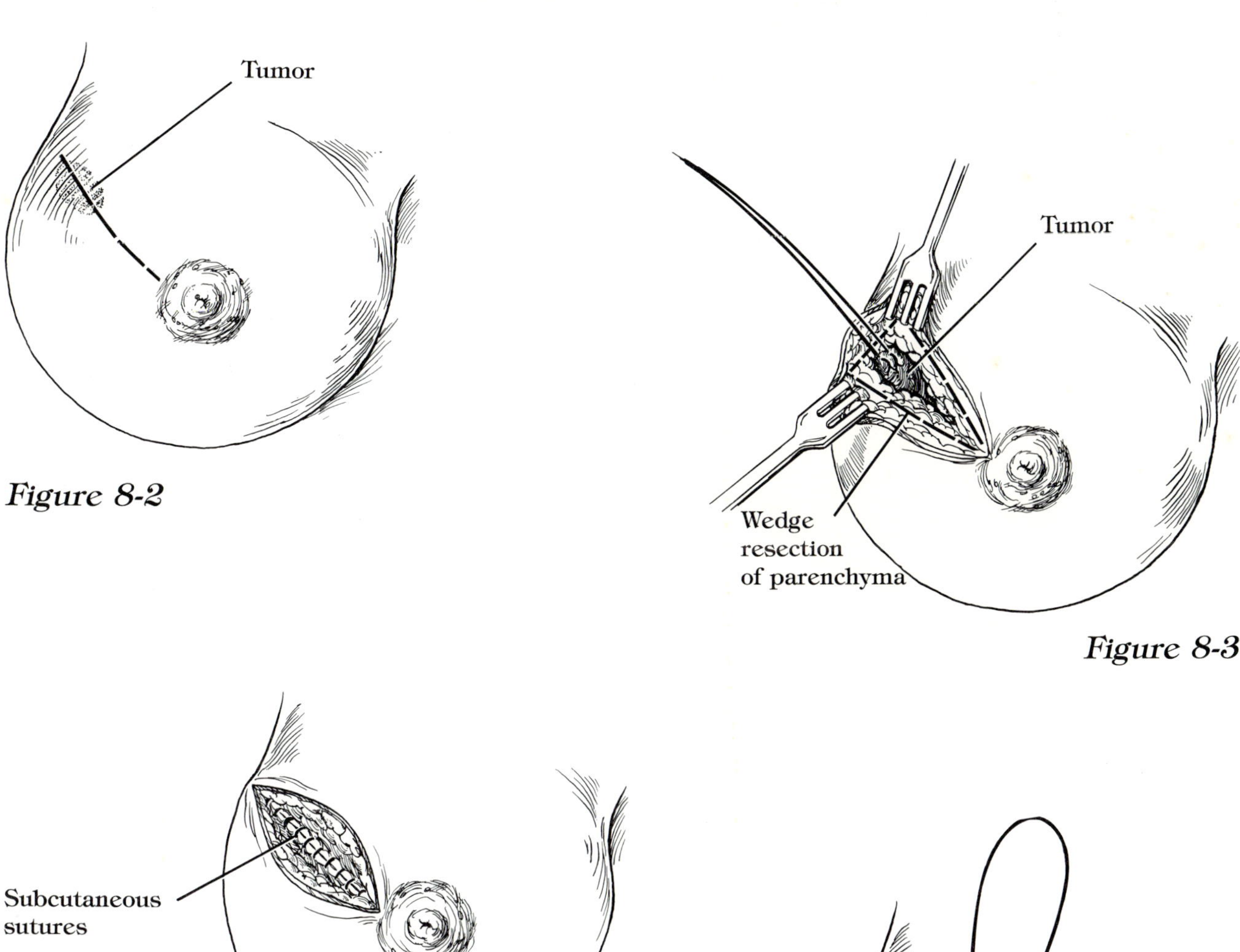

The rationale for the inclusion of an operative procedure that has limited advocacy at present has been defined at the opening of this chapter.

Several different incisions have been suggested for radical mastectomy, and there are variations in the order in which the various steps of the dissection are undertaken. Only one of these is described in the subsequent text and accompanying drawings.

Radical Mastectomy

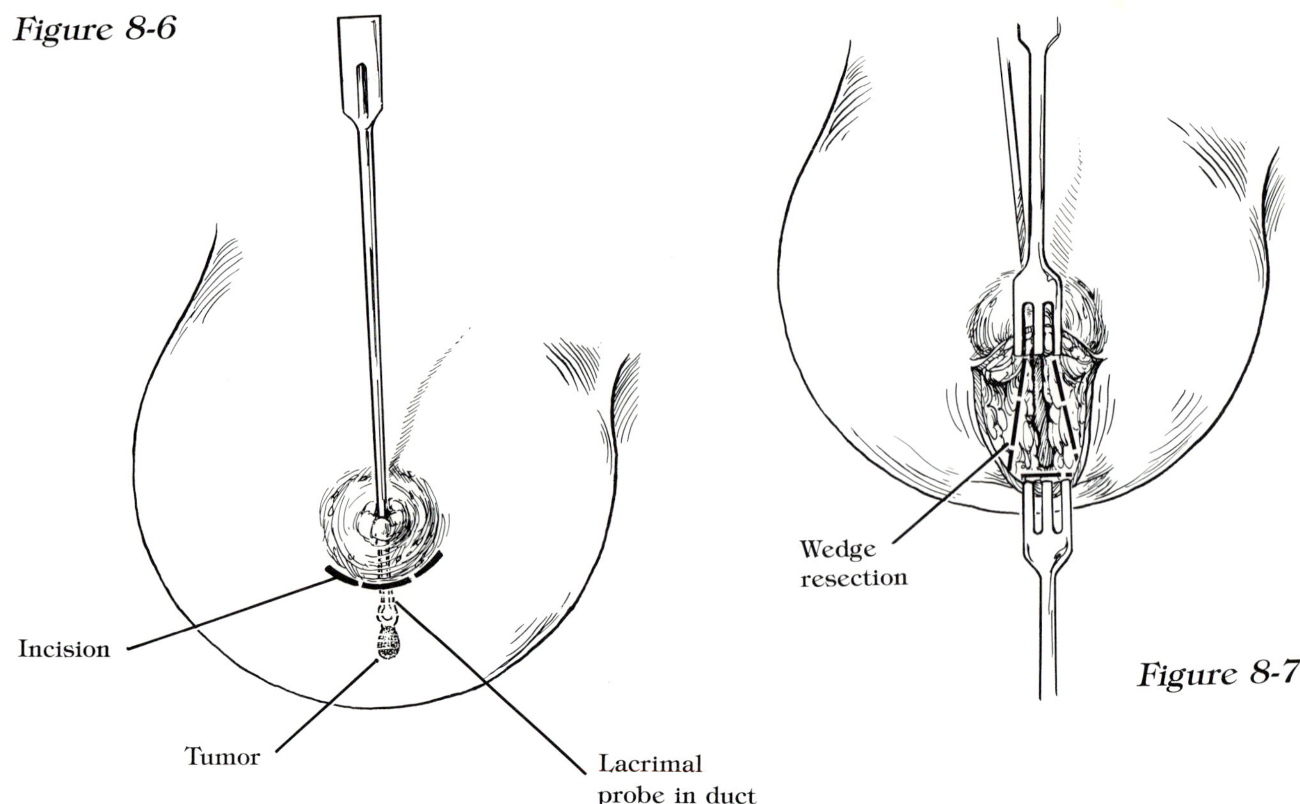

Figure 8-7

The incision is T-shaped. The transverse axillary component begins at the lower border of the clavicle near its midpoint. The course is downward and outward, crossing the free edge of the pectoralis major muscle just below the extension of the axillary hair area. It then continues to the posterior axillary fold at the anterior border of the latissimus dorsi muscle (Fig. 8-8). The downward extension of the incision, which ultimately encompasses the breast, is also shown in Figure 8-8. It begins from a point on the transverse axillary incision near the edge of the pectoralis major muscle, swings first downward then medially toward the sternum around the upper and medial aspect of the breast. The lower component of the breast incision begins at a point in the transverse axillary incision about two inches lower than the upper breast incision. It sweeps downward and then medially around the lateral and inferior borders of the breast to ultimately reach the upper incision on the chest wall well beyond the breast tissue and onto the lateral aspect of the sternum (see Fig. 8-8). The actual placement of these two incisions for the circumferential excision of the breast varies depending on the size of the breast and the location of the tumor.

Skin flaps are then raised from the transverse axillary incision, thus exposing the pectoralis major muscle from its insertion along the line of the clavicle where the fibers of the muscle begin to run parallel to the incision. The insertion of the pectoralis major is then divided close to the humerus. The muscle is split along its fibers of the clavicle, leaving only a few of the lateral fibers of insertion at the upper margin of the incision (Fig. 8-9). If the superior portion of the circumferential breast incision has not already been made, it is necessary to extend this portion of the incision in order to give complete access to the axilla. The cephalic vein, which can be identified as the pectoralis major is divided, should be preserved. After sharp and blunt dissection, the axillary vein can then be identified as it enters the canal behind the subclavius muscle between the clavicle and the first rib. Dissecting distally along the vein, one encounters the medial border of the pectoralis minor muscle, which in turn is divided near its insertion and retracted downward (Figs. 8-9, 8-10), thus giving complete access to the entire axilla. The thoracoacromial vessels and nerves supplying the pectoralis muscles are encountered and divided. If the identity of the nerve is not certain, a gentle pinch with a hemostat results in contraction of the pectoralis muscle and satisfies the surgeon of the exact identity of the nerve, which can then be safely divided. As the lower border of the axilla is reached in the dissection along the axillary vein, the subscapular (or thoracodorsal) nerves and vessels to the latissimus dorsi and subscapular muscles are encountered and should be preserved. Working downward and medially over the surface of the latissimus, one sweeps the axillary contents free from the axilla. The long thoracic nerve can be identified on the chest wall and traced downward to its distribution in the serratus anterior muscle (Fig. 8-11). Beyond this point, there are no nervous or vascular structures to be preserved. When the lower component of the circumferential breast incision is made, dissection can be continued along the chest wall and under the flaps of skin raised from these two incisions until the entire breast, pectoral muscles, and axillary contents are removed (see Fig. 8-11). After hemostasis is secured, the incision is then closed with interrupted silk sutures with suction catheters inserted for drainage. Modified pressure dressing is then applied, although use of the suction catheter has obviated to some extent the need for the heavy pressure dressings utilized in the past (Fig. 8-12).

During the past decade several modifications of the previously accepted procedure of radical mastectomy have appeared. The terminology has not been stabilized because of the numerous individual variations. For the purposes of an atlas, a simple mastectomy with axillary dissection is described, and reference to technical variations on the extent of the latter is included.

    A simple mastectomy or a modified procedure involving some dissection of the axilla can usually be accomplished through a transverse incision that crosses the axilla below the hairline or, depending on the location of the tumor and the re-

SIMPLE OR
MODIFIED RADICAL
MASTECTOMY WITH
AXILLARY
DISSECTION OR
SAMPLING

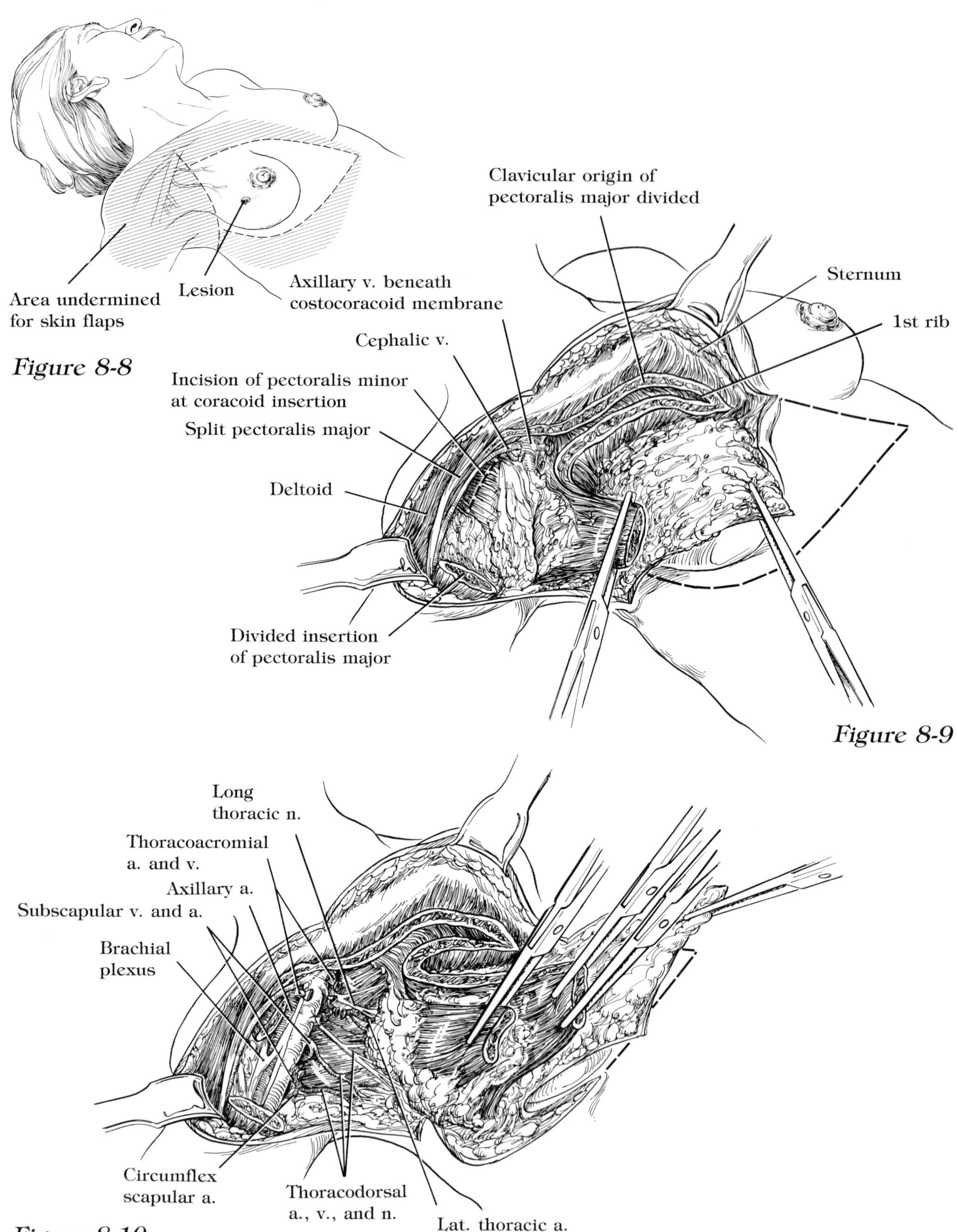

Figure 8-8

Figure 8-9

Figure 8-10

gional anatomy, through a diagonal incision that extends outward and upward over the pectoralis major muscle toward the axilla. Skin flaps with a thin layer of subcutaneous fat are elevated to the extent of the projected resection, which includes all the mammary tissue. This usually carries the flap up to the clavicle superiorly, to the lateral border of the sternum medially, down the chest wall below the lower limits of any extension of the breast tissue, and posteriorly to the lateral border of the pectoralis major muscle. If axillary sampling or dissection is to be included, the incision should be carried across the axilla below the hairline to the anterior border of the latissimus dorsi muscle. Once the flaps have been outlined, an incision is made around the entire area below the flaps vertical to the chest wall and through the superficial fascia overlying the pectoral muscles, which is usually included in the mastectomy (Fig. 8-13). If no axillary procedure is intended, then the breast can be removed as described at the end of this section. If sampling or dissection is to be performed in the axilla, the lateral border of the pectoralis major muscle is identified, dissected free to its insertion, and then retracted superiorly and medially to expose the pectoralis minor muscle and the contents of the midaxilla (Fig. 8-14). The axillary vein is then identified under the retracted edge of the pectoralis major, and the dissection is begun inferiorly to the axillary vein and carried downward toward the midaxilla. In contrast to the historical radical axillary dissection, lymphatic-bearing tissue along the axillary vein should be preserved. The subscapular vessels and nerve should be identified as the dissection proceeds downward; the lateral limits of the operation are thus defined. The axillary fat and node-bearing tissue are then swept inward toward the chest wall and upward toward the retracted pectoralis major muscle with careful identification of the long thoracic nerve, which must be preserved. The axillary contents resulting from this limited axillary dissection are then swept forward. With removal of the pectoral fascia the entire axillary pad and breast can be removed from the chest wall. One individually ligates a number of vessels that traverse the pectoral fascia to enter the breast. The entire breast, the pectoral fascia, and the axillary contents resulting from the limited axillary dissection are then removed (Fig. 8-15). The incision is closed with suction catheters through separate small incisions, and a limited pressure dressing is applied.

Figure 8-11

Pectoralis minor
Pectoralis major
Origin of pectoralis major
from rectus
abdominis
sheath
Origin of
pectoralis minor
Serratus ant.
Subscapular m.
Latissimus dorsi m.

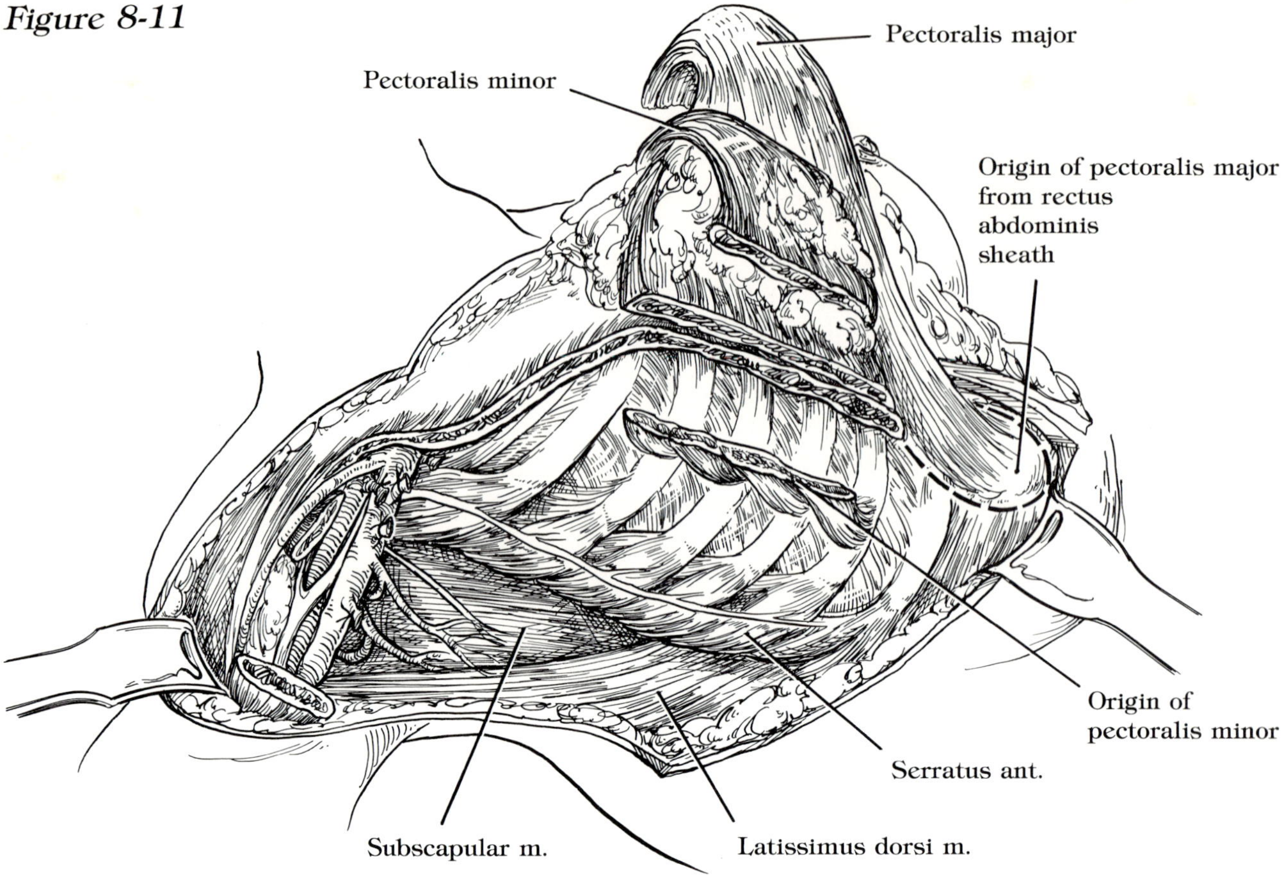

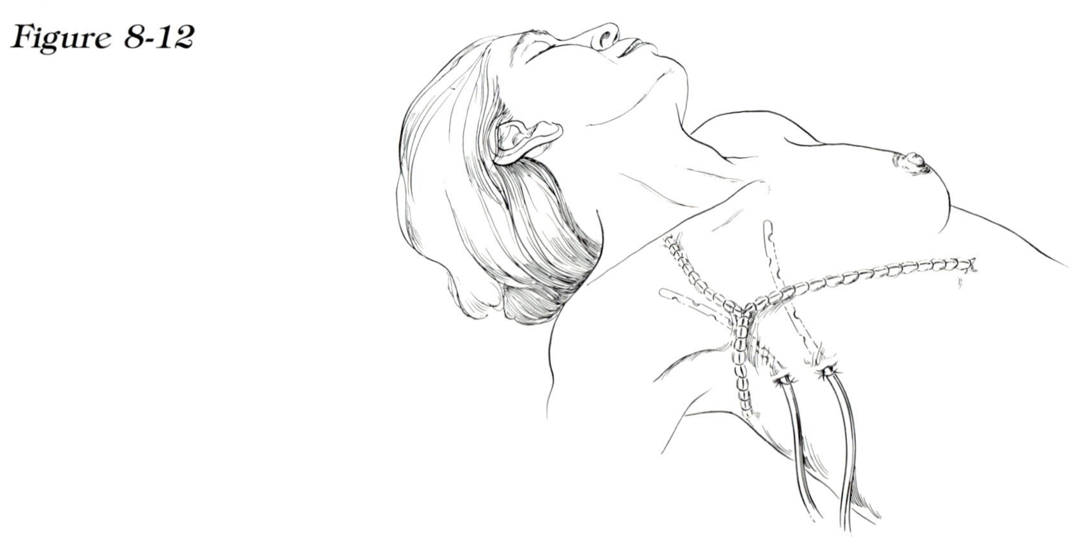

Figure 8-12

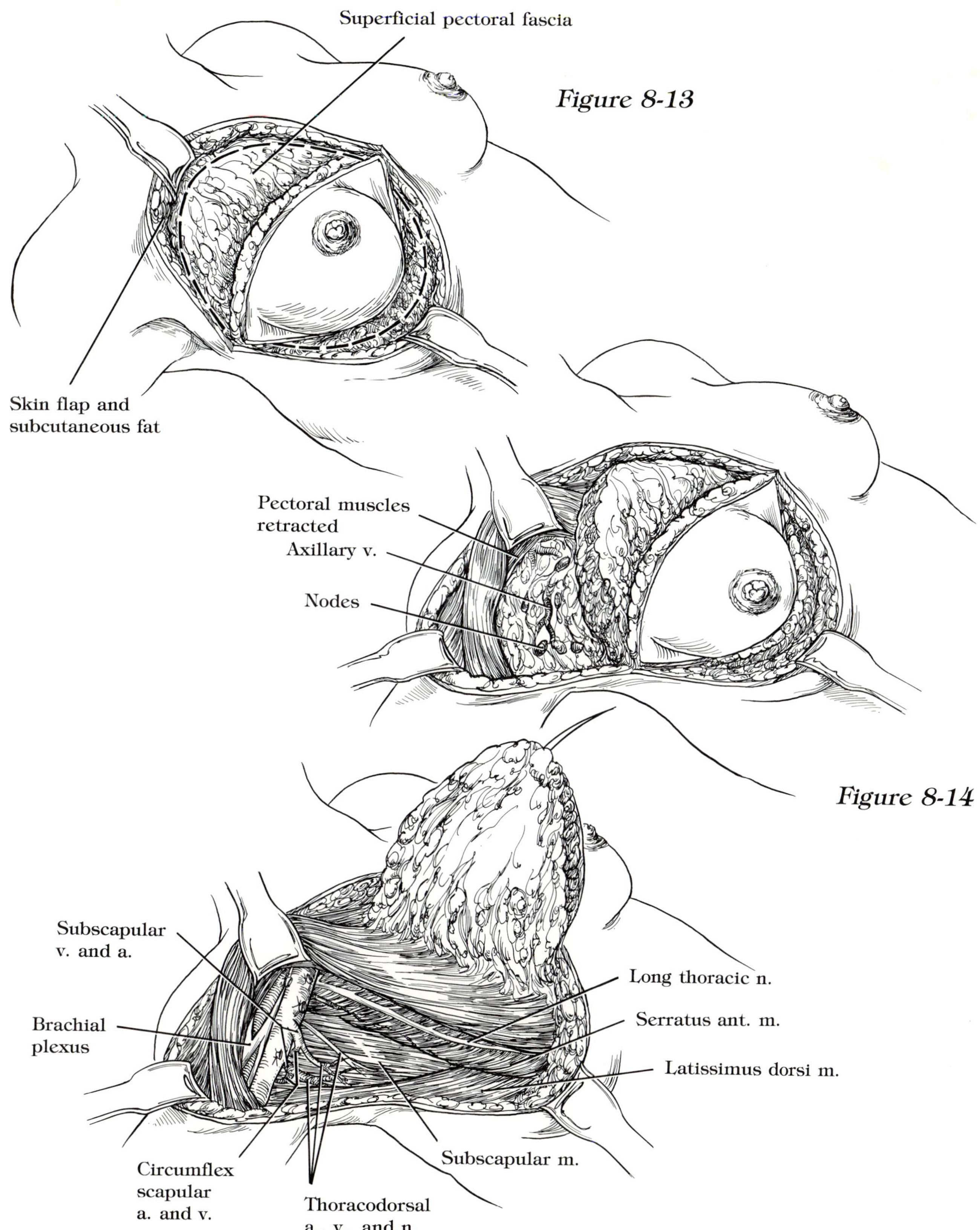

Figure 8-13

Figure 8-14

Figure 8-15

CHAPTER NINE

VASCULAR SYSTEM

ALBERT BOTHE, JR. *and* GARY W. GIBBONS

Arterial Occlusive Disease

This section has been purposely restricted, and no effort has been made to encompass all the corrective and reconstructive procedures available for the treatment of arterial occlusive disease, whether embolic or arteriosclerotic in origin. The more sophisticated details would require a lengthy treatise on the technical surgery, which is available in texts and atlases already available and authored by experts in the field. Rather, this section is limited to a few of the more common procedures likely to be encountered by and managed by surgical residents in training and general surgeons who face the necessity of including some of the more standardized procedures in their ordinary practice.

FEMORAL EMBOLECTOMY

A longitudinal incision is made in the upper thigh over the course of the femoral artery from the inguinal ligament to a point estimated to be distal to the bifurcation of the common femoral artery. Usually the presence of an embolus is apparent both by a bulge in the vessel at the bifurcation and by absence of pulsations distal to this point. When the artery is exposed, the superficial femoral artery distal to the bifurcation is first dissected free and an arterial clamp is applied. The common femoral, superficial femoral, and deep femoral arteries are then dissected, umbilical tapes are passed, and vascular clamps are applied. The use of systemic versus local infusion of heparin is left to the individual surgeon's preference. An arteriotomy is made from the common femoral just above the bifurcation distally over the superficial femoral artery for a total distance of about 3 to 4 cm (Fig. 9-1). The clamp on the superficial femoral artery is then released and this, together with the gentle traction on the clot, results in extrusion of the embolus. The clamps on the deep and superficial femoral arteries are successively released to determine the amount of backbleeding and to flush out any remnants of clot that may have extended down either one of these vessels. A small Fogarty balloon catheter is then inserted distally through the arteriotomy as far as possible down the superficial femoral artery (Fig. 9-2). The balloon is then gently inflated and the catheter withdrawn.

> **CAUTION**
>
> The size of the Fogarty catheter to be used is dependent on the lumen of the artery. One should distend the balloon outside first to appreciate its size and resistance. It is imperative to not inflate the balloon beyond the capacity of the arterial lumen, especially as one is extracting debris or clot proximally or distally.

The distal arterial tree is then flushed with an irrigating catheter and 20 ml of diluted heparin solution. This procedure is then repeated on the deep femoral artery. The clamp on the common femoral artery is released to flush any retained clot. The arteriotomy is then closed with a continuous stitch of 5-0 or 6-0 arterial suture. Just prior to completion of the closure, the clamps on the deep and superficial femoral arteries are released and finally, after completion of the arterial closure, the clamp on the common femoral is released. The incision is closed using interrupted catgut sutures in the femoral sheath and subcutaneous fascia and interrupted nylon sutures in the skin.

SUPERIOR MESENTERIC EMBOLECTOMY

Once the diagnosis of occlusion of the superior mesenteric artery has been established, an upper midline abdominal incision is made. The incision is carried around and below the umbilicus to whatever extent is necessary for adequate exposure. The transverse colon is grasped and retracted firmly upward out of the incision by the assistant, and the first portion of the jejunum is retracted firmly to the left. This maneuver fixes the superior mesenteric artery for identification. An incision is made in the peritoneum just below the estimated duodenal-jejunal junction on the other side of the bowel from the ligament of Treitz (Fig. 9-3). This incision should expose the superior mesenteric artery. With careful, blunt dissection, the midcolic artery can also be identified. The usual embolus lodges just at this point where the superior mesenteric artery narrows. The ligament of Treitz should then be divided and the duodenal-jejunal junction mobilized downward, allowing access to the superior mesenteric ar-

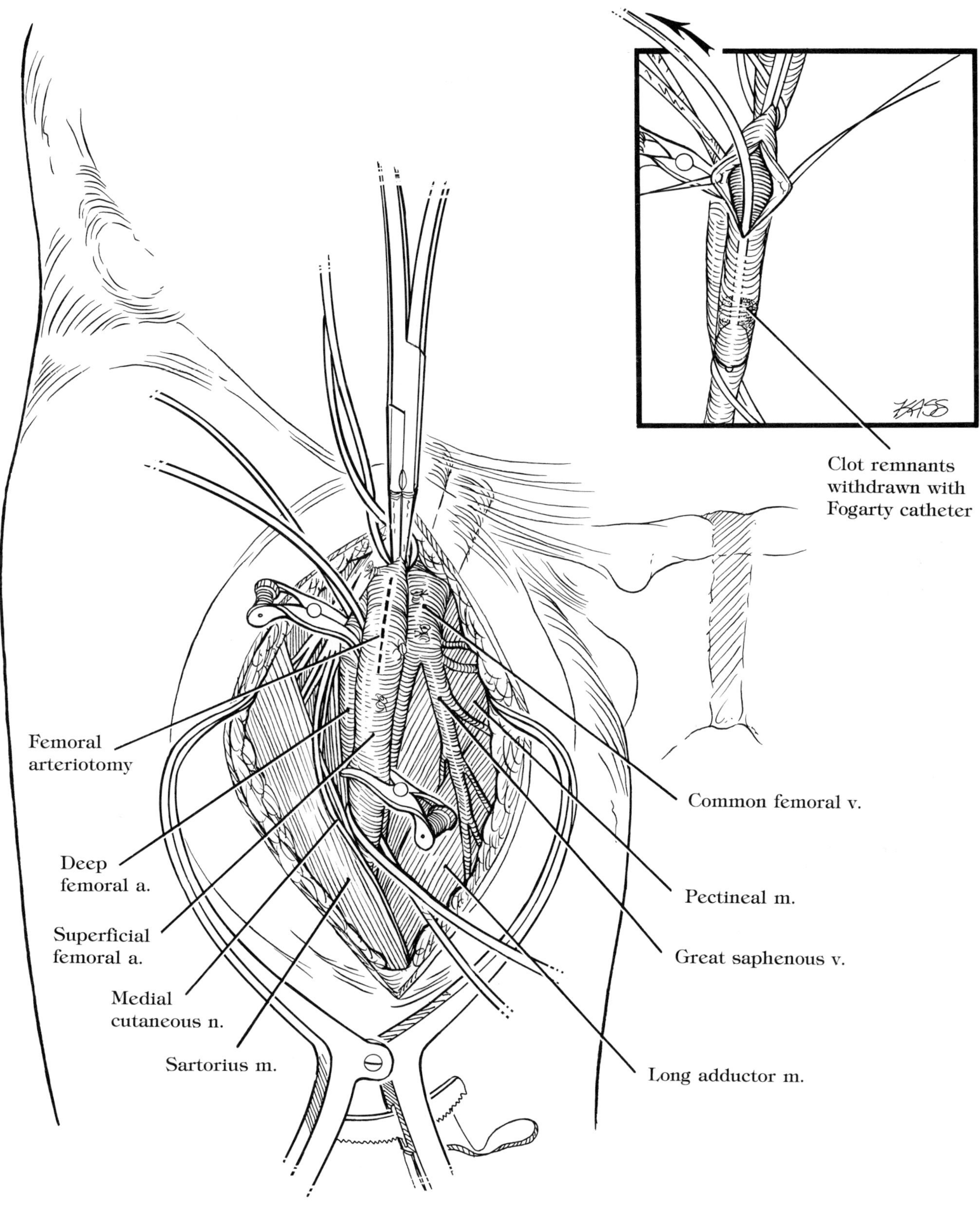

Clot remnants
withdrawn with
Fogarty catheter

Figure 9-1

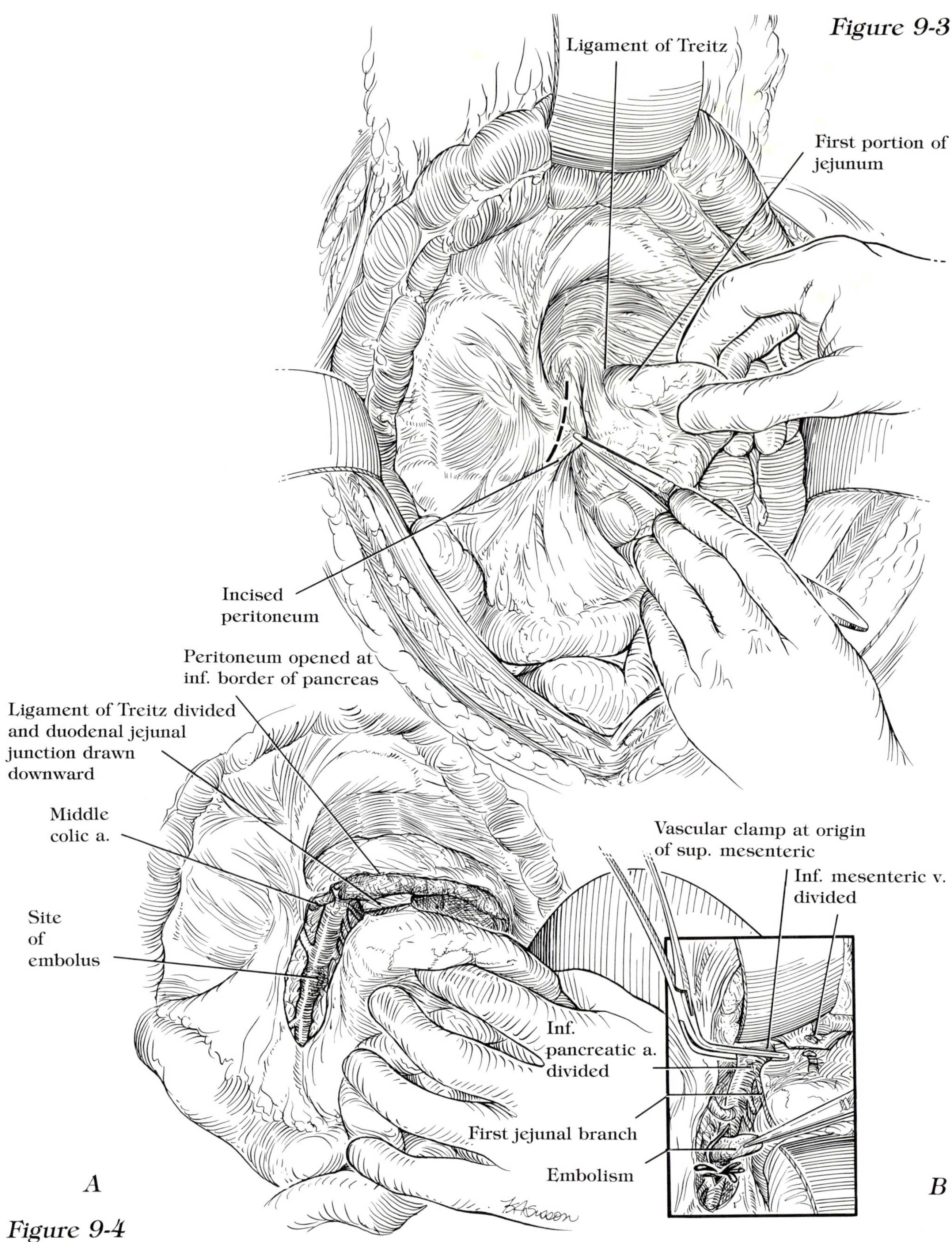

Figure 9-3
Ligament of Treitz
First portion of jejunum
Incised peritoneum
Peritoneum opened at inf. border of pancreas
Ligament of Treitz divided and duodenal jejunal junction drawn downward
Middle colic a.
Site of embolus
Vascular clamp at origin of sup. mesenteric
Inf. mesenteric v. divided
Inf. pancreatic a. divided
First jejunal branch
Embolism
A
B
Figure 9-4

tery as it passes beneath the inferior border of the pancreas (Fig. 9-4A). The pancreas should be dissected free along its border and retracted anteriorly and superiorly to expose the origin of the superior mesenteric artery beneath the pancreas. An arterial clamp is then placed as high as possible along the superior mesenteric artery, and an anterior arteriotomy is performed so that the embolus can be grasped and extracted (Fig. 9-4B). If distal flow is not achieved to the extent necessary to flush out remnants of clot, a Fogarty catheter may be introduced in the fashion described for femoral embolectomy and withdrawn with steady, gentle pressure. The proximal clamp can be temporarily released to ascertain the presence of pulsatile flow. If flow is not adequate, the Fogarty catheter may be introduced proximally upward and into the aorta and then retracted back through the arteriotomy to remove any occluding clot or atheromatous debris. Once pulsatile flow has been reestablished, the arteriotomy is closed with a continuous 5-0 or 6-0 arterial suture.

The abdomen is draped after the skin is prepared with an operative field which extends from the nipples to the mid-thighs bilaterally. The pubic area is covered with a separate drape. An incision is made from midxiphoid to pubis in the midline curving slightly about the umbilicus. The abdomen is explored in the usual manner, and the size and operability of the aneurysm are assessed. Dissection is then begun in the midline over the aorta. One divides the attachments of the third and fourth portions of the duodenum and ligament of Treitz (Fig. 9-5). One then directs the dissection caudad, dividing the peritoneum over the aortoiliac bifurcation in the midline and exposing both common iliac arteries.

RESECTION OF AN
ABDOMINAL
AORTIC ANEURYSM

> CAUTION
>
> It is imperative to discern sexual function preoperatively in male patients undergoing aortoiliac dissection. Extensive dissection in the aortoiliac area may disrupt sympathetic fibers resulting in impotence postoperatively. Careful and minimal dissection of this area is important in young and sexually active males.

The sigmoid mesentery is retracted laterally to expose the left common and external iliac arteries. The inferior mesenteric artery is usually ligated and divided, but the inferior mesenteric vein can usually be preserved as it traverses retroperitoneally upward and disappears under the body and tail of the pancreas. If the cecum, right colon, and portion of the small bowel can be

Divided
ligament of Treitz
Inf. mesenteric v.
Lt. gonadal v.
Aneurysm
Inf. mesenteric a.
Post. parietal
peritoneum
Lt. renal v.
identified
Rt. gonadal
vessels
identified
I.V.C.
Rt. ureter
Inf.
mesenteric
a. divided
Umbilical tapes
on rt. common
iliac a.

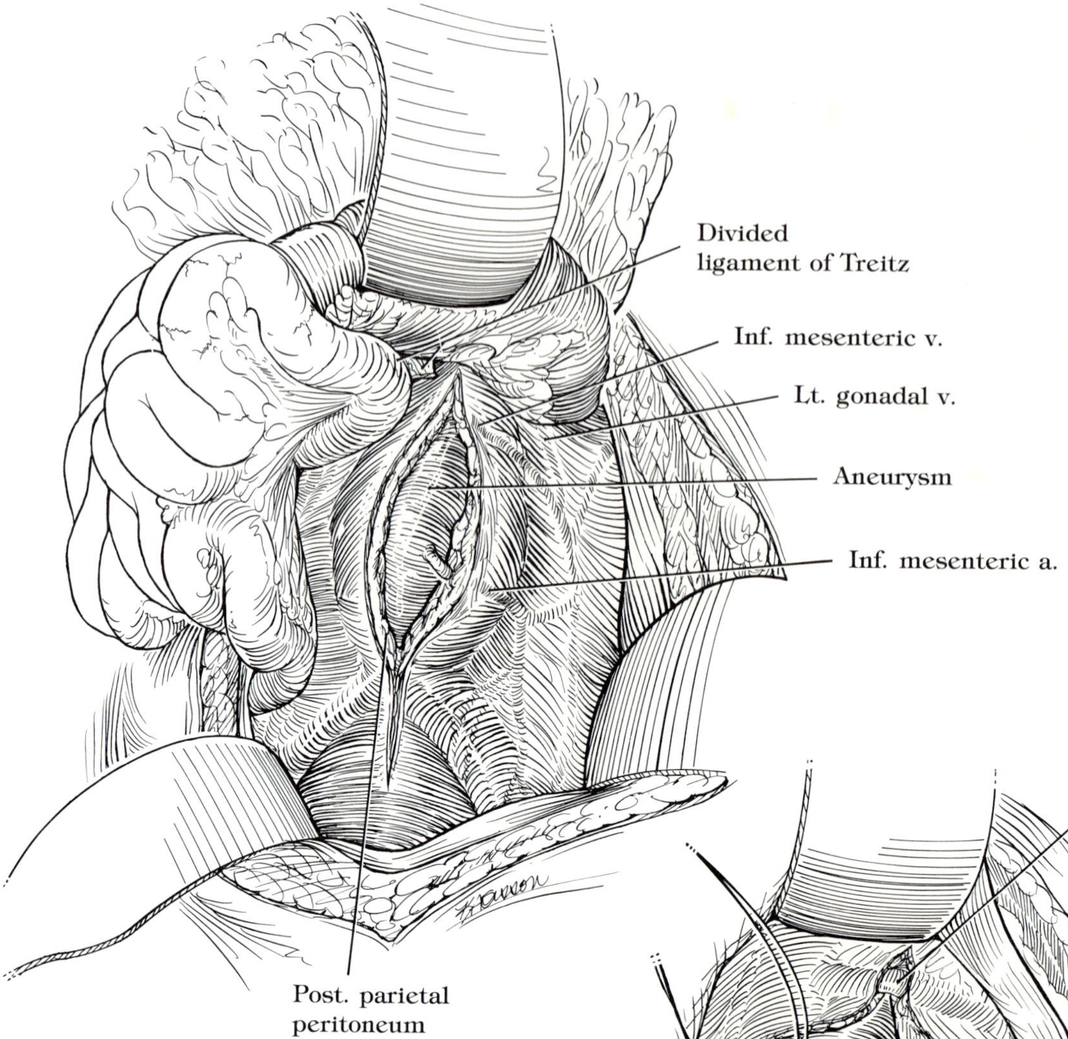

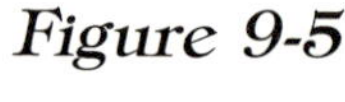

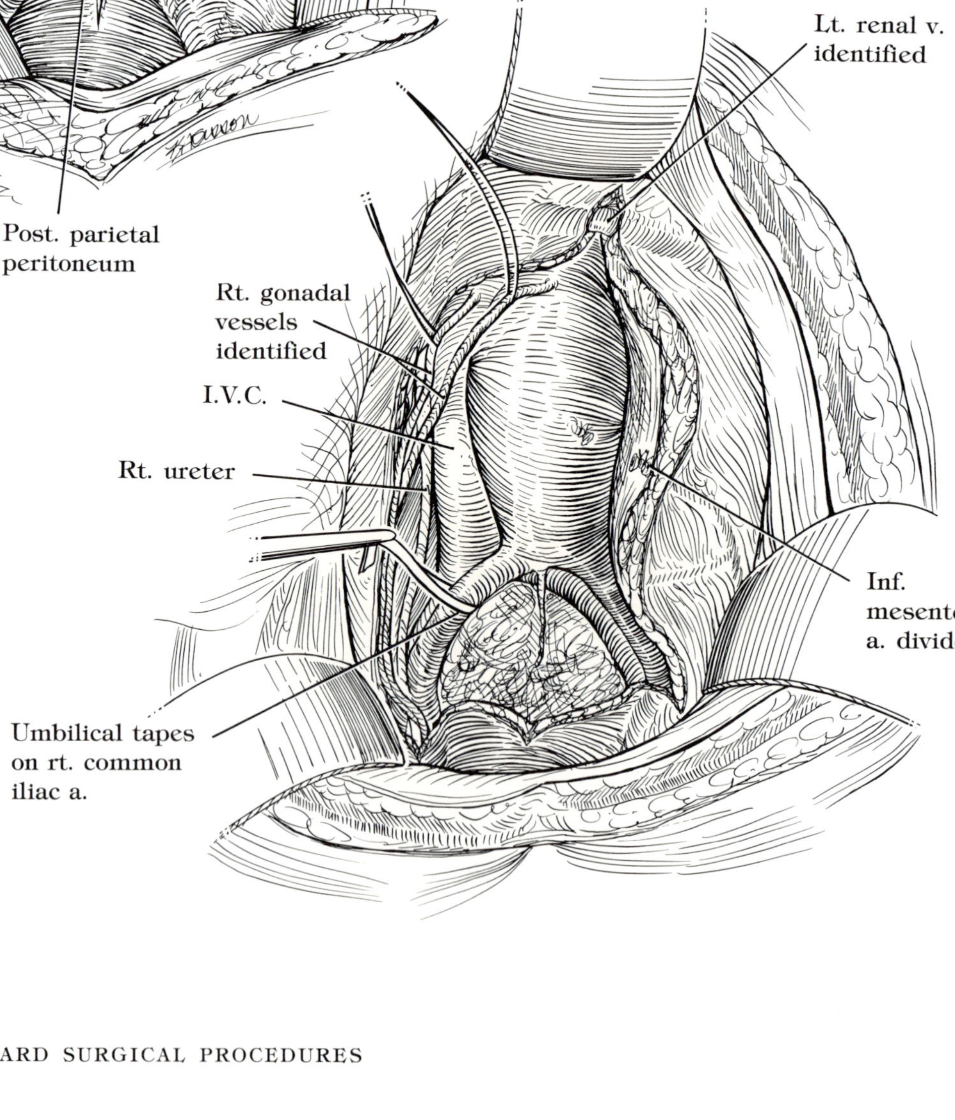

Figure 9-6

packed into the right upper quadrant and the remainder of the small bowel and left colon into the left upper quadrant, then the operation can proceed. Adequate exposure and safety are imperative, however, and the surgeon should not hesitate to eviscerate the entire small bowel into a Lahey bag filled with warm saline solution. One then dissects up the right lateral aspect of the aneurysm, identifying the gonadal vessels and the right ureter. A tape is passed around the common iliac artery in its midportion (Fig. 9-6).

As dissection proceeds superiorly on the right side, many small arterial and venous branches may be encountered in the retroperitoneal area and individually ligated. If a good cleavage plane exists between the aorta and the inferior vena cava, the two vessels are separated by dissection. Often, however, the aneurysm is adherent posteriorly to the vena cava and cannot be safely separated; therefore, the posterior wall of the aneurysm ultimately must be left in situ. Dissection then proceeds up the left side of the aorta so the aneurysm is as free as possible up to the point where the left renal vein crosses what is usually relatively normal aorta. As one dissects posteriorly at this point, a triangular open space usually exists where posterior wall of the normal aorta has been lifted anteriorly by the expansion of the aneurysm. At this point the aorta is cross-clamped. A soft Satinsky or a Crawford vascular clamp is relatively safe and less likely to fracture the aorta than some other instruments. During the dissection, the right and left ureters should both be identified and protected. The choice of systemic versus local infusion of heparin is left to the preference of the surgeon. When proximal and distal control have been obtained, the iliac arteries can then be divided and the proximal ends held with bulldog clamps while soft vascular or bulldog clamps are placed on the distal ends of these vessels (Fig. 9-7). If the aneurysm is not adherent, it can then be turned upward and dissected carefully off the vertebral column and the vena cava. Lumbar arteries and veins are divided and ligated as they are encountered. The proximal aorta is transected, and a bifurcated graft inserted with end-to-end anastomoses (to be described) to the aorta and to the distal ends of the common iliac arteries. If, however, the aorta is adherent to the vena cava, the aneurysm should be entered and the anterior portion resected leaving the posterior wall of the aneurysmal sac adherent to the vena cava with the distal and proximal extent of the disease usually transected. The sac may be sewn over the graft later after any open vessels are stitched and calcium and debris are removed from the lining. In either case, a woven or knitted prosthesis is selected for size and the posterior edge sewn to the posterior wall of the aorta with an everting interrupted mattress suture (Fig. 9-8). A 3-0 arterial suture (preferably braided) is used for this anastomosis. This is continued as an everting over-and-over running

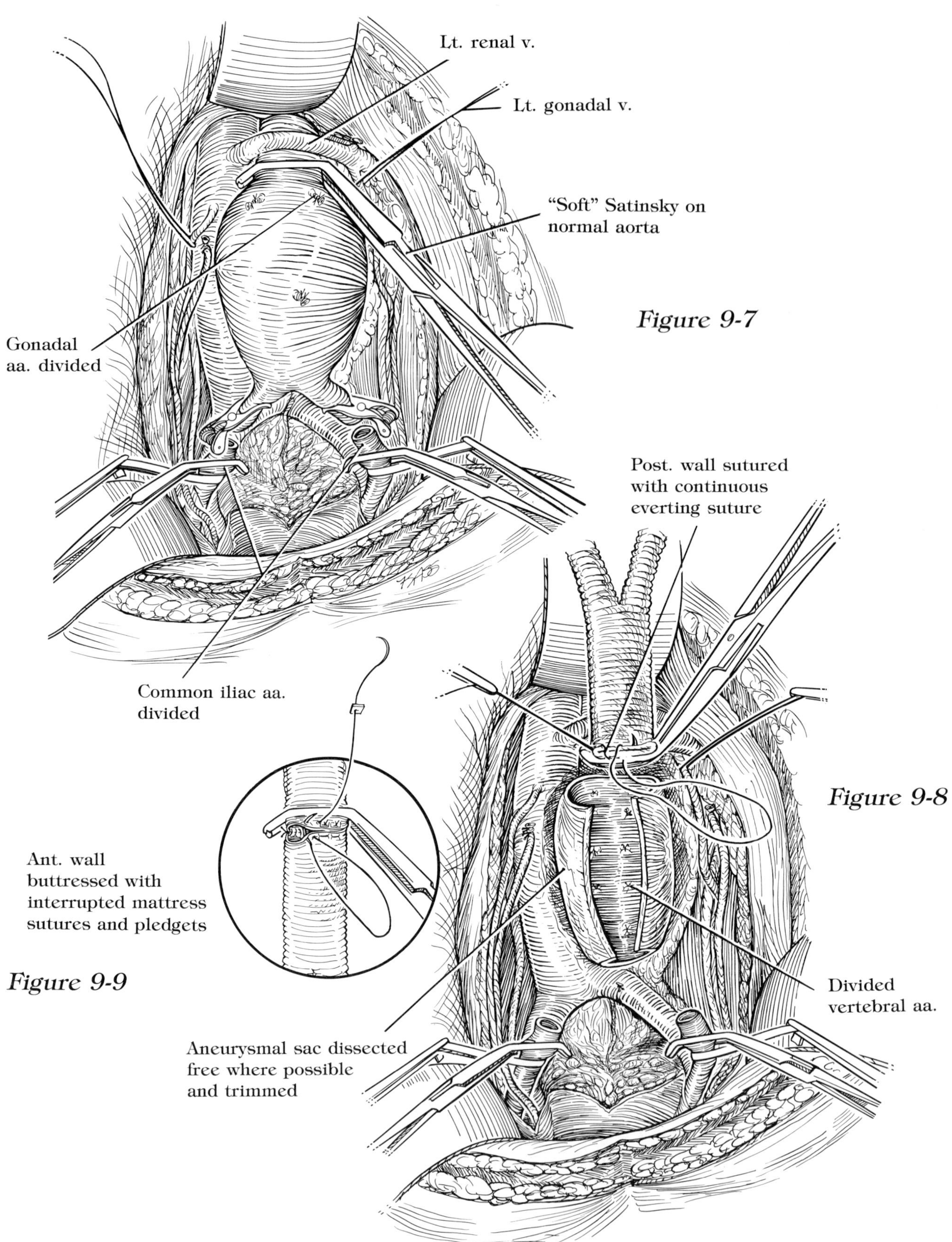

Figure 9-7

Figure 9-8

Figure 9-9

suture to the anterior midportion of the anastomosis where the sutures are tied. The graft is then turned back to a normal position, continuing the anterior row in a similar fashion. If the wall of the aorta is extensively diseased and weak, the entire proximal anastomosis may be performed using interrupted mattress sutures buttressing the outer aortic wall with Teflon pledgets (Fig. 9-9). An over-and-over suture around the outer edges further guarantees a hemostatically secure anastomosis. Whenever possible, the suture should start from the inside of the artery to minimize intimal tearing or fracturing of atherosclerotic plaque.

The distal ends of the bifurcation graft are trimmed to fit the common iliac arteries. End-to-end anastomoses are constructed, again using a 4-0 arterial suture. Prior to final closure of the first distal anastomosis, the common iliac artery clamp is released for back flushing, and then the aortic clamp is released for one or two pulsations to flush out both limbs of the graft. The anastomosis is completed and a soft vascular clamp is placed on the proximal uncompleted limb. Blood flow is reestablished on the completed side. The last distal anastomosis is completed, flushed in a similar manner, and the vascular clamps released. The aortic and iliac clamps should be released slowly in order to avoid sudden hypotension. Transfusions or intravenous fluids should be running at an appropriate rate with careful patient monitoring. The technique as described may prove to be an oversimplification since many technical complications may be encountered, particularly if atherosclerotic disease extends well down into the iliac vessels with calcification sufficient to make anastomosis technically difficult. A more severe problem can be encountered if the length of normal aorta above the aneurysm is limited. Space, however, precludes itemized details of all the variations that may be encountered in abdominal aortic aneurysms and the variations in procedural approach that must be utilized. An atlas specifically devoted to vascular surgery would discuss these variants in more detail.

An abdominal incision from xiphoid to pubis is made for wide exposure. Dissection proceeds as for an aortic aneurysm, and tapes are passed around the aorta and the external iliac and hypogastric arteries. The choice of systemic versus local infusion of heparin is left to individual preference. The aorta is cross-clamped. Soft bulldog clamps are used to temporarily occlude the external iliac and hypogastric arteries. The aorta is then incised, and the incision is extended distally on the side with the most extensive disease (see Caution). The opposite iliac artery is incised, but the incisions are not joined (Fig. 9-10). The plaque is freed up in the aorta. A plane is established between the plaque and the media (Fig. 9-11*B*). The opposite side is treated in a similar fashion, and the entire atheroma is

AORTOILIAC
ENDARTERECTOMY

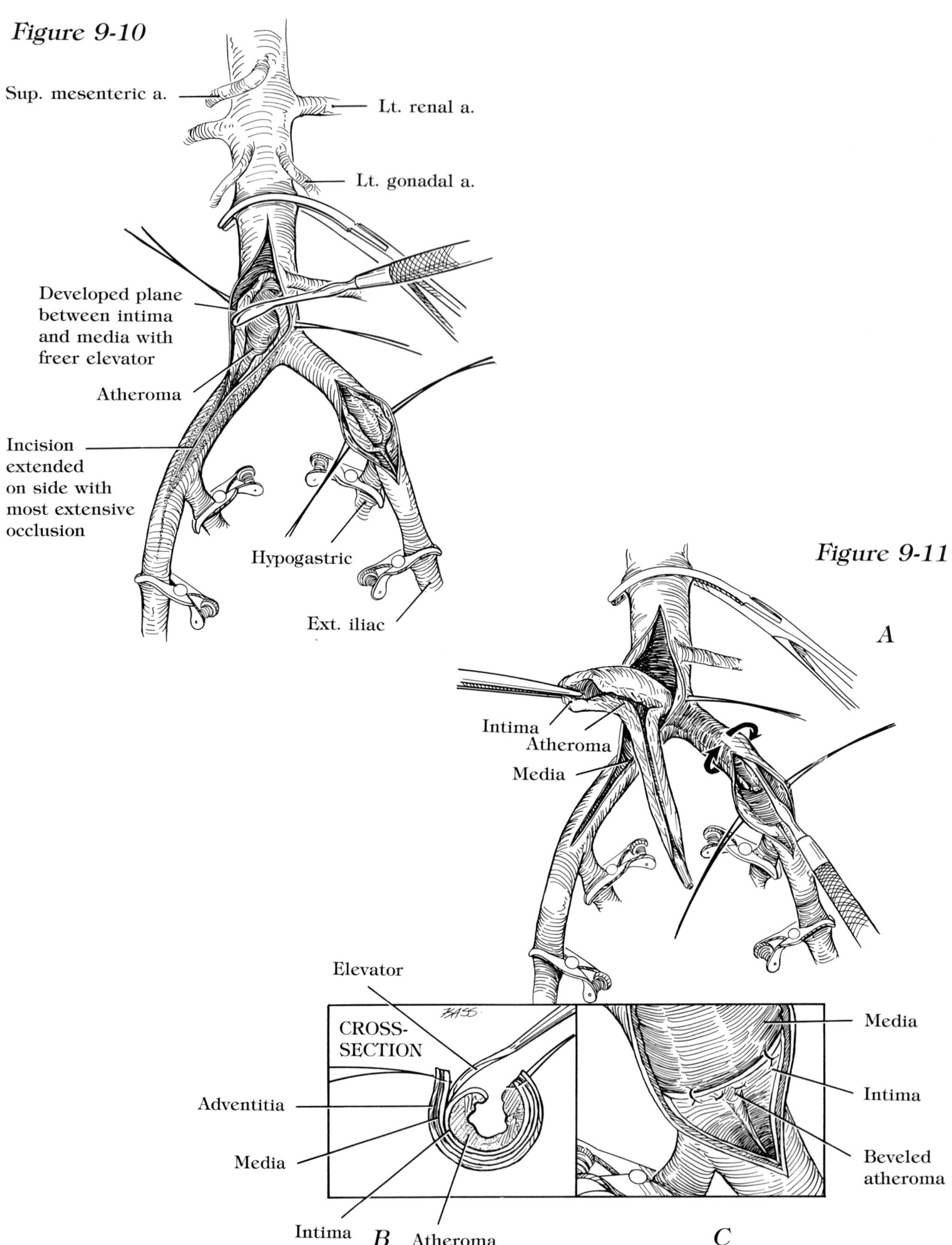

Figure 9-10
Sup. mesenteric a.
Lt. renal a.
Lt. gonadal a.
Developed plane between intima and media with freer elevator
Atheroma
Incision extended on side with most extensive occlusion
Hypogastric
Ext. iliac
Figure 9-11
A
Intima
Atheroma
Media
Elevator
CROSS-SECTION
Adventitia
Media
Intima
Atheroma
B
Media
Intima
Beveled atheroma
C

removed (Fig. 9-11*A*). The distal intimal margins are beveled and tacked with 6-0 arterial sutures (Fig. 9-11*C*). Flow is restored by closing (3-0 or 4-0 arterial suture) the longer arteriotomy to within 1 to 2 cm of the distal end, releasing the hypogastric and iliac bulldogs and aortic clamp sequentially to flush out clots and debris before final closure. Similar closure and flushing procedure are performed on the opposite iliac. Rarely, the endarterectomy must be carried below the inguinal ligament, in which case additional separate incisions and femoral arteriotomies may be necessary.

When aortoiliac occlusions are extensive, a bypass operation is used to restore flow. Depending on the extent of the occlusions, various procedures may be used, one of which is shown in Figure 9-12*A, B.*

On occasion this procedure may be combined with more distal bypass procedures to be described. (Femoral popliteal bypass is depicted in Figures 9-13 through 9-16.) Variations involving the axillary arteries and crossover procedures are not covered in this text.

This operation is predicated on the existence of at least one patent branch of the popliteal artery and the previous correction of any proximal stenoses in the aortoiliac channel. The bypass that is invariably employed today is a long reversed saphenous vein graft. Both the removal and the insertion of the vein graft require meticulous, precise, and gentle handling if the bypass is to be successful. A continuous incision is made over the course of the saphenous vein. If the vein is greater than 4 mm in diameter at its smallest end, the tributaries are ligated with 4-0 silk and the vein graft is placed in cold heparinized blood or solution after removal. The popliteal artery is explored through the distal portion of the incision to determine patency, and tapes are placed around the proximal and distal ends (Fig. 9-13). Through the inguinal portion of the incision, one opens the femoral sheath and dissects the artery proximally and distally, identifying and passing tapes around the common, superficial, and deep arteries.

The incision above the knee is deepened and the sartorius muscle retracted posteriorly, exposing the superficial femoral artery at this level. A tunnel is then made by blunt dissection to the popliteal and common femoral dissections following the course of the superficial femoral artery. The choice of systemic versus local instillation of heparin is left to the individual preference of the surgeon. After heparin is administered, a soft area of the popliteal artery is chosen for the anastomosis, and gentle vascular clamps are applied to the proximal and distal segments. An arteriotomy is made, and the distal clamp is released to allow evaluation of runoff. Varying amounts of heparinized

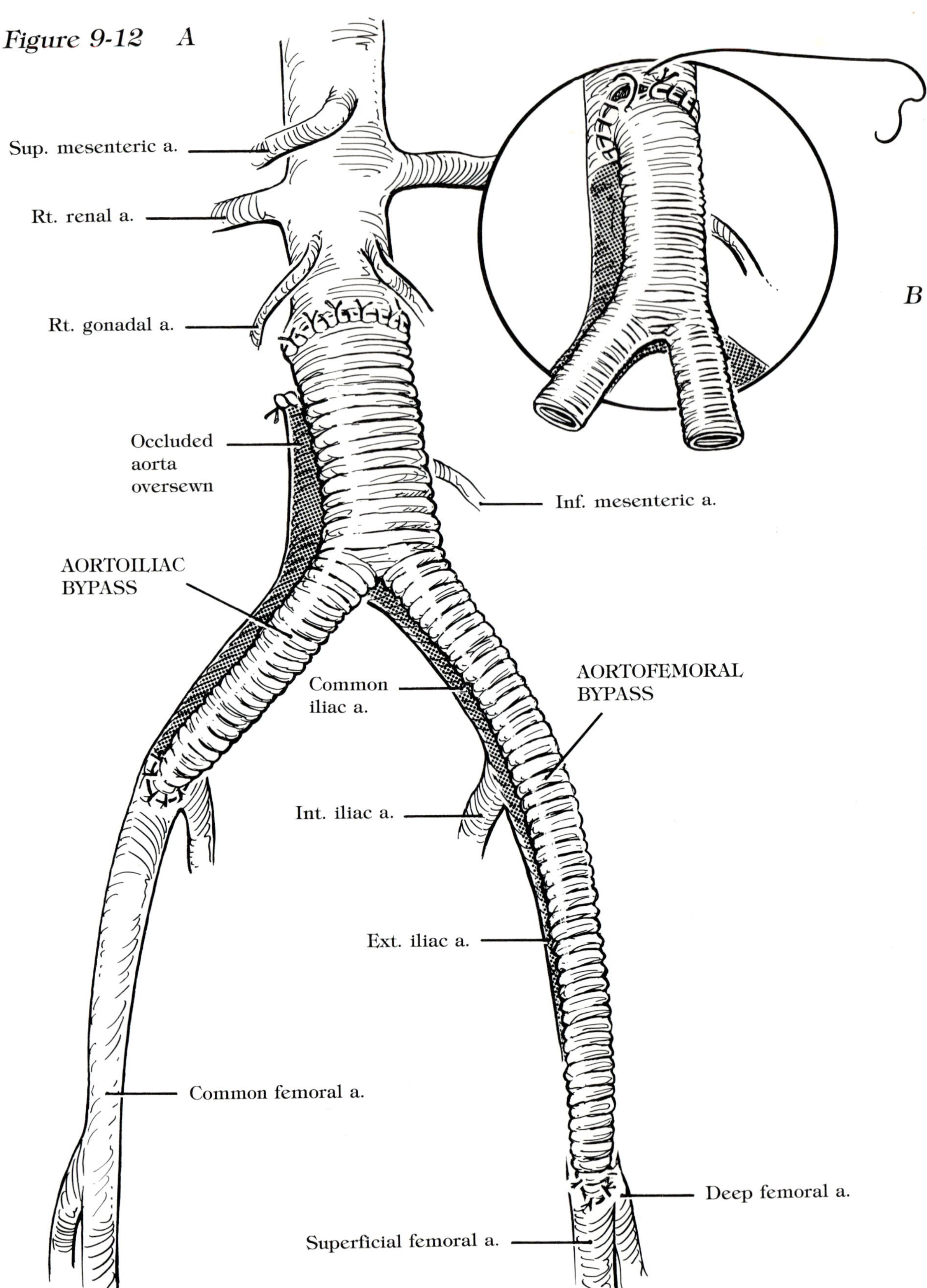

Figure 9-12   A
B
Sup. mesenteric a.
Rt. renal a.
Rt. gonadal a.
Occluded
aorta
oversewn
Inf. mesenteric a.
AORTOILIAC
BYPASS
Common
iliac a.
AORTOFEMORAL
BYPASS
Int. iliac a.
Ext. iliac a.
Common femoral a.
Deep femoral a.
Superficial femoral a.

saline are instilled, depending on prior systemic heparinization. The vein graft is then gently distended again to be sure there are no leaks or constrictions. The vein is reversed and the now proximal end tapered to fit the arteriotomy. The surgeon sews it in place with a running 6-0 arterial suture, beginning with the proximal end of the arteriotomy and sewing from vein to artery distally (Fig. 9-14). The suture is interrupted at the distal end; one must take care not to narrow the lumen at this most crucial

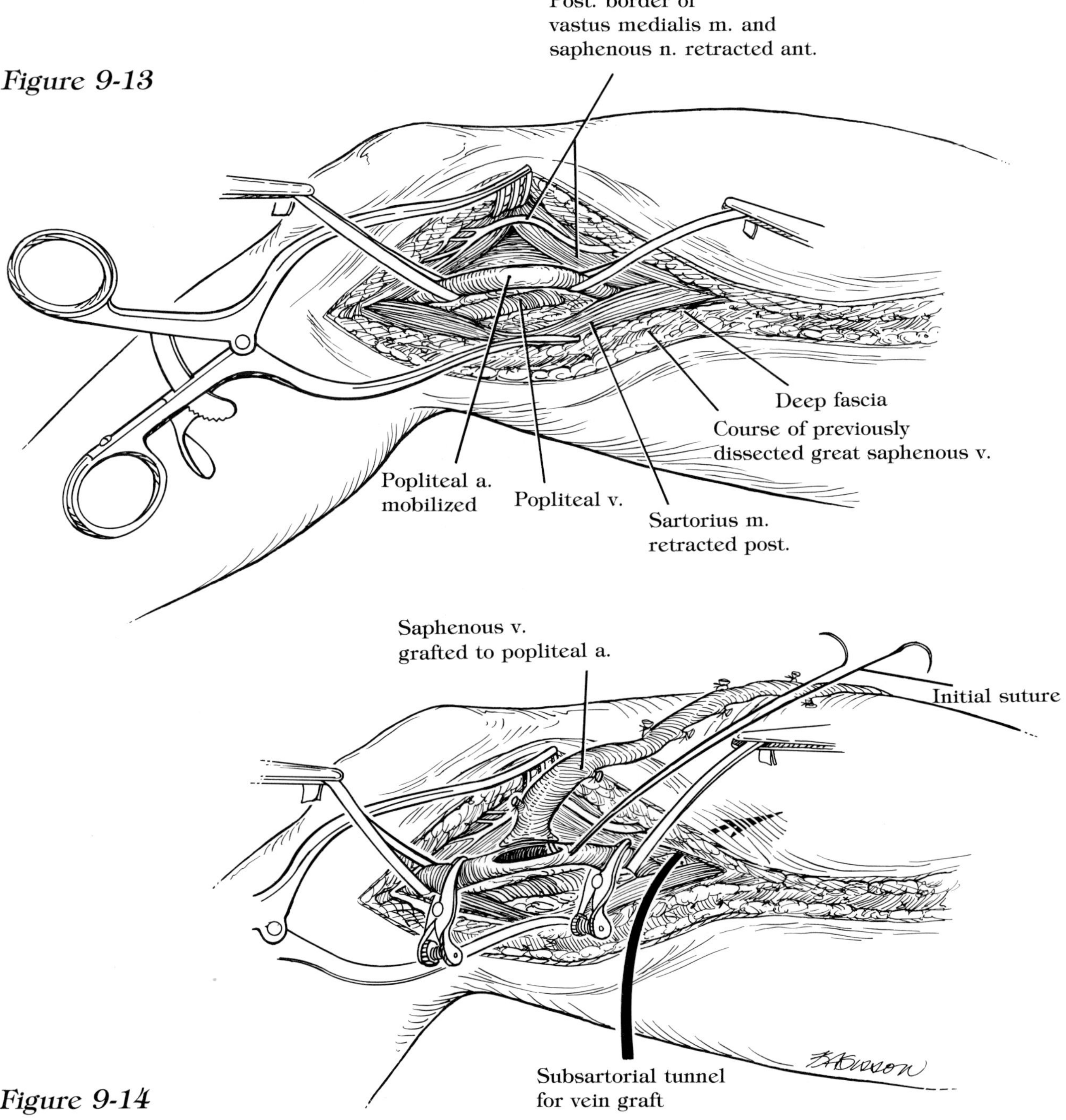

Figure 9-13

Figure 9-14

point. After completing the anastomosis, one gently distends the vein graft again to ensure that the anastomosis is hemostatically secure. One then passes it through the tunnel making sure there are no twists. Gentle vascular clamps are placed on the common, superficial, and deep arteries. An arteriotomy is made in the softest area, as shown in Figure 9-15. Heparinized saline is instilled proximally and distally, the amount varying with the type of previous heparinization. After the appropriate tension is determined, the vein graft is tapered and sutured with 5-0 or 6-0 arterial suture. One begins the anastomosis at the distal end of the arteriotomy, taking care not to narrow the vein graft lumen (Fig. 9-16). The anastomosis progresses proximally. One sews from vein to artery, interrupting the suture line at the apex. The arteriotomy is flushed proximally and distally prior to final closure. The clamps are released and tapes removed after one insures hemostasis and good flow into the distal arterial tree. The deep fascia is closed carefully to prevent possible constriction of the graft. The subcutaneous tissue and skin are closed in a conventional manner.

Amputations General principles of, indications for, and variations on amputations of the lower extremity are more extensively covered in atlases and texts concerned entirely with vascular surgery. In this section, only three types of amputations are considered. These are approached as if each procedure were elective, closed, and definitive.

ABOVE-KNEE AMPUTATION A circular incision is made in the skin just above the superior border of the patella and is carried directly down to the bone anteriorly without undermining (Fig. 9-17). A malleable retractor is inserted between the femur and the posterior portion of the thigh structures. The bone is transected with a saw (Fig. 9-18) after the periosteum is divided and stripped distally for 1 to 2 cm. The point of transection is determined by the natural retraction of the skin, soft tissues, and muscles, but is generally 1½ to 2 inches proximal to the skin incision. After the femur is divided, the proximal popliteal artery and vein can be identified at the medial side of the upper popliteal fossa. These are clamped, cut, and doubly ligated (Fig. 9-19). The sciatic nerve, which can be visualized on the lateral side of the fossa, is crushed. A chromic catgut ligature is applied with the nerve on tension so that it will retract well up into the thigh after division (Fig. 9-19, inset). The deep fascia is closed without tension with 3-0 chromic catgut sutures, and the skin is approximated with interrupted nonreactive suture material.

BELOW-KNEE AMPUTATION The nature of the skin incision varies considerably with the size of the lower extremity and the degree of muscular fullness. As a generalization, the anterior skin incision is usually located

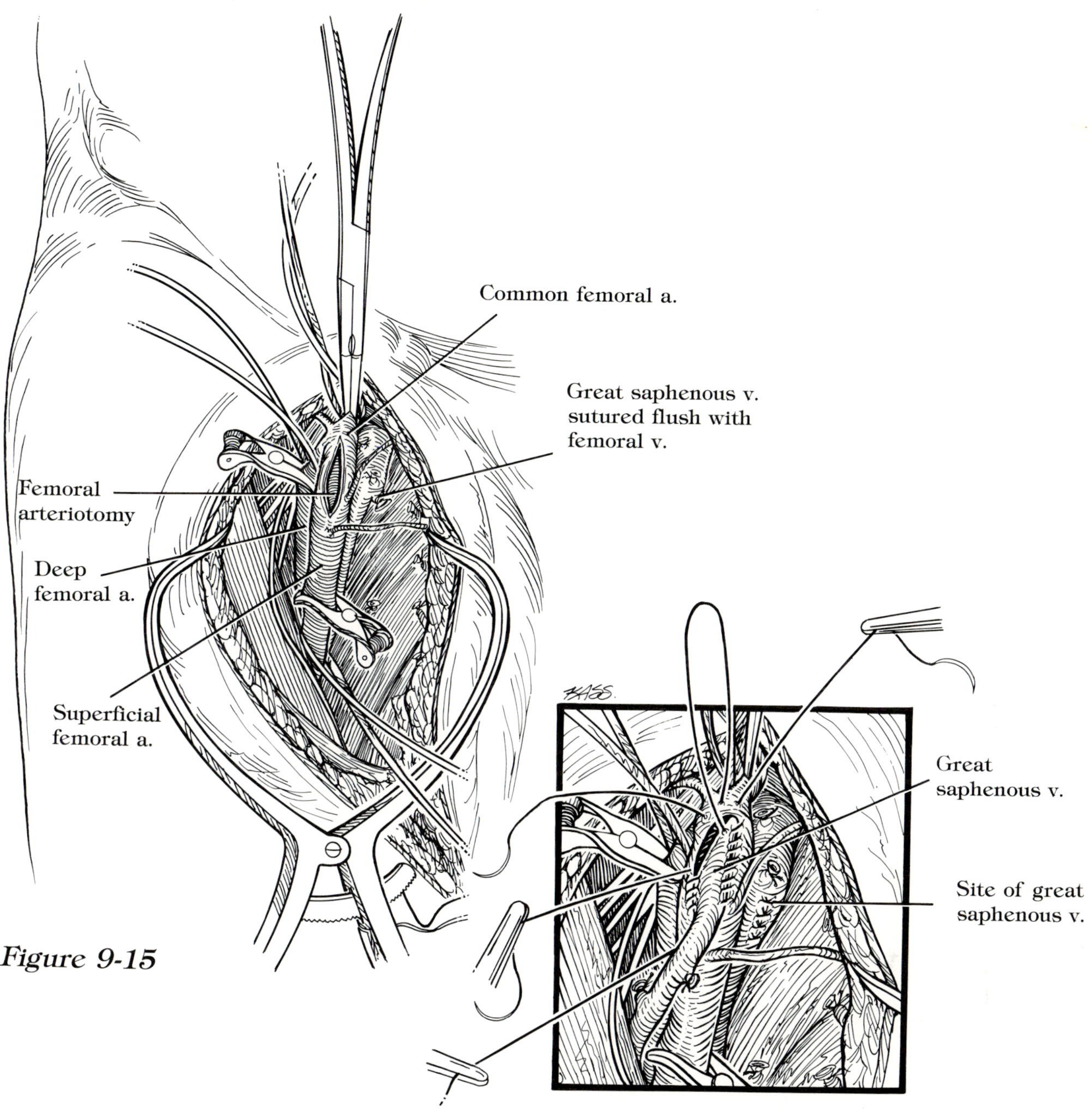

Figure 9-15

Figure 9-16

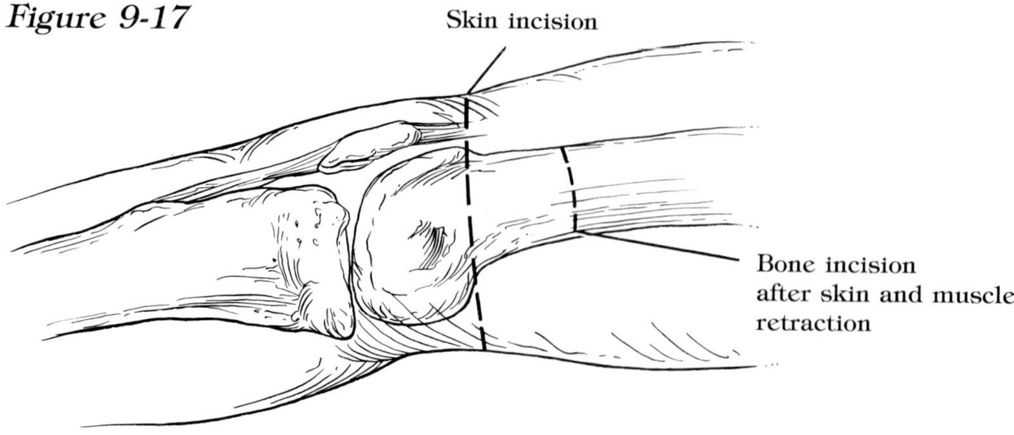

Figure 9-17

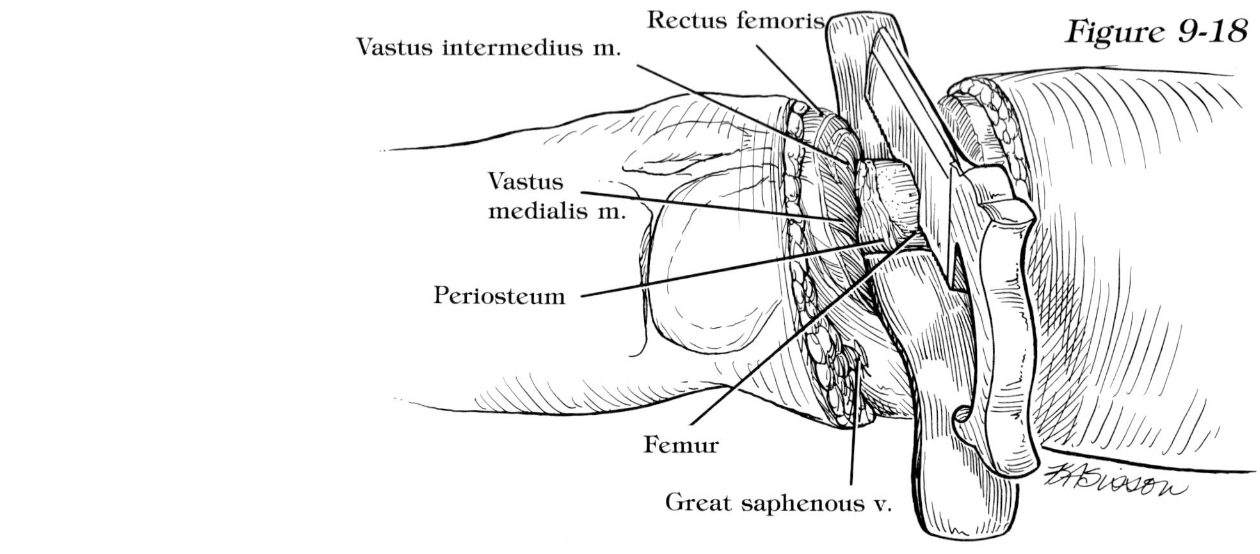

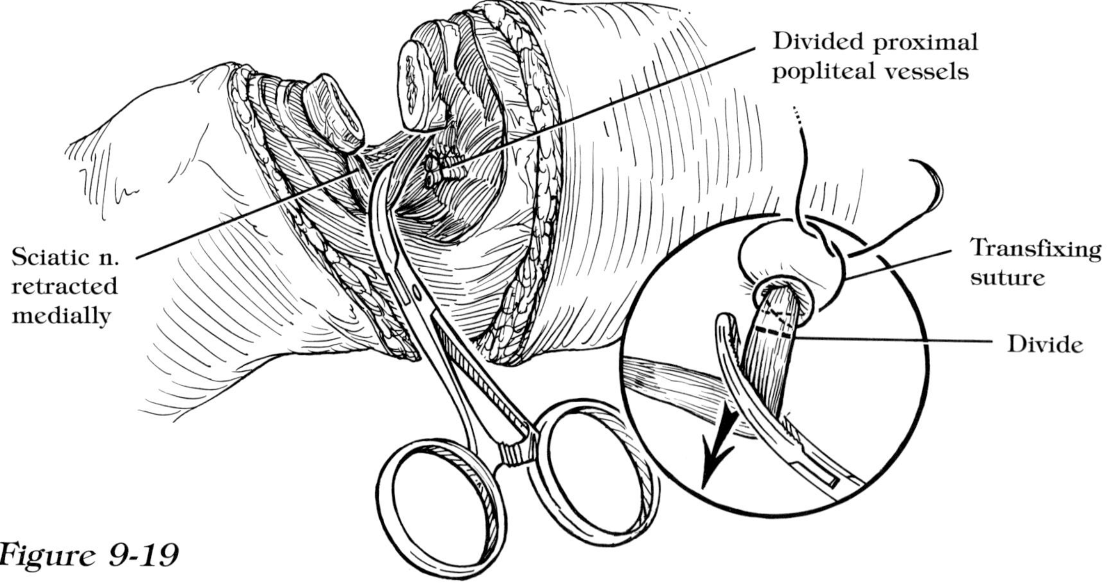

Figure 9-19

about 5 to 6 inches below the anterior tibial tubercle. The incision is carried down through the skin and subcutaneous tissue in a circumferential manner encompassing about one half of the total circumference of the calf. The posterior flap is then outlined so that there is a gentle curve posteriorly and distally toward a point in the posterior calf approximately equal in size to the anterior partially circumferential incision. This incision has a curving component posteriorly (Fig. 9-20). As the anterior incision is continued to the bone, the soft tissue is allowed to retract. The point of transection of the tibia selected is just under the maximum retraction point of the subcutaneous tissue and musculofascial layer (usually 1 to 2 inches proximal to the skin incision). The anterior tibial artery, vein, and nerve coursing on the anterior surface of the interosseous membrane are ligated with 2-0 chromic catgut and divided. The periosteum of the proposed site of tibial transection is then stripped distally for 1 to 2 cm. The surgeon transects the tibia with a saw, using again a malleable retractor inserted behind the tibia to protect the posterior structures. The fibula is transected (1½ inches proximal to the tibial transection) with a Gigli saw or double-action bone cutter. The divided tibia is angulated and beveled anteriorly to minimize pressure on the thin anterior flap. The posterior musculofascial bundles are exposed, and a long, sharp knife or scalpel is used to incise distally at an angle through these tissues. Individual bleeding points are ligated with 4-0 chromic catgut as they are encountered. The posterior tibial nerve is drawn downward with traction as it is encountered, ligated with 2-0 catgut, crushed and cut sharply with a scalpel, and allowed to retract well up into the soft tissues. This should avoid an uncomfortable neuroma near the stump. The peroneal and posterior tibial arteries and veins are appropriately ligated with 2-0 chromic catgut and divided as they are encountered (Fig. 9-21). When the incision through the posterior muscle mass is completed, the severed distal extremity is removed.

CAUTION

Many surgeons prefer completing the entire soft-tissue dissection prior to dividing the fibula and tibia.

The posterior and anterior flaps are tailored to fit loosely but neatly over the stump of the tibia. The deep fascial layers are approximated with interrupted 3-0 catgut sutures. The skin is then closed without tension with nonreactive suture material, and the operation is completed (Fig. 9-22).

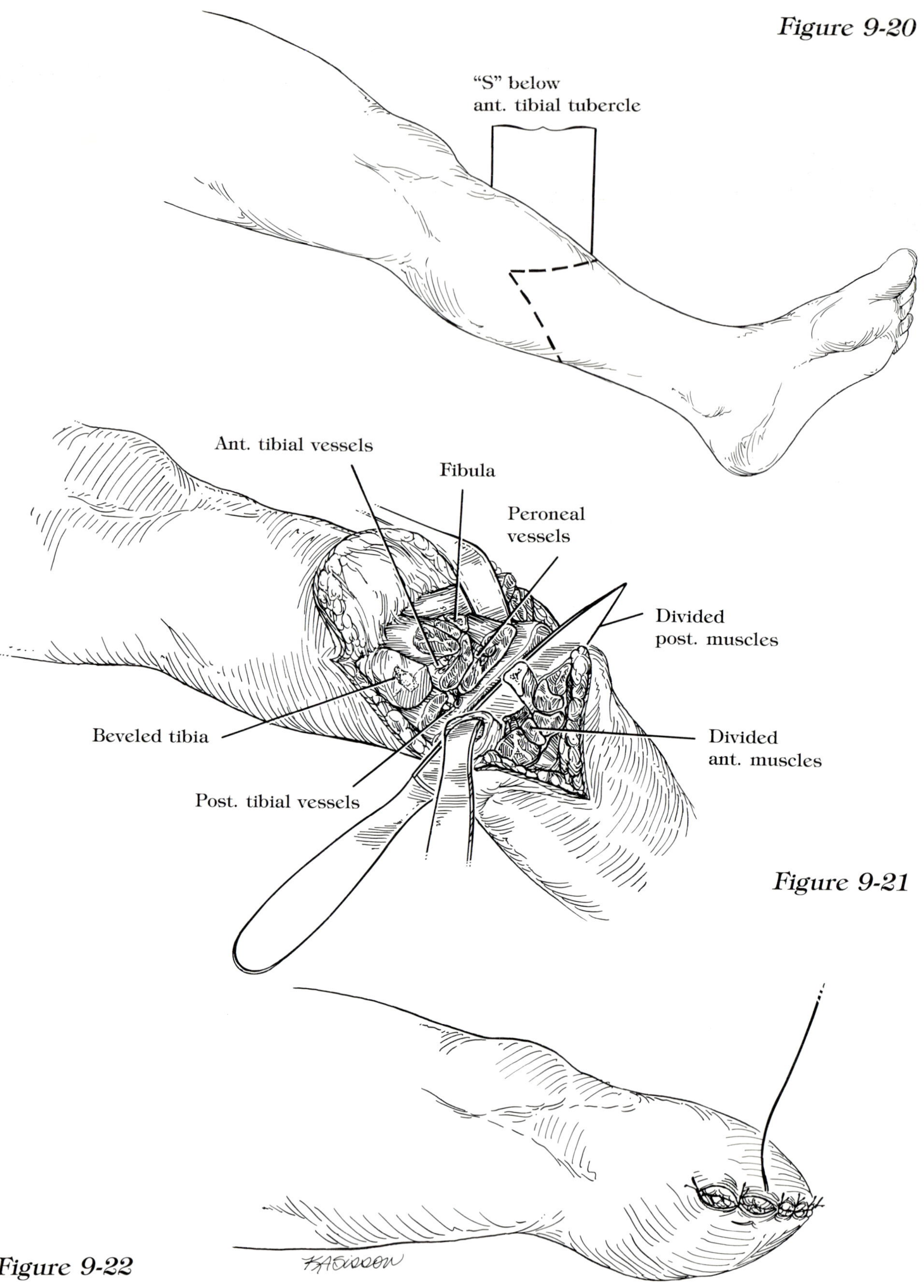

Figure 9-20

Figure 9-21

Figure 9-22

An incision is made across the dorsal aspect of the foot at the same level as a proposed division of the metatarsals (usually about 1 cm behind the first and fifth metatarsal heads) (Fig. 9-23). A curved plantar incision is then made extending distally from the medial end point of the dorsal incision and extending laterally across the sole of the foot about a centimeter behind the flexion crease of the toes (Fig. 9-24). A plantar flap is developed and carried back beneath the metatarsals to the level of the transection determined by the location of the dorsal incision and the junctions of the metatarsal heads with the shaft of these bones. With the toes held down, the dorsal incision is deepened through the tendons and soft tissues until the bones are reached. Small vessels are ligated with fine plain catgut (Fig. 9-25). The toes are then held up and the flexor tendons are stretched so that, when divided, they will retract beneath the flap. The surgeon transects the first metatarsal at the point of the incision with a double-action bone cutter, taking care not to damage the soft tissues. The other four metatarsals are then divided with a small bone cutter (Fig. 9-26*A*). After irrigation of the wound, the exposed tips of the metatarsals are rongeured to achieve smooth surfaces without spicules (Fig. 9-26*B*). The plantar flap is approximated to the dorsal flap with interrupted 5-0 nylon or 6-0 wire sutures and Steri-strips (Fig. 9-27).

CAUTION

    During the course of the operation, it is imperative to handle the soft tissues delicately. One should avoid using forceps or other instruments on the skin flaps.

The leg should be prepared carefully from the toes to the iliac crest circumferentially and draped to exclude the foot, the perineum, and the area above the inguinal ligament.

    In addition, better access to the groin is attained by abducting the hip slightly and flexing the knee after placing it on two or three folded half sheets.

    The exact placement of the proximal incision should be determined by the position of the fossa ovalis which is located on a line that is directly lateral to the pubic tubercle and directly over the femoral vein. At this point the femoral vein lies slightly medial and posterior to the femoral artery. The incision is then made parallel to the inguinal ligament and saphenous vein and about 1 cm inferior to the fossa ovalis (Fig. 9-28).

    Once the saphenous vein has been carefully identified as it enters the fossa ovalis, it should be dissected distally as far as possible. All tributaries should be ligated between clamps. At-

Division and Stripping of the Long and Short Saphenous Veins

Figure 9-23

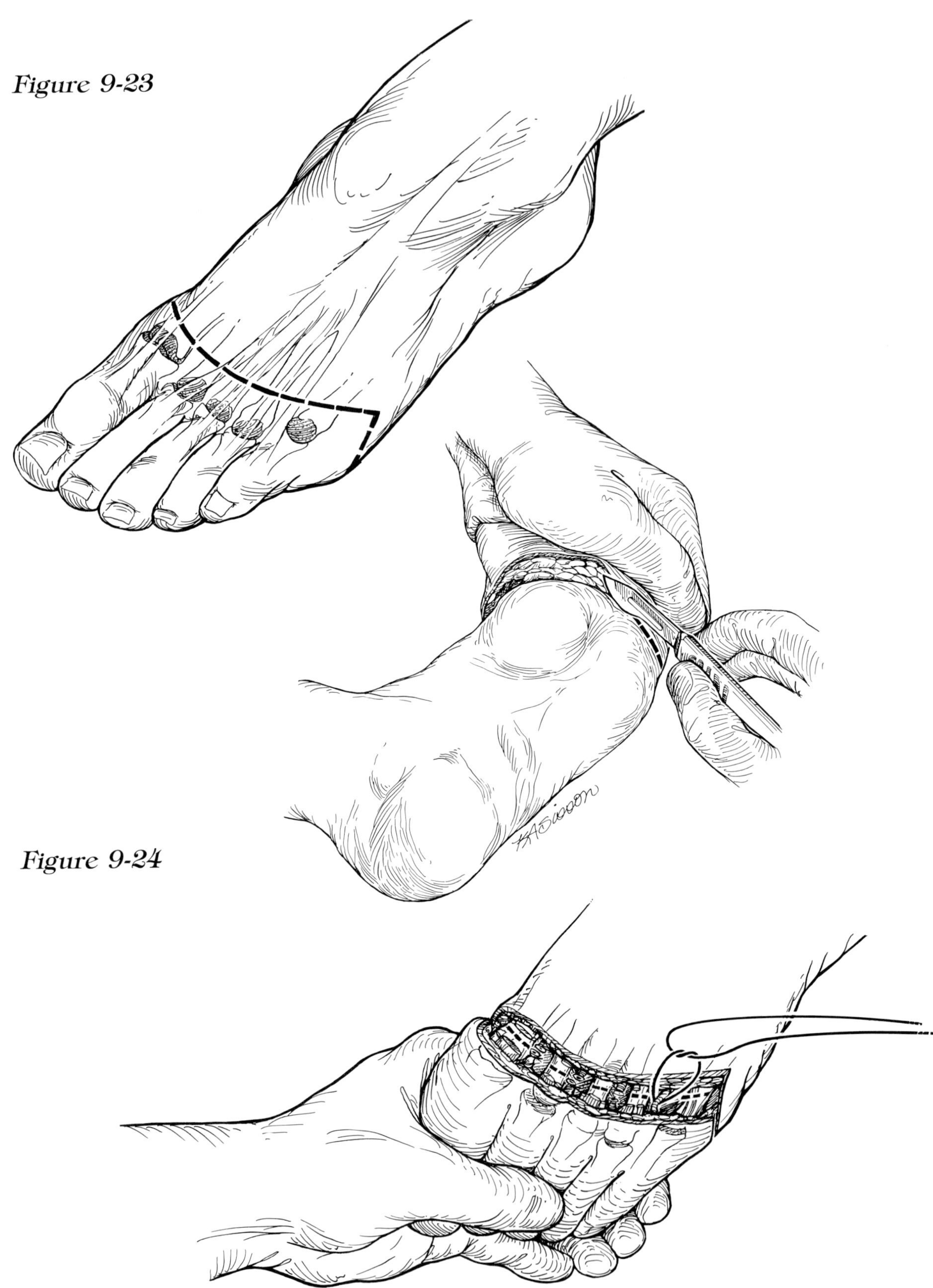

Figure 9-24

Figure 9-25

Figure 9-26

Metatarsal bones divided
with double-action
bone cutter
A
B
Long plantar flap
approximated to
dorsal flap

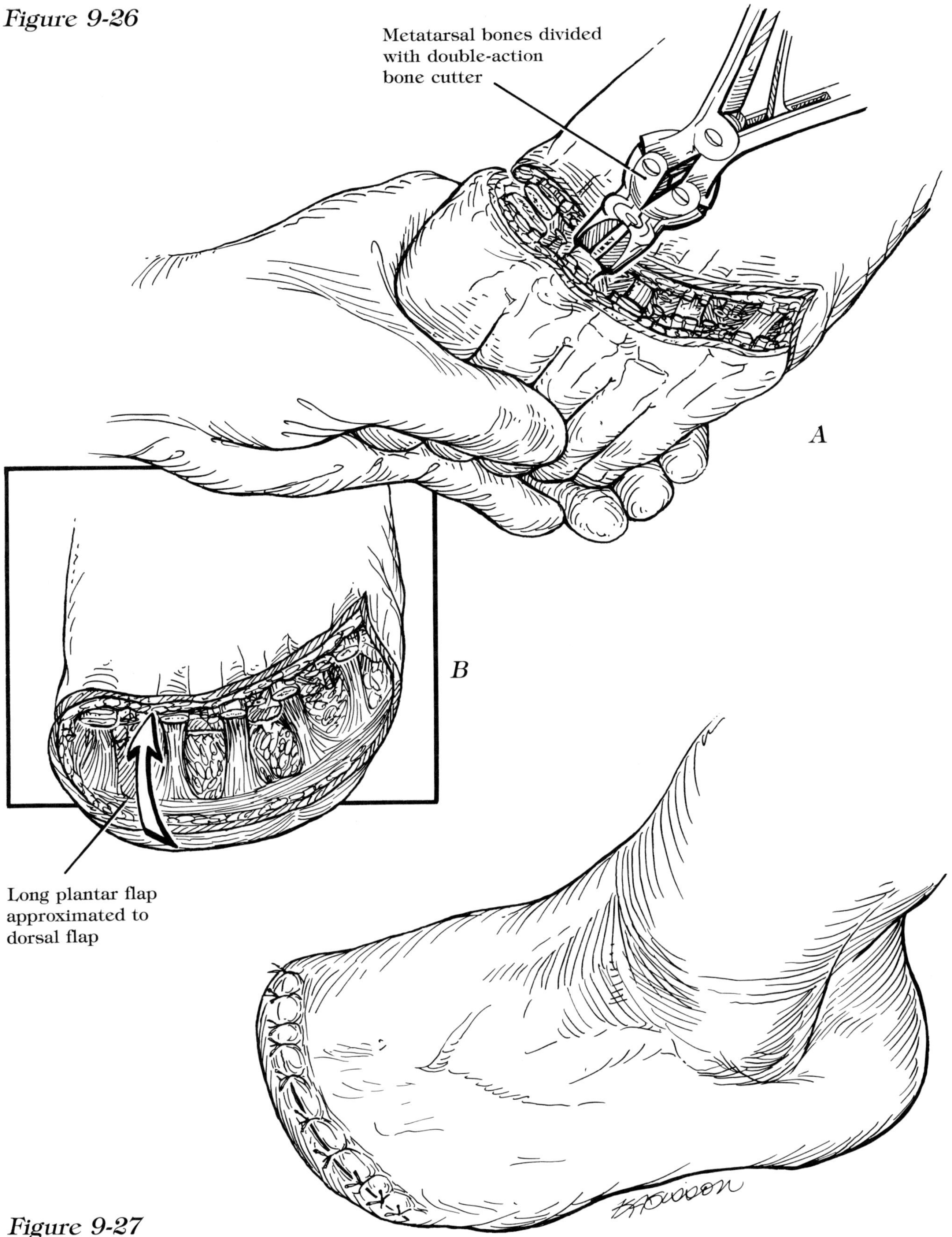

Figure 9-27

Fossa ovalis
Superficial epigastric v.
Pubic tubercle
Superficial circumflex iliac v.
Great saphenous v.
Superficial femoral v.
Superficial femoral a.
Superficial pudendal v.
Med. superficial (femoral) v. (accessory saphenous)
Lat. superficial (femoral) v.
Proximal ligature tied flush with femoral v.
Fascia lata
Scarpa's fascia
Fascia of Camper
Transfixing ligature
Saphenous v. divided between clamps

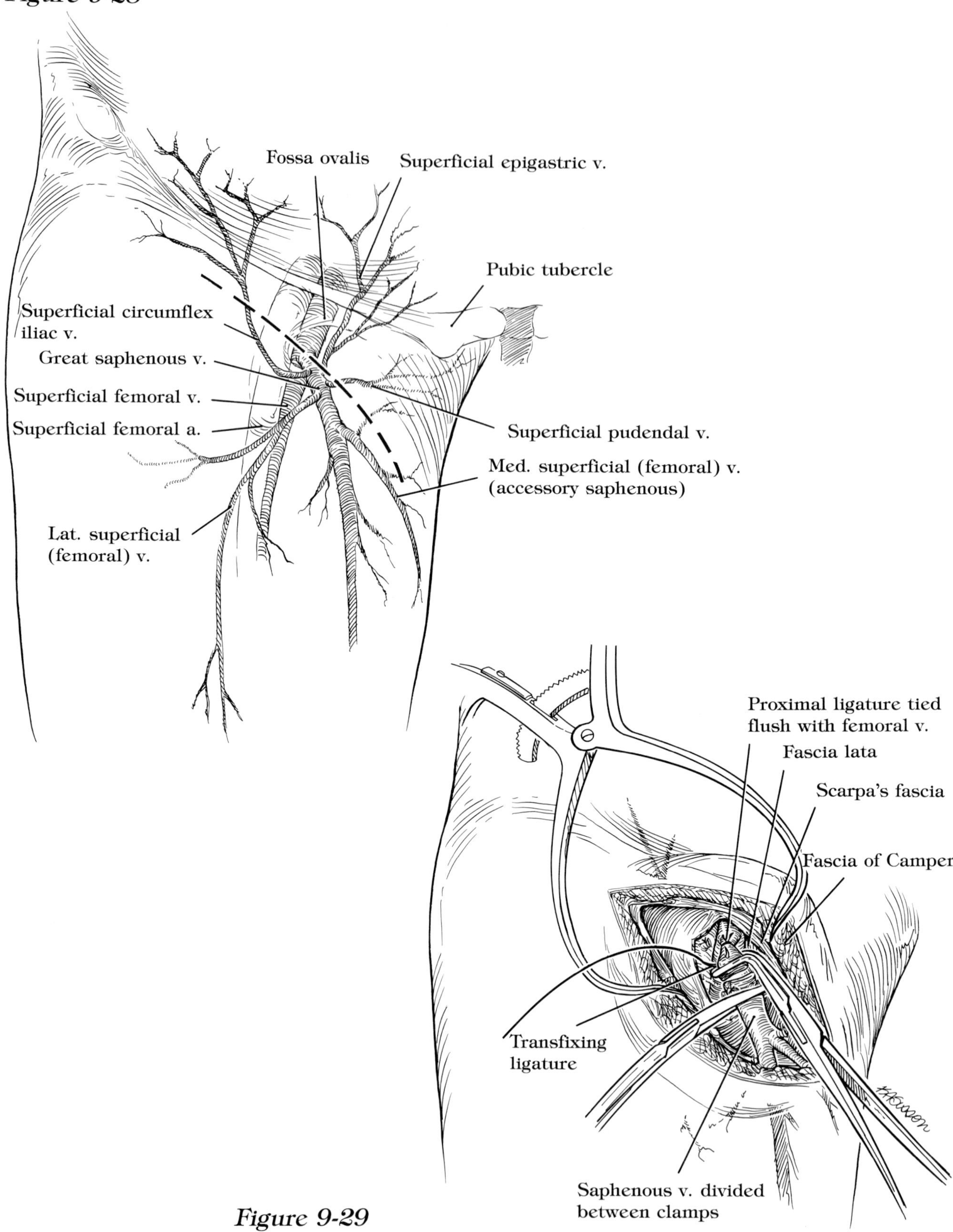

Figure 9-29

tention is directed to the upper segment which leads to the fossa ovalis. Dissection of this portion of the vein should proceed carefully, and every branch should be isolated and divided between clamps until all branches have been divided. During dissection of the proximal saphenous vein, the surgeon should recognize that tenting up the femoral vein in a thin patient might lead to damage of the femoral vein itself. To avoid this, the tension should be released from time to time to allow the surgeon to observe the true anatomic relationships and to decide more accurately when the dissection is complete. A right-angle clamp is then applied and the vein transected and doubly ligated (Fig. 9-29).

At the ankle, the saphenous vein is identified by palpation through the skin. A 2-cm vertical incision is made directly over the vein at a point slightly superior and lateral to the medial malleolus (Fig. 9-30). By combination of blunt and sharp dissection, the saphenous vein is isolated and a ligature passed around it for more careful identification.

> CAUTION
>
> At this point, the vein must be dissected away from the adjacent saphenous nerve in both directions to avoid accidental avulsion at the time of stripping.

Once this has been accomplished, the distal saphenous vein is divided and ligated. The proximal stump is then grasped with three mosquito hemostats and the lumen exposed. If necessary, the lumen can be dilated slightly by either a probe or a mosquito clamp. The surgeon then manipulates the smaller tip of the stripper up the vein with one hand while directing the course by palpation through the skin (Fig. 9-31). Once the stripper has been passed into the groin (Fig. 9-32A), it is brought out through the open end of the vein. The bleeding from the stump of the saphenous vein is controlled by means of either a loose ligature or a simple twisting of the vein around the stripper. The actual stripping of the vein is accomplished by tying the lower vein segment to the stripper with a long catgut ligature (Fig. 9-32B) and exerting steady traction from above while manipulating the head through the skin. If the stripping cannot be accomplished in one maneuver from below, the procedure can be reversed and the remaining segment removed, beginning from above. Additional incisions may be necessary, especially when the saphenous vein is unusually tortuous.

To minimize extravasation of blood along the course of the saphenous vein after stripping, a pressure dressing should be

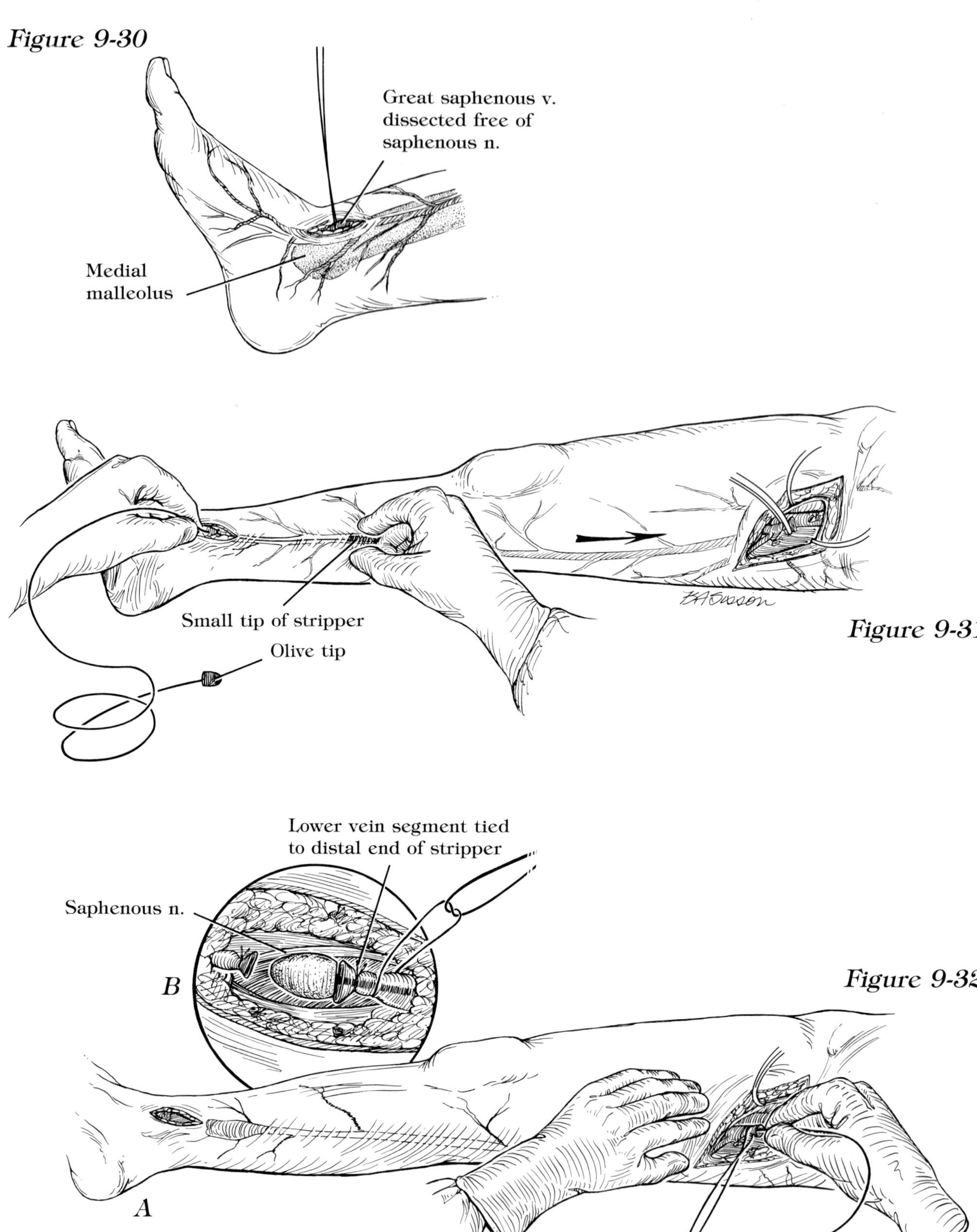

Figure 9-30
Great saphenous v.
dissected free of
saphenous n.
Medial
malleolus
Small tip of stripper
Olive tip
Figure 9-31
Lower vein segment tied
to distal end of stripper
Saphenous n.
B
A
Figure 9-32

Femoral a.
Femoral v.
Tibial n.
Post. femoral
medial
cutaneous n.
Common
peroneal n.
Site of
great saphenous v.
Deep fascia
Short saphenous v.
ligated at
popliteal n.
Med. sural
cutaneous n.
Lat. sural
cutaneous n.
Sural n.

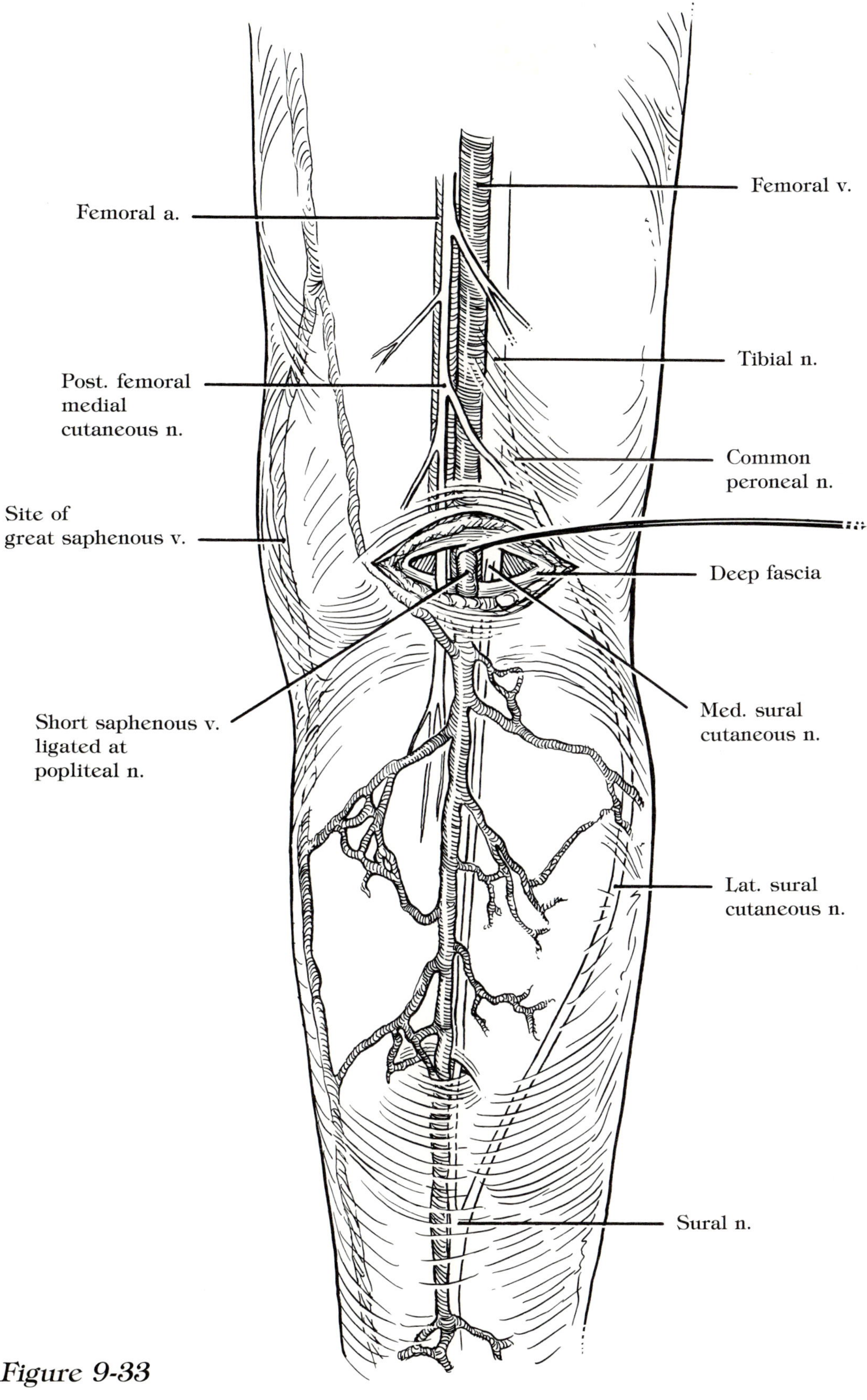

Figure 9-33

applied. Once the ankle wound has been closed, therefore, a gauze roll is placed over the course of the saphenous vein. Beginning with the foot, one applies an Ace bandage over the newly applied dressing at the ankle and over the gauze roll to the groin. The upper wound can then be closed.

SHORT SAPHENOUS VEIN

Varicosities of the short saphenous vein must be treated more carefully because of the intimate presence of the sural nerve. Under normal circumstances, this nerve lies immediately adjacent to the short saphenous vein. In conditions of chronic inflammation, such as chronic varicosities, it may be closely bound to the vein and can be stripped out with the vein inadvertently. This results in annoying hypoesthesia along the lateral aspect of the foot down to and including the fifth toe.

If the short saphenous vein is the site of symptomatic varicosities, it may only be necessary to ligate and divide the vein as it plunges into the popliteal fossa just below the popliteal crease (Fig. 9-33). If removal of the vein is necessary, then it is preferable to remove it in segments with multiple incisions under direct vision rather than strip it blindly.

CHAPTER TEN

KIDNEY TRANSPLANTATION

ANTHONY P. MONACO

A chapter is included on transplantation of the kidney because it has become such a standardized procedure in most large urban hospitals involved with residency training programs. Although the principles of management and control of rejection represent a specialized area of surgery, the resident staff so frequently becomes involved with kidney transplantation that a description of the techniques is appropriate for this atlas.

The patient is placed in the supine position with a thin rolled blanket under the iliac crest to elevate the iliac fossa, which will receive the transplant. A Foley catheter is placed in the bladder after anesthesia induction preparation. The bladder is inflated with 150 to 200 ml of a sterile bladder irrigant solution and the Foley catheter is clamped. In the past, right donor kidneys were placed in the left iliac fossa and left donor kidneys were placed in the right iliac fossa. Depending upon the donor kidney available and previous operation in either iliac fossa, strict adherence to this rule is not essential. Indeed, many surgeons place kidney transplants in the right iliac fossa if possible to avoid retraction of the sigmoid colon on the left side.

The iliac fossa is entered by a curved groin incision (Fig. 10-1) made parallel to the inguinal ligament, extended up over the iliac crest, and carried down through external and internal oblique muscle layers. The fascia over the rectus muscle is incised, and the pyramidal attachment to the rectus is divided. The peritoneum is exposed and retracted medially to enter the

Kidney Transplant
Operation

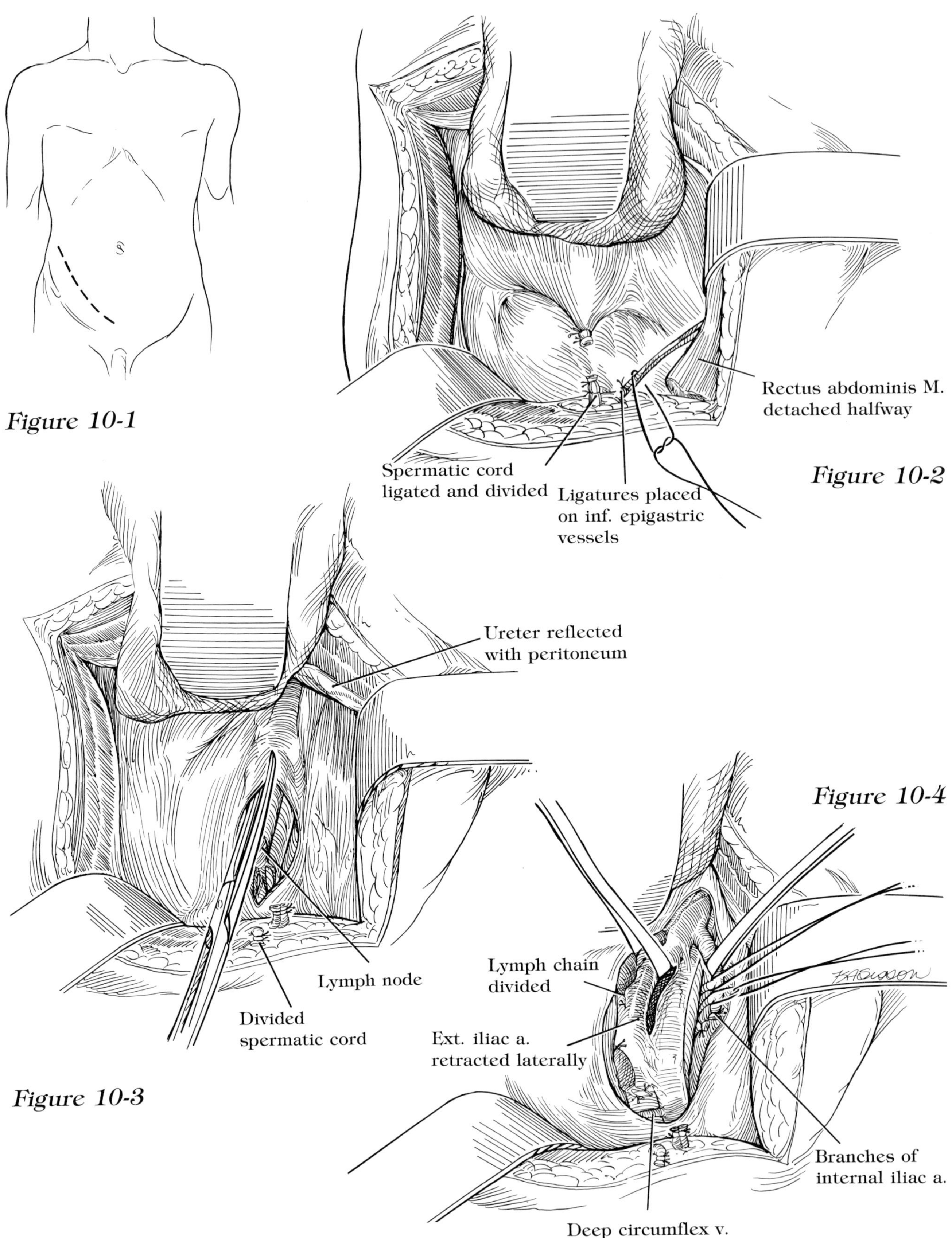

Figure 10-1

Figure 10-2

Figure 10-3

Figure 10-4

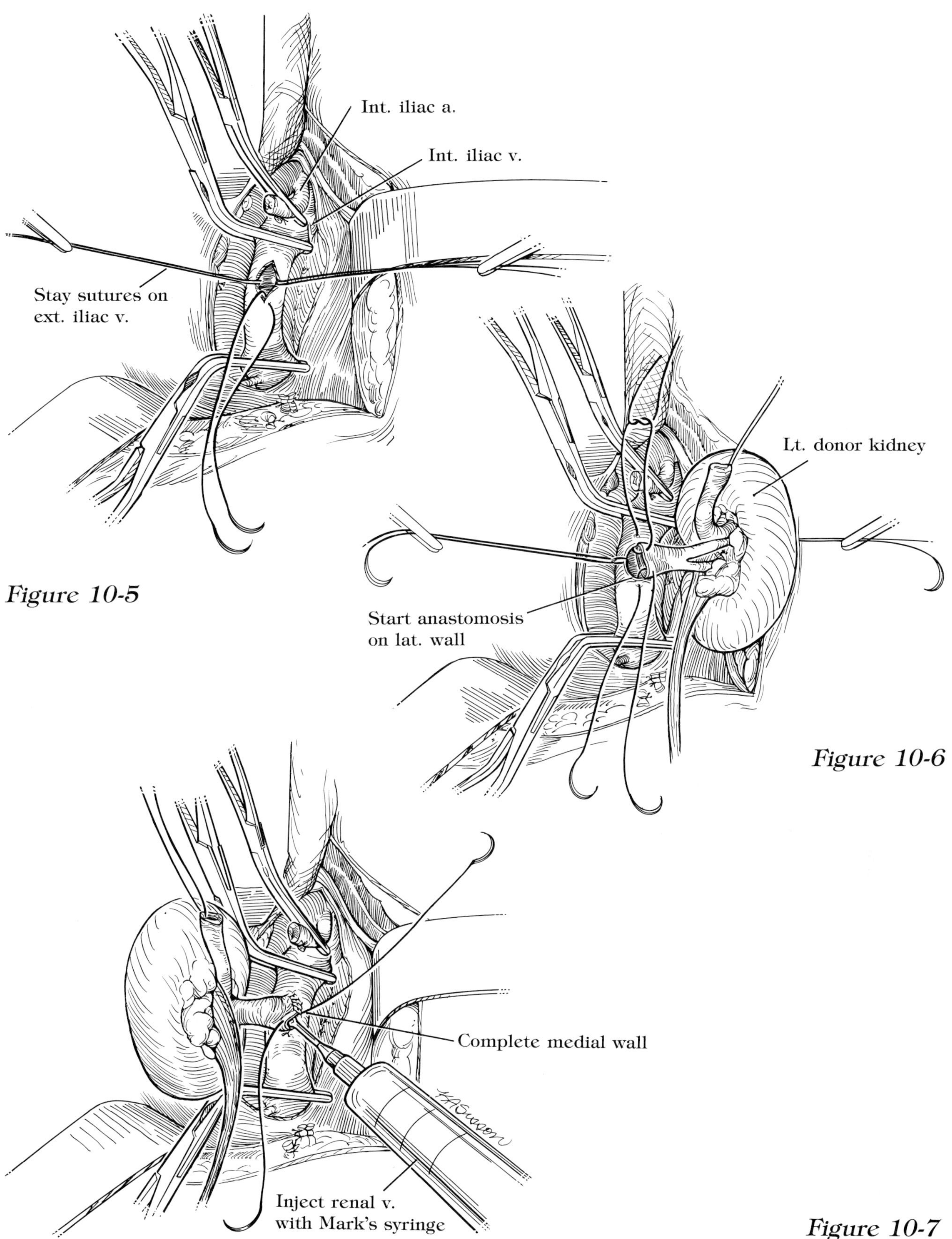

Figure 10-5

Figure 10-6

Figure 10-7

retroperitoneal space. In females, the round ligament is divided. Depending upon the surgeon's preference in males, the spermatic cord is divided. Avoidance of division of the spermatic cord usually prevents postoperative scrotal edema and hydrocele formation. The epigastric vessels are always divided and ligated (Fig. 10-2).

The internal iliac artery is mobilized from the common iliac bifurcation down to its bifurcation or trifurcation. Likewise, the common iliac bifurcation and a portion of the external iliac are also mobilized completely (Fig. 10-3). When the internal iliac artery is divided, it can be rotated upward and laterally without kinking. This procedure is done in preparation for a donar renal artery to internal iliac artery end-to-end anastomosis. If a donor renal artery to external iliac artery end-to-side anastomosis is to be constructed, only the external iliac artery is mobilized.

The external iliac vein is then approached with sharp and blunt dissection. Some surgeons prefer only enough dissection to permit application of a Satinsky clamp with safety. Others prefer to mobilize the external iliac vein, ligating all its tributaries up to and frequently including the hypogastric vein on the operated side. When this latter procedure is followed, the external iliac vein is extensively mobilized. Either separate occlusive clamps at either end or occlusive tapes can be utilized rather than the Satinsky clamp (Fig. 10-4). When the vein and artery have been mobilized, a bulldog clamp is placed on the proximal portion of the internal iliac artery, and then the internal iliac is divided at its trifurcation or bifurcation after suture ligation distally. After division the clamp is released briefly to flush the artery out, and the distal hypogastric arterial stump is flushed with heparinized saline solution. Proximal and distal occlusive clamps (or the Satinsky clamp) are placed on the vein.

The donor kidney is then brought into the operative field. Prior to this, a living donor kidney would have been irrigated with approximately 500 ml of cold Ringer's solution containing heparin, lidocaine (Xylocaine), and methylprednisolone sodium succinate (Solu-medrol) (125 mg/L). Cadaver kidneys are usually taken directly off the perfusion apparatus. Two techniques may be utilized to put the kidney in place. In the first technique, a venotomy is made. In addition, an end-to-side donor renal vein to external iliac vein anastomosis is constructed using double-ended 5-0 Mersilene running suture (Figs. 10-5, 10-6, 10-7). After the venous anastomosis is completed, an end-to-end anastomosis of the donor renal artery to the recipient internal iliac artery is made, again using double-ended 5-0 Mersilene suture running from opposite corners. In general, it is not necessary to use a triangulation or four-quadrant technique for the arterial anastomosis since it is usually quite large (Figs. 10-8, 10-9, 10-10, 10-11). An alternate method is to make the arterial anastomosis first and the venous anastomosis second. After both

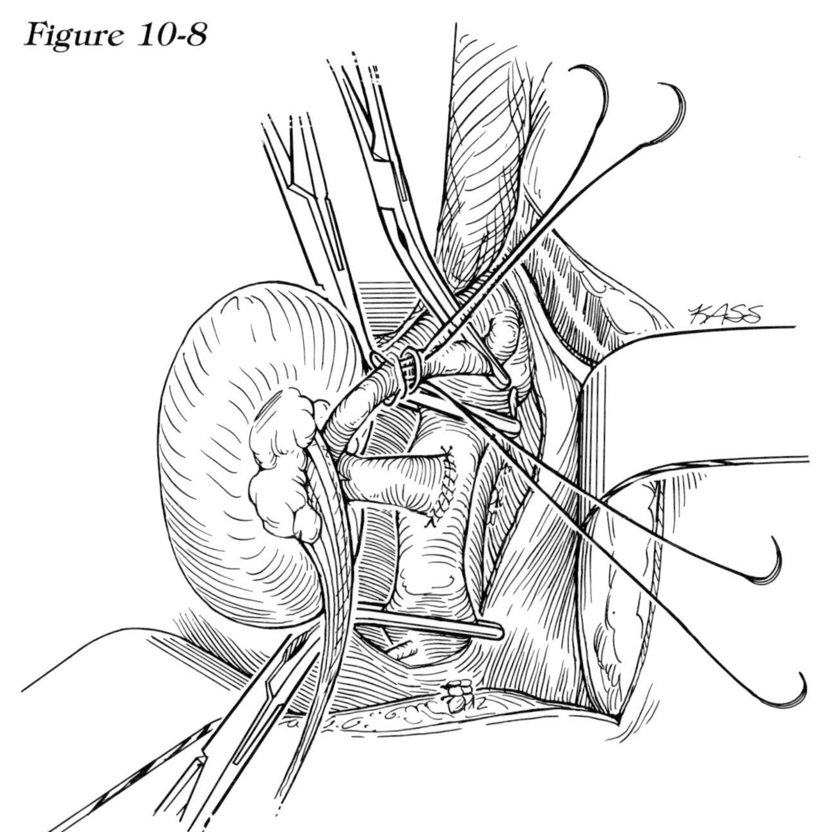

ARTERIAL SURFACES TWISTED BACK TO FRONT

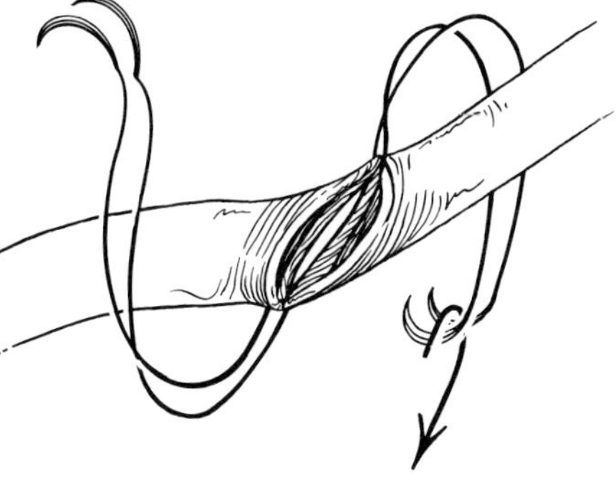

POSTERIOR WALL SUTURED

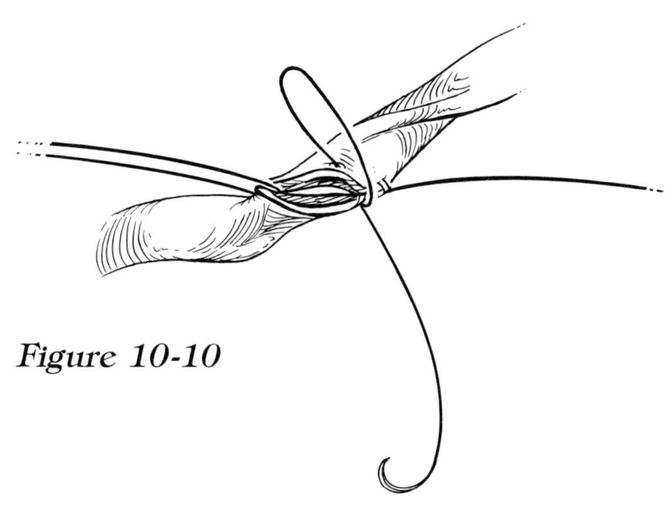

Figure 10-10

POSTERIOR WALL COMPLETE;
ANTERIOR WALL BEGUN

Figure 10-11

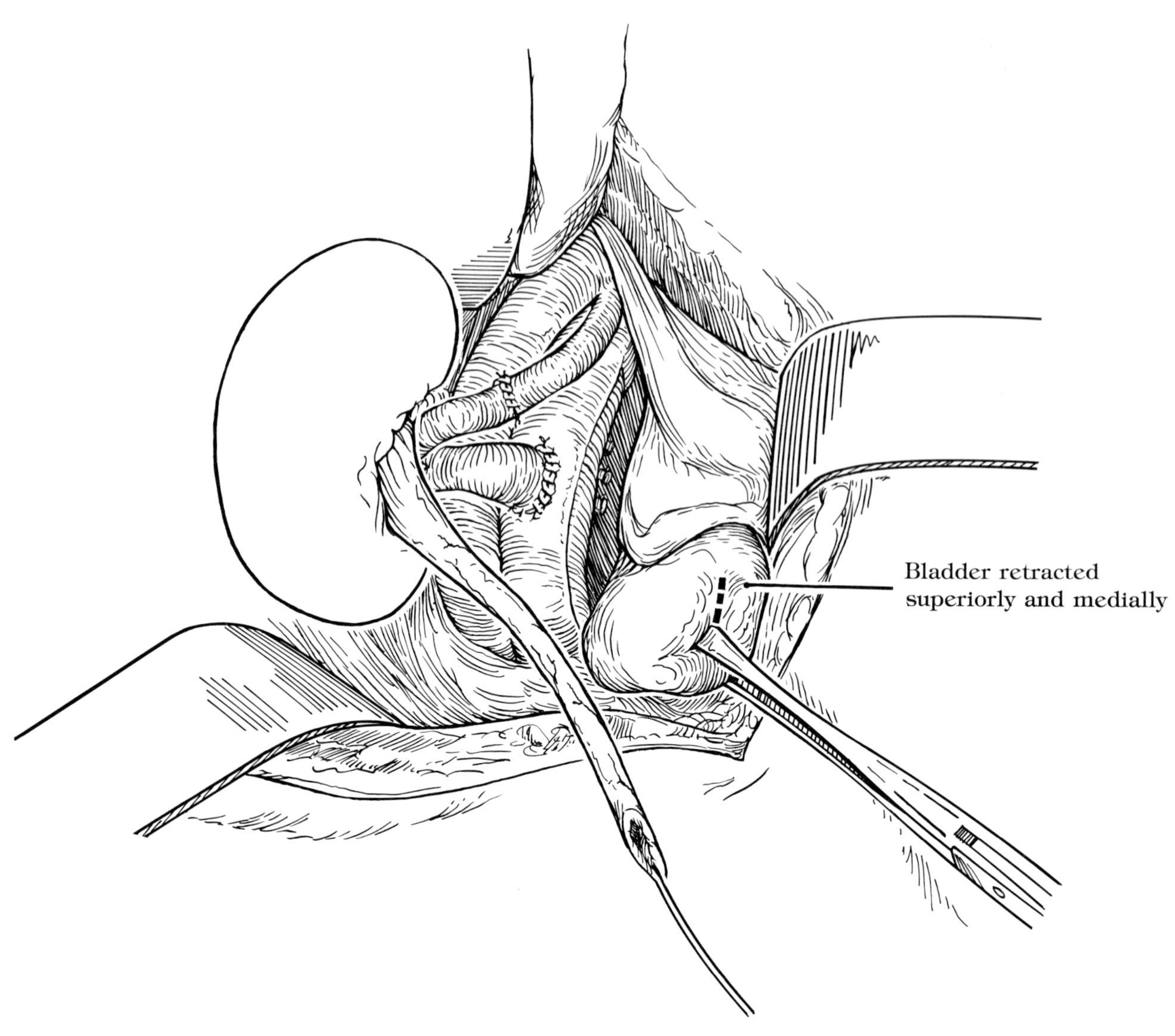

Figure 10-12

anastomoses are completed, the clamps are removed. In general, perfusion is rapid and the kidney becomes firm and pink almost immediately. A kidney that becomes pink and firm and then flaccid and bluish is frequently undergoing a hyperacute rejection. This is relatively rare with modern pretransplant crossmatch techniques. A kidney that becomes extremely distended and purplish may be undergoing a renal vein technical occlusion.

The ureters can be reconstructed by at least two methods. In the standard method (ureteroneocystostomy), the bladder is visualized. (Prior to operation, 200 ml of an antibiotic solution have been instilled in the bladder through a Foley catheter, which remains clamped during the procedure.) The bladder is opened through a midline cystotomy. A standard Politano-Leadbetter ureteral implantation is made, usually 1 cm above and lateral to the ureteral orifice on the side of the kidney transplant.

The bladder mucosa is incised transversely for 1.5 cm at this point (Fig. 10-12), and a gently curving clamp is passed upward and laterally submucosally for 2 to 3 cm. The clamp is then pushed out through the bladder muscle (Fig. 10-13). The ureter is pulled through the tunnel, care being taken not to twist it (Fig. 10-14). The ureter is shortened appropriately. The ureteral artery is ligated, and the anterior surface of the ureter fishmouthed approximately twice the width of the ureter. The ureteral mucosa is sutured to the bladder mucosa with interrupted 5-0 chromic sutures (Fig. 10-15). An adequate, unobstructed ureteral orifice for the new ureteral implant should be constructed (Figs. 10-16, 10-17). The bladder mucosa and muscle layers are then closed with interrupted 4-0 and 3-0 chromic catgut respectively.

An alternate method preferred by this author is the external implantation technique requiring no cystotomy. This is particularly important since patients who have repeated transplants may undergo a bladder slough from repeated bladder cystotomies utilizing the standard Politano-Leadbetter technique. In the external ureteral implantation technique (Coffey procedure), the distended bladder is visualized. The bladder musculature is incised laterally and low toward the bladder neck. The bladder muscle is incised down to the mucosa, which will pout out with the distended solution in it (Fig. 10-18). The distal half centimeter of mucosa is then incised and the fluid evacuated from inside the bladder (Fig. 10-19). The donor ureter is measured down to this opening and excess ureter is amputated. The ureteral vessel is located and ligated. A fishmouth approximately twice the width of the distal ureter is created. The fishmouthed ureter is then sutured to the opened bladder mucosa using interrupted 4-0 or 5-0 chromic catgut (Fig. 10-20). Some surgeons prefer to have a polyethylene ureteral catheter placed in the bladder prior to operation. This catheter is fished out of the bladder through the mucosa opening and passed up the ureter into the ureteral pelvis as a stent. When the ureteral bladder mucosa anastomosis has been completed externally, then the bladder muscle is sutured over the ureter with interrupted 4-0 catgut. An excellent tunnel is thus achieved (Figs. 10-21, 10-22, 10-23).

Hemostasis is secured. The surgeon puts the kidney back into position, taking care that the arterial and venous anastomoses are not occluded by placement of the kidney in the iliac fossa. The wound is irrigated and drained by closed-system (Hemovac or Davol) suction catheters.

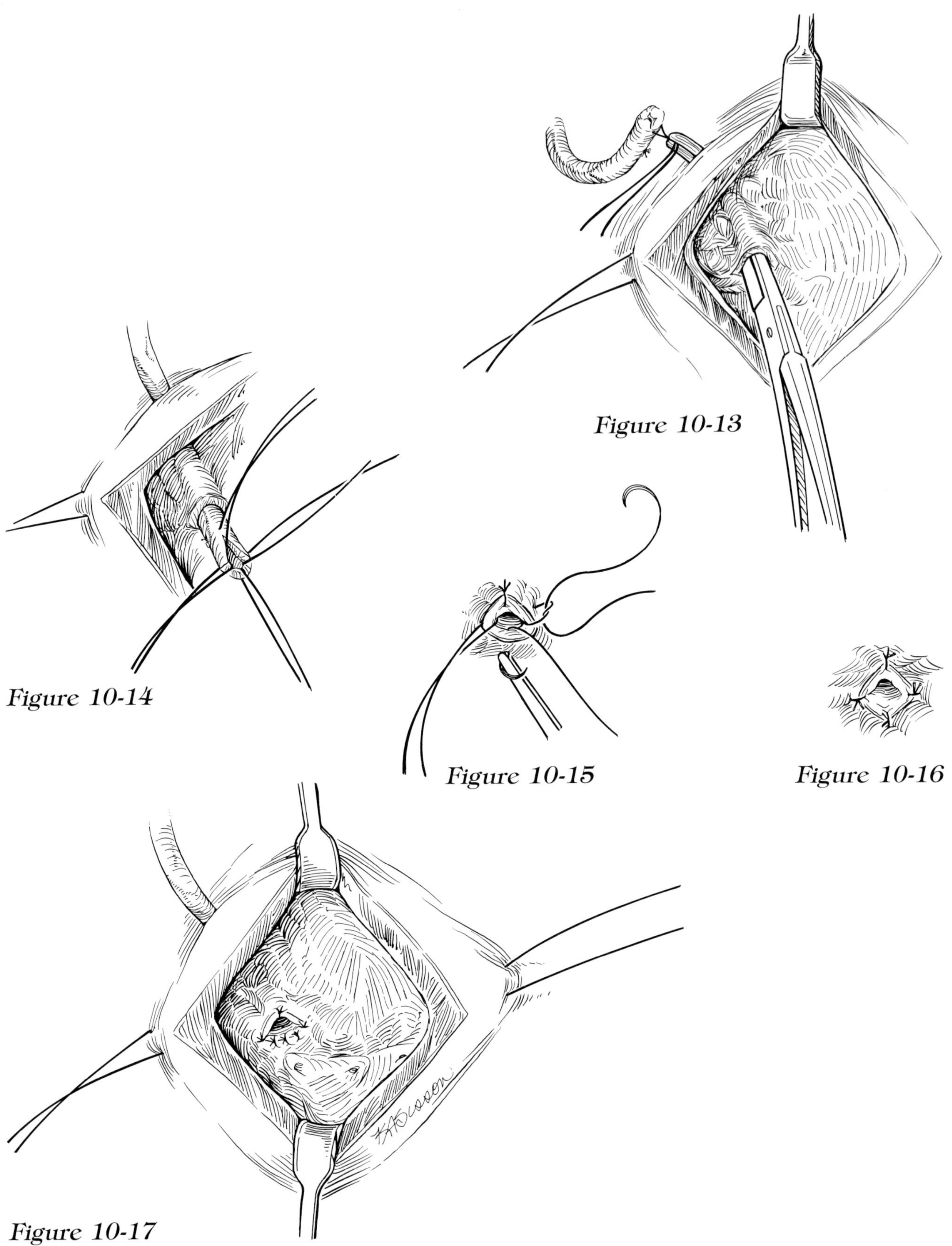

Figure 10-13

Figure 10-14

Figure 10-15

Figure 10-16

Figure 10-17

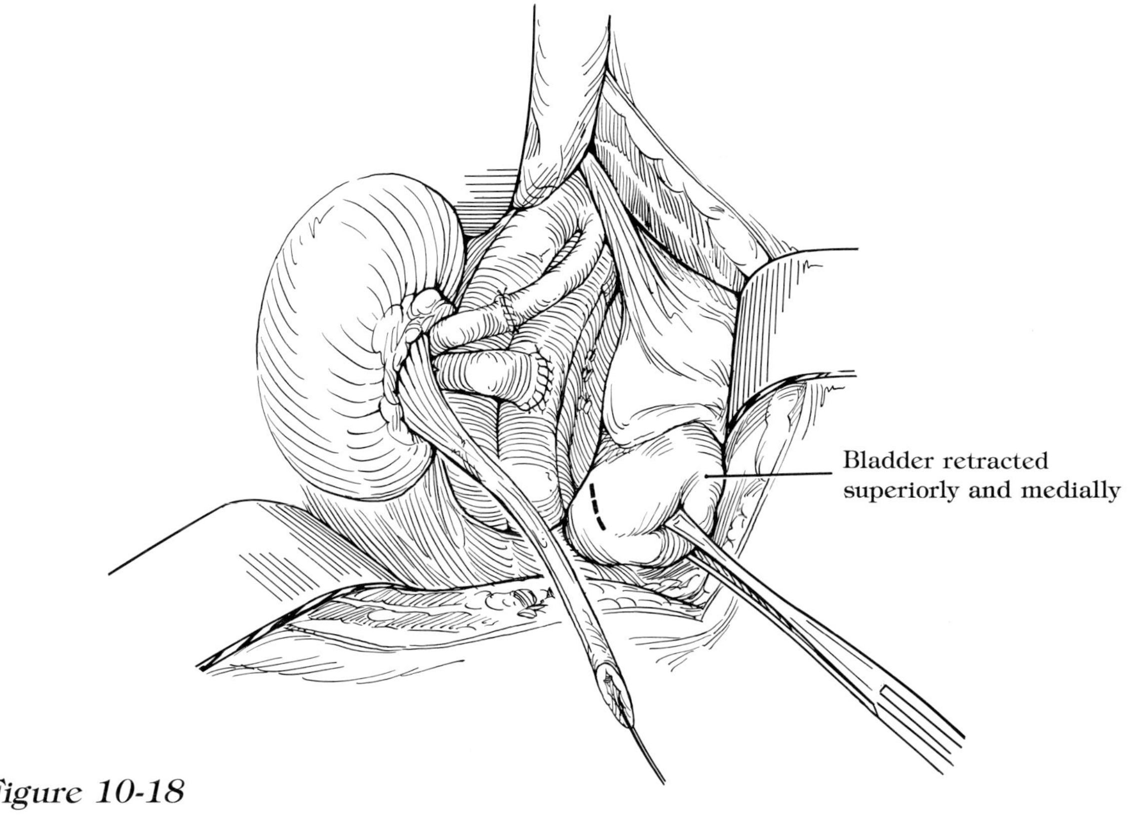

Figure 10-18

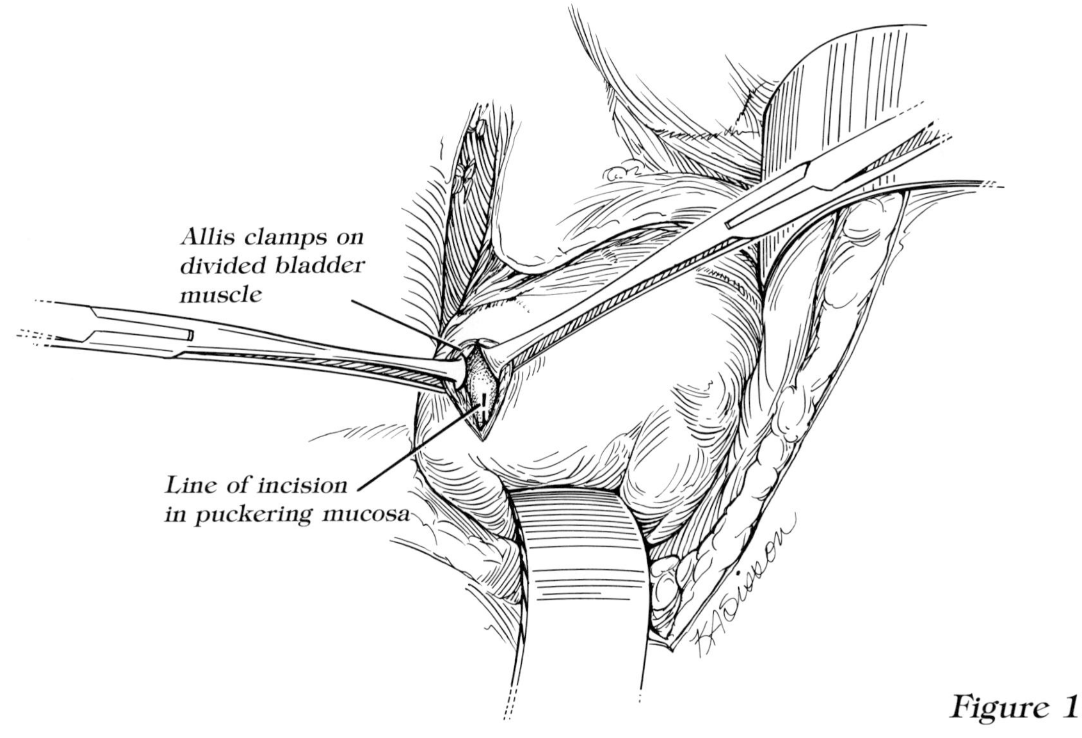

Figure 10-19

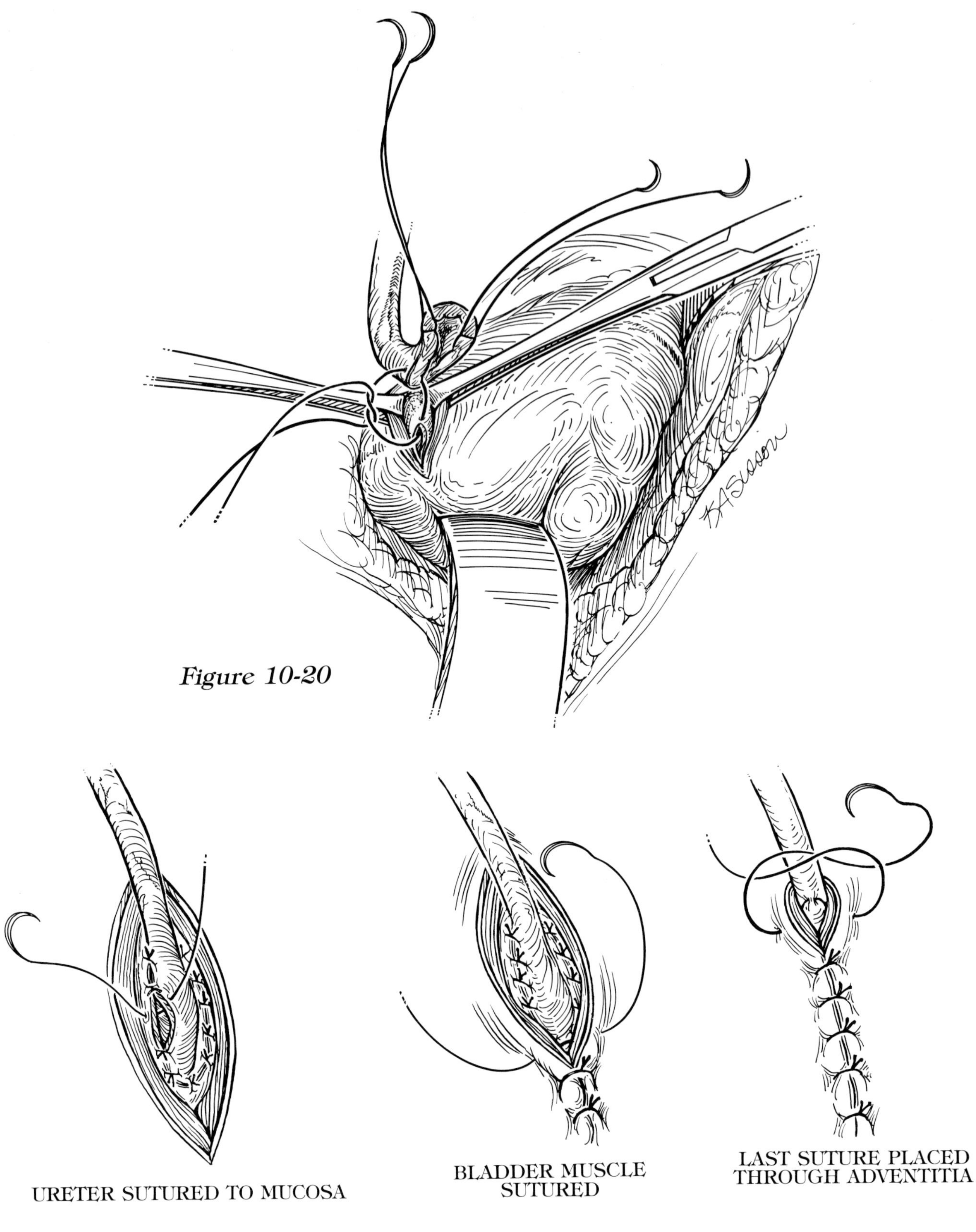

Figure 10-20

URETER SUTURED TO MUCOSA

BLADDER MUSCLE
SUTURED

LAST SUTURE PLACED
THROUGH ADVENTITIA

Figure 10-21

Figure 10-22

Figure 10-23